Professional Ethics in Athletic Training

Professional Ethics in Athletic Training

Gretchen A. Schlabach, PhD, ATC, LAT
Associate Professor
Director, Athletic Training Education Program
Department of Kinesiology and Physical Education
Northern Illinois University
DeKalb, Illinois

Kimberly S. Peer, EdD, ATC, LAT
Associate Professor
Coordinator, Athletic Training Education Program
School of Exercise, Leisure and Sport
Kent State University
Kent, Ohio

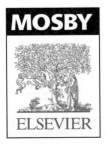

MOSBY

ELSEVIER

11830 Westline Industrial Drive
St. Louis, Missouri 63146

PROFESSIONAL ETHICS IN ATHLETIC TRAINING   ISBN: 978-0-323-04017-4

Notice

Library of Congress Control Number: 2007934622

Vice President and Publisher: Linda Duncan
Acquisitions Editor: Kathryn Falk
Senior Developmental Editor: Melissa Kuster Deutsch
Publishing Services Manager: Julie Eddy
Project Manager: Laura Loveall
Design Direction: Karen O'Keefe Owens

Printed in United States of America

Last digit is the print number: 9 8 7 6 5 4 3 2 1

Working together to grow
libraries in developing countries

www.elsevier.com | www.bookaid.org | www.sabre.org

ELSEVIER   BOOK AID International   Sabre Foundation

This book is dedicated to my parents, Tom and in loving memory of Ruth, who by moral example taught me many of life's greatest lessons. Your love and support have given me courage, strength, and direction in this wonderful, yet amazingly complex, world.

—Gretchen Schlabach

I would like to thank my family for their constant support and inspiration. You remind me on a daily basis why it is so important to do the right thing personally and professionally. You are my compass and reflect all that is right in the world.

Dedicated with love to my parents, Sandra and Eben Arista Peer II.

—Kimberly Peer

These individuals contributed portions of this book:

Catherine Grove, PhD, LAT, ATC
Clinical Associate Professor of the Department of Kinesiology
Undergraduate Athletic Training Curriculum Director
Assistant Athletic Trainer
Indiana University
Bloomington, Indiana

Richard Ray, EdD, ATC
Professor and Chair of the Department of Kinesiology
Program Director, Athletic Training Education
Assistant Athletic Trainer
Hope College
Holland, Michigan

Regis Turocy, DHCE, PT, ECS
Clinical Director
B.O.A.R. Physical Therapy
Bethal Park, PA

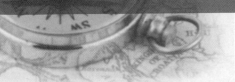

Athletic training has been understandably challenged by the world's rapid complexity relative to health care formalities, cultural diversity, and educational reform. Our colleagues clearly are equally perplexed by the swift current of the ever-changing, multifaceted advancements in health care and its specific effects on our profession of athletic training and the education of our future members. We needed more than the NATA Code of Ethics to help us practice ethically.

Since the inception of the athletic training profession (1950), the norms, values, and traditions of athletic training have been passed down by word of mouth. Furthermore, given that the number of athletic training professionals has grown significantly over the last 2 decades, perhaps a better way of passing down the professional ethical legacy exists. Without a doubt, we were convinced that writing the first textbook on professional ethics in athletic training was the right thing to do, and now was the time.

WHO WILL BENEFIT FROM THIS TEXTBOOK

This textbook is for all athletic trainers. Athletic trainers are in a position to make and act on many value-laden decisions. As health care providers, athletic trainers are not involved with headline-grabbing issues such as the right to life or stem cell research. Yet they are involved in subtle, gray, value-laden problems in everyday practice, whether interacting with a patient-athlete, a student, or another professional. Athletic trainers can benefit from an ethical framework to reflect on dilemmas and, from that position, weigh and consider multiple perspectives before concluding what one ought to do—the right decision.

WHY IS THE BOOK IMPORTANT TO THE PROFESSION?

No other book is dedicated to professional ethics in athletic training. This book is unique in that it allows for appropriate developmental and curricular progression as the student matriculates through the athletic training education program.

CONCEPTUAL FRAMEWORK AND ORGANIZATION

Given the depth, breadth, and complexity of professional ethics, as well as the novelty of such a text in athletic training, the text clearly had to be simple, appropriately sequenced, and complete. After thoughtful deliberation, the conceptual framework evolved into three levels.

- **Level I: Introduction to Professional Ethics in Athletic Training.** This introduction provides the athletic training student with a brief understanding about the profession, being a professional, professionalism, and professional enculturation. A succinct analysis of the history of athletic training sheds light on the important values, beliefs, norms, customs, and traditions that served to shape the profession. Furthermore, a pedagogical perspective regarding how to learn about ethics is coupled with strategies and assessment tools.
- **Level II: Professional Enculturation.** This is the core of the text and consists of three sections. It assists the student to transition from a novice to a skilled professional. Thoughtful progression related to pedagogy and maturation threads throughout six themes (awareness, development of moral behavior, ethical approaches, foundational behaviors of professional practice, conflict and transformation, and learning activities linked to practice). Each section builds on the previous one, culminating in robust insights regarding the moral dimension of the athletic training professional.
- **Level III: Professional Application.** This level provides an opportunity for the athletic training student to use a variety of ethical approaches to think

critically and reflect morally on ethical issues that evolve from professional practice by using case studies in prevention, clinical evaluation and diagnosis, immediate care, treatment and rehabilitation, organization and administration, and professional development.

DISTINCTIVE FEATURES OF THIS BOOK

As the first text dedicated entirely to ethics in athletic training, this book has numerous distinctive features that set it apart from other ethics books in the allied health care fields. This book has the following features:

- Rich applications to the athletic training profession by linking theory to practice
- A progressive approach to ethical discovery through carefully structured stages that align with professional development of the athletic training student
- Breadth and depth of ethical theory, ethical approaches, and ethical decision making to encourage full immersion in the ethical discovery process through scaffolding of material rooted in the ethics literature
- Challenging, engaging learning activities that link directly with the theoretical content to frame each concept in real-life applications specific to athletic training
- "Good to Know" boxes that highlight important concepts and facts relevant to ethical discovery from personal and professional perspectives
- Broad use of case narratives to engage the student in critical thinking
- Specific applications for each component of the *Role Delineation Study* (fifth edition) to challenge students in each domain of the profession
- Cultural awareness threads that encourage the student to reflect on ethical dilemmas from multiple perspectives
- A detailed glossary to assist the student in understanding key terms
- A conceptual framework that transcends each section and ties together all components of the book
- Rich resources to use for ethical discovery and innovative rubrics to use for assessing student progress throughout the ethical journey

LEARNING AIDS (PEDAGOGICAL FEATURES)

As a one-of-a-kind textbook on ethics in athletic training, this engaging text guides the student along a journey toward ethical discovery through the use of the personal and professional compass. Pedagogical features facilitate this journey and include the following:

- Specific learning objectives for each chapter and each learning activity
- "Good to Know" that highlight critical information for young professionals
- Learning activities specifically linked to each chapter that encourage individual and group activity
- Liberal use of case narratives that promote critical thinking with direct application to the domains of athletic training
- Threaded narratives throughout the text to scaffold previous information to new information

NOTE TO THE STUDENT

In athletic training, you will be faced with many challenges—both personal and professional—that will require moral courage. As you journey through this text, you will see that it is deliberately designed to help you move through the content in a progressive manner—one that will allow you to evolve each step of the way. Your professional identity will be crystallized and your professional commitment will become authentic. This text is unlike any other you will use; it will help you embrace the real-world challenges that lie ahead in this exciting, complex profession by helping you understand the broad-reaching role of ethics. As you emerge at the end of your educational program and embark on your professional career, you will be reminded of the importance of the foundational behaviors of professional practice that you convey. This book will serve as a significant resource for you now and in the future. We encourage you to use it regularly to reflect on things that are important to you and to the profession. This book will help you decide what ought to be done while understanding why we choose to act the way that we do. The ethical journey never ends, and in this ever-changing profession a compass such as this book will provide guidance and direction.

May you always keep your footing and balance on the high road of your professional life!

We would like to thank our families, colleagues, students, and friends, who provided us with patient encouragement throughout this entire journey. Furthermore, we thank our mentors, Marje Albohm, John Schrader, John Faulstick, Robert Moss and Jonathon Rakich, who taught us about professional ethics by example and gave us invaluable insights.

Additionally, we would like to thank the hardworking, masterminds of Elsevier/Mosby, especially Linda Duncan, who was our constant "go-to-person" during the staff changes. Many thanks to Kathy Falk and Melissa Kuster Deutsch, we appreciate your courage to direct our textbook midway through the project. Laura Loveall, thanks for directing us through the final edits. We are grateful to Marion Waldman and Margory Fraser, who believed in us and determinedly convinced us from the very beginning that we could, indeed, write a textbook.

Furthermore, we greatly appreciate the support we received from the leaders of the Great Lakes Athletic Trainers' Association (GLATA), more specifically Marje Albohm, Katie Grove, and Mark Gibson, for helping us initiate the professional values research to include in the text. Of equal importance, we are grateful for the participation and support of the GLATA members, themselves, in this research endeavor that led to the discovery of important professional values.

To our reviewers: 1) Clint Thompson, retired ATC and residing in Mukilteo, Washington; 2) Jackie Williams, Assistant Professor at Slippery Rock State University, Pennsylvania; 3) Kathleen Stroia, Director of the Women's Tennis Association; 4) Carrie Graham, Clinical Coordinator and Instructor at the University of Connecticut; 5) Sheri Hedlund, Kent, Washington High School Athletic Trainer; 6) Mary Kirkland, Supervisor, Kennedy Space Center RehabWorks; 7) Ray Castle, Louisiana State University Program Director; and 8) Mark Smaha, retired athletic Trainer residing in Keyport Washington, your diverse and immeasurable professional experiences provided us with significant feedback. We greatly appreciated your time and energy in the review. Your thoughts and comments helped us to sharpen the focal points of this text. Also, we thank our NATA Hall of Fame Inductees, Clint Thompson, Mark Smaha, Kathy Schniedwind, Julie Max, and Bob Behnke, who provided "real-world" professional pearls. Your moral perspective relative to professional life added value.

Many thanks to those athletic trainers, who shared their "real-life" experiences with us, which called into question, professional ethics. We trust that we carefully captured the essence of your stories as we folded them into our case scenarios.

Last, but certainly not least, huge gratitude goes to our three contributors: Rich Ray, Katie Grove, and Rege Turocy. Rich, thanks so much for Maria's descriptive, true-to-life narrative, it truly captures many of the thoughts, feelings, and anxieties of newly admitted students. Katie, your "Good-to-Know" boxes added real-world spice, and Rege, your significant knowledge relative to health care ethics and principles added depth and greater understanding. Beyond your contributions, your light-hearted humor and unwavering support and enthusiasm for this project motivated us through the challenging times. Many Thanks! The three of you define what it means to be both a friend and a colleague.

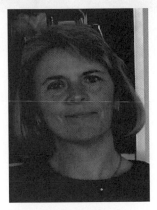

Gretchen Schlabach, PhD, ATC, LAT

Gretchen is an associate professor and athletic training program director at Northern Illinois University. After graduating from Indiana University in athletic training with a Master's degree, Gretchen served the profession over the last 30 years as an assistant athletic trainer at Western Michigan University (1 year), head women's athletic trainer at the University of Mississippi (8 years), and athletic training program director at Northern Illinois University (16 years). She was recognized in 2000 as one of NATA's Most Distinguished Athletic Trainers. Also, Gretchen has served her profession as a member of the NATA Ethics Committee, NATAREF Research Committee, GLATA Research Committee, NATA and GLATA Women in Athletic Training Committee, and NATAEC Post Certification Graduate Education Committee.

Her research is related to the discovery of professional values, and its influence on clinical practice, professional behavior, and ethics. Recent collaborative research with Kimberly Peer has examined professional values in the Great Lakes Athletic Trainers' Association (GLATA), more specifically, professional values among program directors and head athletic trainers, professional values among NATA Hall of Fame Inductees, who have worked in GLATA, and professional values among athletic training students in Ohio and Illinois. Future research will discover professional values at the national level including the professional values of 1) athletic trainers engaged in the NATA leadership and 2) athletic trainers employed in a variety practice settings (clinical/hospital, sports, industrial) across the nation.

Recently, Gretchen became the Chair of the NATA Ethics Committee and a member of the Ethics and Professional Standards Committee of the Commission on the Accreditation of Athletic Training Education (CAATE). She admires the thoughts of one, who wrote, "reputation is what the world thinks a man is; character is what he really is."

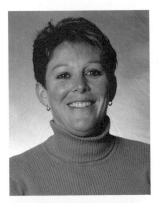

Kimberly S. Peer, EdD, ATC, LAT

Dr. Peer is the ATEP coordinator and an associate professor at Kent State University where she has been a faculty member since 1999. Kimberly graduated from Kent State University with a degree in Physical Education/Athletic Training and then pursued a Master's degree in Athletic Training at Western Michigan University. After working as an instructor/assistant athletic trainer at Mount Union College and as a clinical athletic trainer at the Rehabilitation and Health Center, she commenced her journey toward her doctorate. In 2001, Kimberly graduated from the University of Akron with an EdD in Higher Education Administration with a cognate in Health Care Management. While pursuing her doctorate, Dr. Peer collaborated with the Ohio Department of Education to create and validate the College Tech Prep curriculum while directing an advanced study program in Sports Medicine at the Portage Lakes Career Center. Following the approval of the state curriculum, Dr. Peer returned to her alma mater, Kent State University, to direct the athletic training education program.

Her areas of research are professional ethics and athletic training education. She has presented at the national, district, state and local levels on ethics and athletic training education. In addition, Dr. Peer serves on the Editorial Board for the *Journal of Athletic Training* and the *Athletic Training Education Journal,* the Research Committee of the NATA REF, as Chair of the Standards Committee of the BOC, and as a member of the Ethics and Professional Standards Committee of the CAATE. She is currently serving as President for the Ohio Athletic Trainers' Association. For her contributions to athletic training, Dr. Peer has received the NATA Service Award, GLATA Outstanding Educator Award, and the OATA Athletic Trainer of the Year Award (College/University).

Over the past three years, Dr. Peer has committed herself to a collaborative effort with Dr. Gretchen Schlabach to educate athletic training professionals at all levels about professional values and pedagogical approaches for developing foundational behaviors of professional practice. This journey has resulted in multiple research projects which have culminated in the writing of this text. We hope this journey will be as enlightening for you as it was for us!

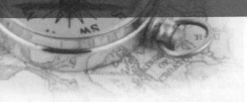

CONTENTS

LEARNING ACTIVITIES

Introduction: Maria's Story

Maria Trusk joined her father at the table for breakfast as she had every Saturday since she was a little girl growing up near the city limits of Detroit. Maria's father, a Polish immigrant who escaped Communism in his native country before it collapsed of its own weight, could tell that something was on his eldest daughter's mind.

"Sorry I couldn't come to your basketball game last night," he said as he scanned the sports page of the local newspaper. "The foreman offered me some overtime and we need the money. How did the game go?"

Maria shrugged and responded, "We won by 10 points. It was a pretty good game, but I didn't get to play very much. I love basketball, but I don't think I'm going to be making a career out of it. I'm just not good enough."

"There are more important things than basketball," her father mumbled through the newsprint.

"Papa," said Maria, "I want to talk to you about what I want to do when I graduate from high school in the spring. You know I want to go to college, but every time I bring it up you seem reluctant to talk about it. I know that you and Mama didn't go to college, but this is America. If I'm going to have any chance of getting ahead I'll need a college education. Money is tight, I know. But I have all As and had the best ACT score at my school. I think I might be able

to get a good scholarship. But I'll never have a chance unless you allow me to apply and unless you'll help by filling out the financial aid forms."

Maria's father lowered the newspaper, took a swallow of his dark, strong coffee, and sighed. "Maria, I'm sorry if I haven't seemed supportive. I want you to have all the best things—things I never had when I was growing up. Your mama and I have worked hard to provide you and your sisters with the best things we could. It was a real sacrifice, you know, to send five girls to the parish school. I wouldn't have had it any other way, but it was expensive. I still have quite a few years of tuition to pay for your sisters. Maria, I'll do everything I can to help you pay for college, but it won't be much. I'm a simple man with a modest income trying to raise my children with the same values I had growing up. What do I know about college? In my country, you finished high school, served your time in the army, and then went to work in a factory. Oh sure, some kids went to the university, but not many from our class of people. I love you, Maria. Bring me the papers."

Maria graduated from her Roman Catholic parish's high school a few months later and was admitted to the school of health sciences at the regional state university 50 miles from her home. True to his word, her father helped her complete the required applications for financial aid. Maria was

Continued

(Case narrative continued)

thrilled to open a letter from the university one day in June informing her that she was the recipient of a scholarship that would pay more than half of her college expenses. She would still have to work very hard to pay the rest of her fees, and she'd probably graduate with some debt, but the scholarship put college in reach.

On the day the scholarship letter arrived her mother sat down with her. "So, my daughter will go to college—the first one in her family! We're so proud of you, Maria. Girls today have so many chances my friends and I didn't have growing up. What will you study at the university?"

Maria considered her answer carefully, knowing that her parents, with their traditional ways and thinking, would have certain expectations regarding her choice of a college major. "Well," she began, "You know how much I enjoy science. And I've always wanted to help people. The stories you told me about Grandma Katya and her nursing career make me think I want to do something in the health care area. But I also really love sports. I've been an athlete all my life, and I honestly can't imagine a life apart from sports. The athletic trainer at school and I have been talking I think I'd like to investigate what it might take for me to become an athletic trainer."

Maria's mother responded, "Well, it's true that the athletic trainer at your school is a fine person, and she was very kind to you when you injured your knee last year. All I ask is that you don't jump into this decision too hastily. You're a talented young woman who could do anything you put your mind to."

"Don't worry, Mama," said Maria. "The School of Health Sciences at the university requires us to investigate a variety of health care professions before settling on just one. I'll be careful."

Maria arrived at the university in September. In addition to a variety of liberal arts courses that all first-year students take, Maria also signed up for *Introduction to Health Professions*. The purpose of this course was to provide prospective health professionals with an overview of the health care system and the various disciplines that comprise it. The course had a field placement component that required each student to spend 4 hours per week shadowing a variety of health care professionals in their work settings. Because Maria indicated that her primary area of interest was athletic training, she was assigned to spend the first half of the term observing the work of four athletic trainers. Her first 2 weeks would be with the athletic trainer who worked with the university's soccer programs. This would be followed by 2-week stints with athletic trainers at the local hospital's sports medicine center, a large high school across the street from the university, and at a local auto manufacturing plant. The second half of the term would be spent with a physical therapist, nurse, occupational therapist, and a physician's assistant. She hoped that she would enjoy the athletic training rotations because the application for the athletic training program would be due during the second semester. What if she did not feel athletic training was a good fit for her? What if the people she observed were not like her high school's athletic trainer? While she was hopeful that her predisposition toward athletic training would be confirmed during her field placements, she was glad that she would also have experiences with the other disciplines—just in case.

As the semester drew to a close, Maria met with her academic advisor, a nurse practitioner who served as a faculty member in the nursing department, but who, like all School of Health Sciences faculty, also advised first-year students until they declared their majors. "How is everything going for you, Maria?" she asked as Maria entered her office and sat down. "Are you enjoying your *Intro to Health Professions* course?"

"Absolutely!" Maria responded. "It's my favorite class."

"Terrific. What do you especially like about the course?" asked Maria's advisor.

(Case narrative continued)

Maria considered the question for a second and then responded, "Well, first of all, the field experiences have convinced me that I want to become an athletic trainer. I really love the way the athletic trainers I've shadowed used their specialized knowledge to help their patients get back to their previous level of activity. And all the patients seem to really appreciate everything the athletic trainers do for them."

"OK, that sounds great," responded Maria's advisor. "But didn't you also observe some other health professionals? How did that go?"

"Oh, I liked each experience very much," answers Maria. "It's interesting, though. Each place I visited seemed different in some ways. For example, the athletic trainers I observed all seemed to push their patients a bit harder than either the physical therapists or occupational therapists did. I think I also enjoyed the athletic training experiences more than the physician's assistant and nursing observations because the athletic trainers seemed to be more 'hands-on' in some way. I mean, the nurse and physician assistant were both great and really helped their patients, but their work environments seemed more static and unvaried than those of the athletic trainers, who did a wide variety of tasks in quite a few different settings. I have to admit that I didn't realize how many different places employ athletic trainers. And their patients were easily the most motivated to get better of all the patients I encountered in any of my rotations."

"It seems that you've really gotten quite a bit out of this course," said Maria's advisor. Did you notice any differences between the various athletic training settings you visited?"

"Oh yes," Maria responded. "The pace in the sports medicine clinic was a bit more relaxed since the athletic trainer in that setting typically worked with just one patient at a time. The university and high school athletic trainers were the busiest. But I think I also enjoyed those settings the best because you have to really know your patients extremely well to be effective. I mean, those trainers are with all those athletes every day. Plus, I liked the fact that these settings had the most athletic activity associated with them. I liked the industrial setting more than I thought I would, to be honest. It was almost exactly like the university and high school settings except there weren't any sports. The athletic trainer at the factory seemed to relate to her patients in the same way the high school and university athletic trainers did to theirs. The auto workers seemed just as comfortable with her as the university soccer players did with the athletic trainer in the campus athletic training room. The auto plant talked to the foreman in much the same way as the high school trainer did with the coaches."

After discussing her first-semester experiences with her parents during the Christmas vacation, Maria decided to apply for the university's athletic training program. If accepted, she would begin the clinical part of the program in the fall semester of her sophomore year.

Level I: Introduction to Professional Ethics in Athletic Training

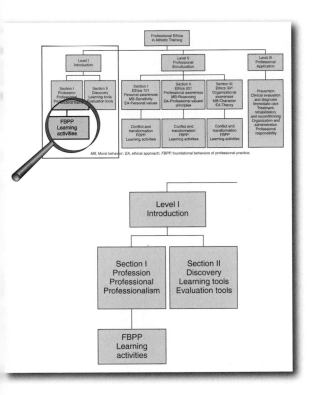

Athletic training has undergone significant transformation and transition as a profession over the past 50 years. During this time of change, we have expanded our employment opportunities, enhanced our professional organization, and developed critical positioning in the health care arena. However, before you can embrace the significant changes that have impacted and shaped this profession, it is crucial that you understand the foundations upon which this profession has evolved.

Part I of this textbook, Introduction to Professional Ethics in Athletic Training, is composed of two fundamental sections that introduce you to the profession as a whole and also introduce you to existing literature relative to ethics in allied health care. Section I provides a straightforward, easy-to-understand glimpse of the profession as it has evolved over time. It frames the concept of "profession" in the context of "athletic training" and makes critical links to the unique services and skills offered by athletic training professionals. Addressed within this section are the fundamental regulatory and codified components that guide our profession and the impact this has on the profession as a whole. Within this framework, the evolution of the athletic training professional is also addressed. Factors such as professional enculturation, beliefs, and values are introduced to help you embrace the role of self-discovery as you journey through the ethical discovery process. Specific learning activities are included to assist you in making connections between theory and practice. Following a brief introduction to current literature regarding ethics training, you are challenged by completing a series of active learning activities that begin to take you along the journey of understanding yourself. Emphasizing the roles of critical thinking and self-reflection, these activities provide a foundation for understanding not only where we are as a profession, who we are as professionals, and what it means to display professionalism—but more important, who we are personally and how this guides our behaviors.

Section II provides a rich review of literature regarding ethics education. Since athletic training literature is very limited relative to ethics education, these chapters frame the relevance, need, and specific strategies for learning about ethics. In order to fully embrace the journey on which you are about to embark, it is critical to conceptualize key components related to ethics education so that you can understand that it transcends all aspects of what we do didactically and clinically.

At the beginning of this section, Chapter 3 introduces key literature relative to the value of ethics education and how it will enrich athletic training as a profession. Pulling on literature from other allied health care professions such as nursing, medicine, physical therapy, and occupational therapy as well as business and education literature, this chapter makes essential links to the profession of athletic training and the importance of ethics education to our profession. Emphasizing the need to go beyond the code of ethics, this chapter introduces professional enculturation as an imperative to ethical discovery. It further introduces the role of moral character as one chooses to do what is right after discerning what is wrong. This chapter addresses ethical sensitivity and emphasizes the role it plays in ethical dilemmas facing athletic training professionals. Additionally, Chapter 3 details the reasons why we need to integrate ethics education into the profession and addresses the rationale for the content and structure of ethics education models. Lastly, this chapter will help you to understand the processes associated with ethical discovery and stimulate thinking as we journey through the ethical discovery processes to come in the latter parts of this book.

Chapter 4 builds on the previous chapter by providing specific literature related to specific approaches for learning about ethics. This chapter goes into great detail on the various learning strategies that will help you along your journey. Deeply rooted in the literature, this chapter provides multiple perspectives on ethical discovery. Because we all learn in different ways, this chapter integrates theory and practice by encouraging you to fully embrace the richness of each approach. Fundamental to each approach is the notion of active learning and engagement. As we embark upon the journey toward ethical discovery, we cannot be passive. Providing concrete strategies and activities that encourage engagement in the process is the focus of Chapter 4. Specific emphasis is placed on the role of individual activities and group activities so that the learner can fully embrace the tenet that ethics education does not occur in a vacuum. It is based on interactions with others and is situated in complex professional settings encountered along the journey. Emphasizing the value of collaboration and communication in the process, this chapter highlights the multiple dimensions of each approach. From fun, stimulating gaming approaches to more serious, Socratic approaches, Chapter 4 covers a broad range of approaches to ethics education and makes direct links to the profession of athletic training. Through this multiple-lens approach, you will be able to gain an appreciation for the breadth and depth of strategies available to you as you continue through the remainder of the book.

Chapter 5 consists of a thorough review of literature on ethical decision making models. Intended to frame ethical decision making from multiple perspectives, this chapter provides advantages and disadvantages of each model. Although the intent of the chapter is to provide a rich background in ethical decision making processes, the intended outcome of Chapter 5 is to have you fully identify with one or several models for ethical decision making so that when you are placed in a professional situation that requires a prompt, effective decision, you will have some basis for decision making. Internal and external factors affecting decision making are introduced to promote reflection as you continue along the ethical discovery journey. A broad range of models derived from allied health care, medicine, and business are presented in the context of facilitating logical sequencing as one processes ethical dilemmas. Framed contextually, each model is addressed relative to the profession of athletic training.

Chapter 6 provides engaging learning activities that stimulate critical thinking as you are challenged to process the theory and content addressed in Chapters 3 through 5. These learning activities provide a variety of activities from multiple perspectives that facilitate integration and application of the content. Through rational processing and full engagement in the learning activities, you will begin to see the direct relevance of the rich theoretical introduction to this text. Each activity helps guide you along your journey toward ethical discovery while tying directly back to the athletic training profession.

CHAPTER 1

Aspects of the Profession

ETHICAL CONCEPTS

Athletic Trainer Certified (ATC)
Board of certification (BOC)
Code of ethics
Profession
Professional
Professional ethos
Professionalism
Role delineation study
Standards of professional practice

LEARNING OBJECTIVES

After reading this chapter, the student should be able to do the following:

1. Define *profession*, and list four unique characteristics of the concept.
2. List the unique knowledge and skills that athletic trainers possess.
3. List the unique services that athletic trainers provide.
4. Describe how athletic training services are managed.
5. Discuss regulatory control.
6. Describe the concept of professionalism, and list its important characteristics.
7. Describe the concept of professional ethos.
8. Compare the static and dynamic components of professional ethos.
9. Compare the NATA Code of Ethics and the BOC Standards of Professional Practice.

Today, a lack of integrity coupled with self-interest has resulted in a number of stunning newspaper headlines, reflecting an erosion of values and ethics in society at large. The world's view relative to the decorum of a business, organization, and/or profession can have a significant positive or negative effect on that entity. The examination of professional ethics in athletic training begins with a closer look at the terms *profession, professional,* and *professionalism.*

PROFESSION

The term *profession* is a challenging concept to define. In the late seventeenth century, industry had become highly specialized and working societies began to organize into secular professions. By the early twentieth century, the traditional fields of law and medicine held a distinctive status and recognition as professions among the middle class.[24] Today, the sociological literature identifies unique characteristics of a profession, including (1) a unique knowledge and skill base, (2) a unique service, (3) management of that service, and (4) regulatory control. In sum, society recognizes the unique services that are outlined in the knowledge and skills of the profession.[25] Reciprocally, the profession is awarded special authority.[6] Figure 1-1 illustrates the concepts of profession, professional, and professionalism.

Unique Knowledge and Skill Base

Professions are distinguished from one another by the educational preparation and the knowledge and skills contained within each. The profession of athletic training has a unique set of cognitive competencies and clinical proficiencies. The fifth edition of the Board of Certification (BOC) *Role Delineation Study* identified competency areas as outlined in the following domains:

- Domain I—prevention
- Domain II—clinical evaluation and diagnosis
- Domain III—immediate care
- Domain IV—treatment, rehabilitation, and reconditioning
- Domain V—organization and administration
- Domain VI—professional responsibility

Within each domain, the study identifies the unique knowledge and skills in athletic training.[4] Furthermore, the National Athletic Trainers' Association (NATA) has highlighted unique knowledge and skills that an athletic trainer must possess (Box 1-1).[15]

Unique Service

The profession of athletic training provides a service that specializes in the prevention, assessment, treatment, and rehabilitation of injuries and illnesses that

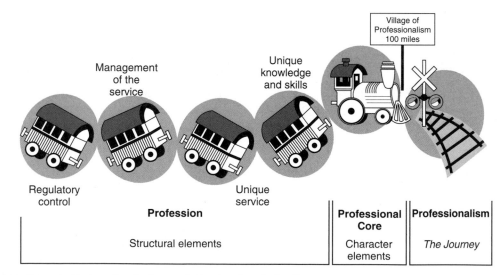

Figure 1-1 ■ Conceptualization of profession, professional, and professionalism.

UNIQUE KNOWLEDGE AND SKILLS

NATA recommends 10 reasons why ATCs are essential in sports:

1. ATCs are first responders who specialize in injury prevention, recognition, assessment, immediate care, treatment, rehabilitation, and reconditioning.
2. As part of the complete health care team, the ATC works under the direction of a licensed physician and in cooperation with other health care professionals, athletic administrators, coaches, and parents. ATCs can treat injuries more effectively because they are part of the health care team from start to finish.
3. ATCs are qualified to make the ultimate call on how soon—due to injury—a player returns to the game, a worker returns to his job, or a serviceman goes back in the line of duty.
4. ATCs are the final word regarding participation in extreme heat and cold conditions and inclement weather forces, such as lightning.
5. Patient satisfaction ratings are greater than 96% when an ATC provides treatment.
6. ATCs have specific knowledge of the musculoskeletal system and can maintain vital signs in any situation that warrants urgent care.
7. ATCs can decrease the odds against something going wrong at events, thus decreasing event or corporate liability issues.
8. The American Medical Association recognizes athletic training as an allied health care profession; through their expertise, ATCs can help prevent trips to the emergency department.
9. ATCs must receive certification from the NATA BOC, attend an accredited athletic training curriculum, and experience rigorous hands-on training to ensure they are qualified professionals.
10. ATCs act as a voice of reason in injury prevention.

Modified from National Athletic Trainers' Association: *Top 10 reasons why athletic trainers are a necessity for the physically active* [news release], Dallas, 2002, National Athletic Trainers' Association. Retrieved April 12, 2005, from http://www.nata.org/newsrelease/archives/000014.html.

result from physical activity. The exclusive skills offered by credentialed members of the athletic training profession were recognized nationally by Congressman Pete Session (R-Tex.) on March 6, 2001. Congress passed a resolution that declares March as National Athletic Training month.[14] Box 1-2 distinguishes the unique services of athletic trainers.

Management of Service

The BOC provides certification for entry-level practitioners, thereby protecting the public by awarding the athletic trainer certified (ATC) credential to qualified candidates. The ATC credential is the acknowledgement that an individual has met an acceptable level of competence in the athletic training profession.

UNIQUE SERVICES PROVIDED BY ATHLETIC TRAINERS

- Quality health care is vital for individuals engaged in physical activity.
- ATCs, based on knowledge and skills acquired through nationally regulated educational processes, have a long history of providing quality health care for athletes and other individuals engaged in physical activity.
- ATCs provide prevention, recognition, evaluation, immediate care, and rehabilitation for injuries and offer education, guidance, and health care administration.
- Athletic training was recognized by the American Medical Association in 1990 as an allied health care profession.
- More than 20,000 ATCs nationwide are employed in high schools, colleges, universities, clinics, and hospitals and in professional sports and corporate and industrial settings.
- Leading organizations concerned with athletic training and health care have joined together to raise public awareness of the importance of the athletic training profession and quality health care for athletes and other individuals engaged in physical activity.

National Athletic Trainers' Association: *U.S. Congress resolves: certified athletic trainers play vital role in health care* [news release], Dallas, 2001, National Athletic Trainers' Association. Retrieved April 12, 2005, from http://www.nata.org/publications/press_releases/congress.html.

However, many states require a license to practice athletic training, and state governments manages the licensing requirements to practice athletic training.[2]

Regulatory Control

The cognitive and psychomotor components of the profession are regulated by the BOC and NATA's Educational Council. Regulatory control requires the athletic training profession to self-assess and set standards for high-quality professional practice. The BOC is a national credentialing agency, and the purpose of its role delineation study is to assess essential com-petency areas in knowledge and skill that a certified athletic trainer must demonstrate. Furthermore, the role delineation study provides content requirements for athletic training education programs accredited by the Commission on the Accreditation of Athletic Training Education (CAATE) and content validity of the BOC examination that leads to the credential ATC.[19]

Ethical components of professional practice and conduct are regulated by the NATA Codes of Ethics[18] and the BOC Standards of Practice.[13] Codes of ethics are statements of aspiration, provide rules of conduct and a framework for ethical decisions, and are considered the hallmark of a profession.[11,20] The profession of athletic training developed its first Code of Ethics in 1958. It has been modified, containing a preamble, four principles, and procedures to report a violation. Furthermore, each state licensing agency outlines acceptable professional behavior and conduct for professional practice. Thus NATA, BOC, CAATE, and each state licensing agency serve to standardize the athletic training profession.

THE PROFESSIONAL

A health professional commits to competence within a trustworthy relationship devoted to protecting, advocating, and caring for the patient and society at large. Essentially, the professional measures his or her worth through external and internal parameters. The external parameter of a professional reflects objective qualifications (e.g., academic professional preparation, the ATC credential, and a state license) that a person has attained to demonstrate adequate competence in providing a service to the patient.

The internal parameter of a professional consists of core character elements: norms, values, and beliefs. In essence, the internal parameter is the extent to which a person has acquired the character of the profession and predictably, enthusiastically, and passionately commits to exceptional competence in providing responsible service. Values such as caring, truth telling, accountability, promise keeping, integrity, courage, and respect provide an internal professional compass to guide and develop a conscience, responsible practice, and a genuine connection with others (e.g., patients, athletes, administrators, and colleagues).[8] Figure 1-1 portrays the professional as the engine of a train. Like an engine, being a professional is an active process characterized by developing core character elements expressed as appropriate values, beliefs, and norms.

PROFESSIONALISM

Because an implicit social contract exists between a profession and the public, professions are given authority and autonomy.[7] Sullivan[23] purported that professionalism hinges on "the moral understanding among professionals that gives concrete reality to this social contract. It is based on mutual trust."[23]

Concepts of professionalism may refer to the profession as a whole or to individual members. Thus professionalism can be viewed by using external (profession) and internal (professional) parameters. The external parameters wrapping around the concept of professionalism in athletic training include attaining and maintaining certification and licensing, two important yet distinct elements of professionalism. Athletic training students are eligible to sit for the BOC examination if they have met all the requirements of an accredited athletic training educational program and, in doing so, have been awarded a baccalaureate degree. Students who have successfully passed the BOC examination are then awarded the ATC credential.[16] The BOC examination is voluntary. State regulation (e.g., licensure, registration, certification), on the other hand, is mandatory, and those states that require athletic trainers to be state licensed, registered, or certified determine the requirements the applicant must possess to practice athletic training in that particular state. Each licensed athletic training professional must also abide by the state's standards of competence and ethical practice. Those who have earned the ATC credential awarded by the BOC have reached the highest level of professionalism.[17]

The internal parameter of professionalism is a commitment to the core values, norms, and beliefs of the profession. It is much more than talking the talk; it is walking the walk. It means *being* a professional. Professionalism is a journey. Figure 1-1 illustrates professionalism as a mile marker on the journey. John Schrader, the 1997 NATA Hall of Fame recipient, said it best:

> We should take on professionalism like walking in ankle-deep water. We can walk through it pretty easily. Our feet are always in contact with the ground and people barely recognize that we are wet. It is there. It is necessary and it is not too uncomfortable.
>
> Perhaps some of us take on professionalism like wading in waist-deep water. It is more strenuous to get through. Good choices are harder because the footing is not always predictable. Other people know that choices are being made because we are wet up to our waist.
>
> What if we jumped over our heads and totally immersed ourselves in it? Deep water is frightening. There is no footing, we must swim freely, confidently, and with determination lest we drown. We must be resolute in purpose, our eyes fixed on the shore and let nothing delay us in our efforts. When we arrive, people clearly know where we have been and what we are about. We can arrive on that shore knowing that we arrived there for a purpose, for ourselves as well as those standing on the shore. Those on the shore clearly know that your efforts involved a total commitment, a journey with a purpose.[21]

Box 1-3 outlines some professional behaviors that reflect professionalism.[5]

PROFESSIONAL ETHOS

The profession and its ethos are linked and embedded in our health care system. Professional ethos is the sum of the distinguishing characteristics of a profession

---

Box 1-3

TWELVE POINTS ON PROFESSIONALISM

1. Be civil; treat all people with respect.
2. Be ethical; stand up for personal and professional standards.
3. Be honest; be truthful and forthright; do not participate in gossip, rumor, and deceptive behaviors.
4. Be the best; do the best you can. Understand and admit your limitations. Have the courage to admit mistakes.
5. Be consistent; behavior should coincide with values and beliefs. Avoid being "two faced."
6. Be a communicator; invite ideas, opinions, and feedback from others. Be aware that nonverbal communication behaviors can be unprofessional.
7. Be accountable; take responsibility for your own actions. Do not be afraid to admit your mistakes.
8. Be collaborative; work in partnership with others for the benefit of athletes, patients, students, and colleagues.
9. Be forgiving; everyone makes mistakes; give people a fair chance.
10. Be current; keep knowledge and skills up to date.
11. Be involved; be active at local, state, and national levels.
12. Be a model; what a person says and does reflects on his or her profession. Do not be self-serving.

Modified from Nativio D: Professionalism revisited, *Nurs Outlook* 49:71-72, 2001.

---

and consists of values, norms, and beliefs. The intersection of values, norms, and beliefs represents the distinguishing professional core elements that have stood the test of time. Figure 1-2 illustrates the distinctive core features that interconnect to shape the professional ethos.[22]

Professional ethos evolves over time as internal and external influences affect the professional body's maturation. Thus the professional ethos is shaped and reshaped and provides the form to contour professional enculturation development. Figure 1-3 illustrates how internal (organizational influences) and external (social, historical, and cultural influences) factors affect professional ethos in athletic training. The curved arrows emerging from the outside influ-

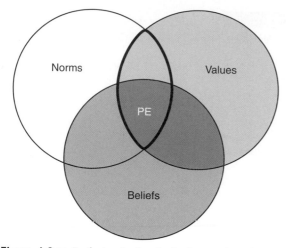

Figure 1-2 ■ Professional ethos is the intersection of norms, values, and beliefs.

ences suggest an indirect effect, whereas the straight arrows emerging from the inside influences suggest a more direct effect on professional ethos in athletic training from 1950 to 2006. Moreover, static and dynamic components also shape professional ethos.

Dynamic Components

The internal and external dynamic components are straightforward and can be scrutinized by using timelines. Table 1-1 identifies the specific internal and external dynamic influences. An examination of NATA's timeline underscores internal dynamic influences that have affected professional ethos.

Figure 1-4 is a historic timeline of NATA over the last 5 decades. The dynamic external influences also are easily viewed in global timelines. Types of athletes and physically active individuals served, litigation, and changes in health care delivery systems are examples of external dynamic influences.

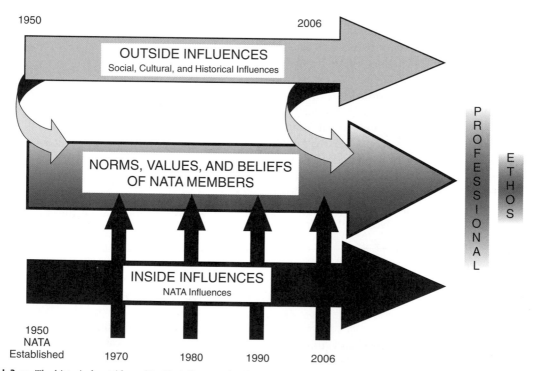

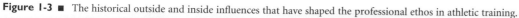

Figure 1-3 ■ The historical outside and inside influences that have shaped the professional ethos in athletic training.

Table 1-1	DYNAMIC INFLUENCES SHAPING THE PROFESSIONAL ETHOS
Type of Influence	**Changes in the Profession**

Internal	Diversification in job setting
	• Professional and amateur sport facilities
	• College, university, community college faculty and staff
	• High school faculty and staff
	• Physical therapy and orthopedic clinics
	• Industrial and corporate facilities
	Membership diversification
	• Increase in female athletic trainers
	• Ethnically diverse athletic trainers
	Education
	• Undergraduate: NATA-approved athletic training education programs (1972-1994)
	• Undergraduate education accreditations
	  • American Medical Association Committee on Allied Health Education Accreditation (1994)
	  • Commission on the Accreditation of Allied Health Education Programs (1994-2006)
	  • Commission on the Accreditation of Athletic Training (CAATE) (2005)
	• Graduate athletic training education programs
	  • CAATE entry level
	  • NATA approval (postcertification: advanced)
	  • Postprofessional education: educational programs reviewed and approved by NATA Graduate Review Committee

External	Levels of sports and athletes served • Professional and amateur athlete • College athlete • High school athlete • Recreational person, the physically active Societal changes • Increased litigation • Expectations of health care Changes in health care delivery • Federal, state, and local mandates • Issues relating to third-party reimbursement • Technology Diversification of athlete and patient population served • Ethnicity • Race • Gender (male athletic trainers working with females and female athletic trainers working with males) • Age

Static Components

The internal static components have not yet been explicitly articulated but are considered the unchanging core elements of the profession. *Far Beyond the Shoe Box* examines the first 50 years (1950-2000) of the athletic training profession. Intuitively, professional preparation, professional leadership and membership, the association, and the NATA journal have stood the test of time and appear to be implicit core elements of the profession (see Fig. 1-4).[9]

PROFESSIONAL ENCULTURATION

Professional enculturation is a process by which newcomers become members of the professional community. Tammivaara and Yarborough[26] first introduced the notion of professional ethos into the physical therapy literature and highlighted the importance of intentionally articulating the values, norms, and culture of physical therapy into the professional curricula.

Athletic training students are the newcomers learning to become members of the athletic training

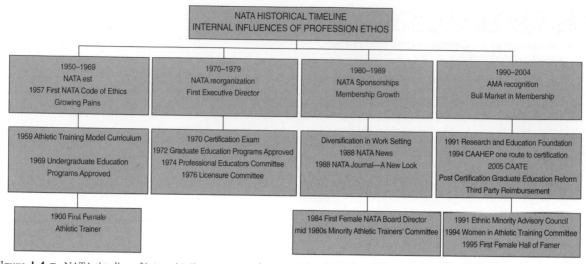

Figure I-4 ■ NATA timeline of internal influences on professional ethos.

profession. Although the role of the athletic trainer is clearly outlined in the cognitive competencies and psychomotor proficiencies, what may not be so apparent are the affective competencies—the core norms, values, and beliefs that are, in effect, the elements that constitute the professional ethos. These competencies are conveyed in the *foundational behaviors of professional practice,* which have been put forth and described by NATA.[19]

Little scientific evidence has addressed norms, values, and beliefs in athletic training. However, Malasarn et al[12] reported personal attributes of expert male National Collegiate Athletic Association (NCAA) Division I certified athletic trainers. The experts identified loyalty, generosity, and a strong work ethic as important core characteristics of expert athletic training professionals. Additionally, the personal philosophies of the participants suggest that out of their strong work ethic evolved a great passion for their work.[12]

CODE OF ETHICS

The professional ethos of athletic training is codified in the NATA Code of Ethics. Historically, societies, including various professions in health care, have had codes that govern behavior. One of the earliest and most recognized codes is the Code Hammurabi. The code originated in the city of Babylon, a diverse community, in 1727 BC. Hammurabi, the exalted prince, intended to make Babylon his metropolis. He attempted to link his vast empire by a uniform system of law. A total of 282 laws were outlined and underpinned the social structure of Babylon, and almost all trace of tribal customs disappeared.[1]

A code of ethics is considered the necessary sociological characteristic and hallmark of a true profession. In essence, the code of ethics is professional agreement with a moral tenor designed to govern the conduct of members when acting alone, interacting with another, and caring for the people they serve. Although the code attempts to guide appropriate professional behavior, it does not offer a specific course to take in terms of moral decisions.[10,13] Knowledge of the code of ethics is not enough to direct the goodness of all who desire to practice athletic training. Codes are important for what they express. Equally important, however, is the character of the professionals, whom the code recognizes. Ideally, professional ethics should be about developing appropriate behavior, not controlling it.

GOOD TO KNOW

Why do professions have a code of ethics? They add layers of responsibility to members in any one group. A code of ethics exists to set boundaries for proper and acceptable behavior. It can increase the probability that an individual will act in a certain way, but it is not a guarantee. Take, for example, sexual harassment. Twenty years ago men interacted with women differently and made comments then that would not be acceptable today. Most organizations have specific rules and regulations about acceptable behavior and how these are handled.

Modified from Lichtenberg J: What's a code of ethics for? In Coady M, Bloch S, editors: *Codes of ethics and the professions*, Melbourne, 1996, Melbourne University Press.

The first NATA Code of Ethics was written by Howard Waite and Pinky Newell in 1957. The preamble stated that "The purpose of this code of ethics is to clarify the ethical and approved professional practice distinguished from those that might prove harmful and detrimental, and to instill into the members of the Association the value and importance of the athletic trainer's role."[22] Pinky Newell was later quoted as stating that "this was the most significant action in the 1950s . . . A professional code of ethics is, in a nut shell, a public statement of expected behavior of any member of the profession."[22] For almost 3 decades, L.F. "Tow" Diehm served as the NATA ethic's chair, and his committee would deliberate on ethical issues relative to the profession of athletic training.

In the late 1980s the NATA and BOC split into two distinct entities, and in doing so a new NATA Code of Ethics and BOC Standards of Professional Practice evolved. Box 1-4 gives the current NATA Code of Ethics,[18] and Box 1-5 provides the BOC Standards of Professional Practice.[3]

Box 1-4

NATA CODE OF ETHICS

Preamble

NATA's Code of Ethics states the principles of ethical behavior that should be followed in the practice of athletic training. It is intended to establish and maintain high standards and professionalism for the athletic training profession.

The principles do not cover every situation encountered by the practicing athletic trainer but are representative of the spirit with which athletic trainers should make decisions. The principles are written generally; the circumstances of a situation will determine the interpretation and application of a given principle and of the Code as a whole. When a conflict exists between the Code and the law, the law prevails.

Principle 1

Members shall respect the rights, welfare, and dignity of all.

1.1 Members shall not discriminate against any legally protected class.

1.2 Members shall be committed to providing competent care.

1.3 Members shall preserve the confidentiality of privileged information and shall not release such information to a third party not involved in the patient's care without a release unless required by law.

Principle 2

Members shall comply with the laws and regulations governing the practice of athletic training.

2.1 Members shall comply with applicable local, state, and federal laws and institutional guidelines.

2.2 Members shall be familiar with and abide by all National Athletic Trainers' Association standards, rules, and regulations.

2.3 Members shall report illegal or unethical practices related to athletic training to the appropriate person or authority.

2.4 Members shall avoid substance abuse and, when necessary, seek rehabilitation for chemical dependency.

Continued

Box 1-4

NATA CODE OF ETHICS—cont'd

Principle 3

Members shall maintain and promote high standards in their provision of services.

3.1 Members shall not misrepresent, either directly or indirectly, their skills, training, professional credentials, identity, or services.

3.2 Members shall provide only those services for which they are qualified through education or experience and which are allowed by their practice acts and other pertinent regulation.

3.3 Members shall provide services, make referrals, and seek compensation only for those services that are necessary.

3.4 Members shall recognize the need for continuing education and participate in educational activities that enhance their skills and knowledge.

3.5 Members shall educate those whom they supervise in the practice of athletic training about the Code of Ethics and stress the importance of adherence.

3.6 Members who are researchers or educators should maintain and promote ethical conduct in research and educational activities.

Principle 4

Members shall not engage in conduct that could be construed as a conflict of interest or that reflects negatively on the profession.

4.1 Members should conduct themselves personally and professionally in a manner that does not compromise their professional responsibilities or the practice of athletic training.

4.2 National Athletic Trainers' Association current or past volunteer leaders shall not use the NATA logo in the endorsement of products or services or exploit their affiliation with the NATA in a manner that reflects badly upon the profession.

4.3 Members shall not place financial gain above the patient's welfare and shall not participate in any arrangement that exploits the patient.

4.4 Members shall not, through direct or indirect means, use information obtained in the course of the practice of athletic training to try to influence the score or outcome of an athletic event, or attempt to induce financial gain through gambling.

From National Athletic Trainers' Association: *Code of ethics,* Dallas, 2005, National Athletic Trainers' Association. Retrieved July 14, 2006, from http://www.nata.org/about/codeofethics.htm.

Box 1-5

BOC STANDARDS OF PROFESSIONAL PRACTICE

I. Practice Standards

Preamble

The Practice Standards (Standards) establish essential practice expectations for all athletic trainers. Compliance with the Standards is mandatory.

The Standards are intended to:

- Assist the public in understanding what to expect from an athletic trainer
- Assist the athletic trainer in evaluating the quality of patient care
- Assist the athletic trainer in understanding the duties and obligations imposed by virtue of holding the ATC credential

The Standards are NOT intended to:

- Prescribe services
- Provide step-by-step procedures
- Ensure specific patient outcomes

The BOC does not express an opinion on the competence or warrant job performance of credential holders; however, every athletic trainer and applicant must agree to comply with the Standards at all times.

Standard 1: Direction

The athletic trainer renders service or treatment under the direction of a physician.

Standard 2: Prevention

The athletic trainer understands and uses preventive measures to ensure the highest quality of care for every patient.

Box 1-5

BOC STANDARDS OF PROFESSIONAL PRACTICE—cont'd

Standard 3: Immediate Care

The athletic trainer provides standard immediate care procedures used in emergency situations, independent of setting.

Standard 4: Clinical Evaluation and Diagnosis

Prior to treatment, the athletic trainer assesses the patient's level of function. The patient's input is considered an integral part of the initial assessment. The athletic trainer follows standardized clinical practice in the area of diagnostic reasoning and medical decision making.

Standard 5: Treatment, Rehabilitation, and Reconditioning

In development of a treatment program, the athletic trainer determines appropriate treatment, rehabilitation, and/or reconditioning strategies. Treatment program objectives include long- and short-term goals and an appraisal of those which the patient can realistically be expected to achieve from the program. Assessment measures to determine effectiveness of the program are incorporated into the program.

Standard 6: Program Discontinuation

The athletic trainer, with collaboration of the physician, recommends discontinuation of the athletic training service when the patient has received optimal benefit of the program. The athletic trainer, at the time of discontinuation, notes the final assessment of the patient's status.

Standard 7: Organization and Administration

All services are documented in writing by the athletic trainer and are part of the patient's permanent records. The athletic trainer accepts responsibility for recording details of the patient's health status.

II. Code of Professional Responsibility

Preamble

The Code of Professional Responsibility (Code) mandates that BOC credential holders and applicants act in a professionally responsible manner in all athletic training services and activities. The BOC requires all athletic trainers and applicants to comply with the Code. The BOC may discipline, revoke, or take other action with regard to the application or certification of an individual that does not adhere to the Code. The

Professional Practice and Discipline Guidelines & Procedures may be accessed via the BOC website, www.bocatc.org.

Code 1: Patient Responsibility

The BOC certified athletic trainer or applicant:

1.1 Renders quality patient care regardless of the patient's race, religion, age, sex, nationality, disability, social, economic status, or any other characteristic protected by law.

1.2 Protects the patient from harm, acts always in the patient's best interests, and is an advocate for the patient's welfare.

1.3 Takes appropriate action to protect patients from athletic trainers, other health care providers, or athletic training students who are incompetent, impaired, or engaged in illegal or unethical practice.

1.4 Maintains the confidentiality of patient information in accordance with applicable law.

1.5 Communicates clearly and truthfully with patients and other persons involved in the patient's program, including, but not limited to, appropriate discussion of assessment results, program plans, and progress.

1.6 Respects and safeguards his or her relationship of trust and confidence with the patient and does not exploit his or her relationship with the patient for personal or financial gain.

1.7 Exercises reasonable care, skill, and judgment in all professional work.

Code 2: Competency

The BOC certified athletic trainer or applicant:

2.1 Engages in lifelong, professional, and continuing educational activities.

2.2 Participates in continuous quality improvement activities.

2.3 Complies with the most current BOC recertification policies and requirements.

Code 3: Professional Responsibility

The BOC certified athletic trainer or applicant:

3.1 Practices in accordance with the most current BOC Practice Standards.

3.2 Knows and complies with applicable local, state, and/or federal rules, requirements, regulations, and/ or laws related to the practice of athletic training.

Continued

Box 1-5

BOC STANDARDS OF PROFESSIONAL PRACTICE—cont'd

3.3 Collaborates and cooperates with other health care providers involved in a patient's care.

3.4 Respects the expertise and responsibility of all health care providers involved in a patient's care.

3.5 Reports any suspected or known violation of a rule, requirement, regulation, or law by him/herself and/or by another athletic trainer that is related to the practice of athletic training, public health, patient care, or education.

3.6 Reports any criminal convictions (with the exception of misdemeanor traffic offenses or traffic ordinance violations that do not involve the use of alcohol or drugs) and/or professional suspension, discipline, or sanction received by him/herself or by another athletic trainer that is related to athletic training, public health, patient care, or education.

3.7 Complies with all BOC exam eligibility requirements and ensures that any information provided to the BOC in connection with any certification application is accurate and truthful.

3.8 Does not, without proper authority, possess, use, copy, access, distribute, or discuss certification examinations, score reports, answer sheets, certificates, certificant or applicant files, documents, or other materials.

3.9 Is candid, responsible and truthful in making any statement to the BOC, and in making any statement in connection with athletic training to the public.

3.10 Complies with all confidentiality and disclosure requirements of the BOC.

3.11 Does not take any action that leads, or may lead, to the conviction, plea of guilty, or plea of nolo contendere (no contest) to any felony, or to a misdemeanor related to public health, patient care, athletics, or education. This includes, but is not limited to: rape; sexual abuse of a child or patient; actual or threatened use of a weapon of violence; the prohibited sale or distribution of controlled substance, or its possession with the intent to distribute; or the use of the position of an athletic trainer to improperly influence the outcome or score of an athletic contest or event or in connection with any gambling activity.

3.12 Cooperates with BOC investigations into alleged illegal or unethical activities. This includes, but is not limited to, providing factual and non-misleading information and responding to requests for information in a timely fashion.

3.13 Does not endorse or advertise products or services with the use of, or by reference to, the BOC name without proper authorization.

Code 4: Research
The BOC certified athletic trainer or applicant who engages in research:

4.1 Conducts research according to accepted ethical research and reporting standards established by public law, institutional procedures, and/or the health professions.

4.2 Protects the rights and well being of research subjects.

4.3 Conducts research activities with the goal of improving practice, education, and public policy relative to the health needs of diverse populations, the health workforce, the organization and administration of health systems, and health care delivery.

Code 5: Social Responsibility
The BOC certified athletic trainer or applicant:

5.1 Uses professional skills and knowledge to positively impact the community.

Code 6: Business Practices
The BOC certified athletic trainer or applicant:

6.1 Refrains from deceptive or fraudulent business practices.

6.2 Maintains adequate and customary professional liability insurance.

From Board of Certification: *Standards of practice*, Omaha, 2004, Board of Certification. Retrieved July 14, 2006, from http://www.bocatc.org/providers/Docs/SI-MR-TAB2-423.htm.

SUMMARY

Professionalism is a journey, and *being* a professional is an active process. Everyday experiences in athletic training have the potential to shape and reshape the professionals in training. Ultimately over time, professional distinctiveness is sculpted and the norms, values, and beliefs of the profession become established and apparent in the professional.

The extent to which new experiences shape a person's professional character depends on a willingness to immerse himself or herself into preprofessional experiences and reflect on them. In the next chapter, the professional in training is introduced to important learning strategies and assessment tools to facilitate greater reflection and greater awareness relative to *being* an athletic trainer.

REFERENCES

1. Barton GA: Ethics of Babylonian and Assyrian religion. In Sneath EH, editor: *The evolution of ethics, as revealed in great religions,* New Haven, Conn., 1927, Yale University Press.
2. Board of Certification: *Certainty for public protection,* Dallas, 2004, NATA (website): www.bocatc.org/partners/Docs/SI-MR-TAB7-414.htm. Accessed July 14, 2006.
3. Board of Certification: *Standards of practice,* Omaha, NE, 2004, Board of Certification (website): www.bocatc.org/providers/Docs/SI-MR-TAB2-423.htm. Accessed July 14, 2006.
4. Board of Certification: *Role delineation study,* ed 5, Omaha, Neb., 2004, Board of Certification.
5. Bruhn JG: Being good and doing good: the culture of professionalism in the health professions, *Health Care Manag* 19:47-58, 2001.
6. Churchill LR, Smith HL: *Professional ethics and primary care medicine: beyond dilemmas and decorum,* Durham, N.C., 1986, Duke University Press.
7. Cruess RL, Cruess SR, Johnston SE: Professionalism and medicine's social contract, *J Bone Joint Surg Am* 82:1189-1195, 2000.
8. Day LJ, Stannard D: Developing trust and connection with patients and their families, *Crit Care Nurse* 19:66-71, 1999.
9. Ebel F: *Far beyond the shoe box,* New York, 1999, Forbes.
10. Gabbard DL, Martin MW: *Physical therapy ethics,* Philadelphia, 2003, FA Davis.
11. Guy M: *Ethical decision making in everyday work situations,* New York, 1990, Quorum Books.
12. Malasarn R, Bloom GA, Crumpton R: The development of expert National Collegiate Athletic Association Division I certified athletic trainers, *J Athl Train* 37:55-63, 2002.
13. Martone M: Building character for a new era, *Health Progress* 80:30-32, 1999.
14. National Athletic Trainers' Association: *U.S. Congress resolves: certified athletic trainers play vital role in health care* [news release], Dallas, 2001, National Athletic Trainers' Association (website): www.nata.org/publications/press_releases/congress.html. Accessed April 12, 2005.
15. National Athletic Trainers' Association: *Top 10 reasons why athletic trainers are a necessity for the physically active* [news release], Dallas, 2002, National Athletic Trainers' Association (website): www.nata.org/newsrelease/archives/000014.html.   Accessed April 12, 2005.
16. National Athletic Trainers' Association: *The ATC credential and professionalism,* Dallas, 2004, National Athletic Trainers' Association (website): www.nata.org/members1/committees/gac/toolkit/benefits_of_boc.pdf. Accessed April 12, 2005.
17. National Athletic Trainers' Association: *Certification vs. licensure,* Dallas, 2005, National Athletic Trainers' Association (website): www.nata.org/members1/committees/gac/toolkit/cert_vs_lisc.pdf. Accessed July 14, 2006.
18. National Athletic Trainers' Association: *Code of ethics,* Dallas, 2005, National Athletic Trainers' Association (website): www.nata.org/about/codeofethics.htm. Accessed July 14, 2006.
19. National Athletic Trainers' Association: *Athletic Training Educational Competencies,* ed 4, Dallas, 2006, National Athletic Trainers' Association.
20. Schank MJ, Weis D: Professional values: key to professional development, *J Prof Nurs* 18:271-275, 2002.
21. Schrader J: Professionalism, one member's perspective, *NATA News,* pp. 20-21, 1997.
22. Stiller C: Exploring the ethos of the physical therapy profession in the US: social, cultural, historical influences and their relationship to education, *J Phys Ther Educ* 14:7-17, 2000.
23. Sullivan M: Medicine under threat. Professionalism and the professional identity, *Can Med Assoc J* 162:673-676, 2000.
24. Sullivan WM: What is left of professionalism after managed care, *Hastings Ctr Rep* 19:7-14, 1999.
25. Swisher LL, Beckstead JS, Bebeau MJ: Factor analysis as a tool for survey analysis using a Profession Role Orientation Inventory as an example, *Phys Ther* 84:784-800, 2004.
26. Tammivaara J, Yarborough P: In transition: perspectives on physical therapy and competent physical therapists. In *Physical therapy education and societal needs,* p. 1927, Alexandria, Va, 1984, American Physical Therapy Association.

Learning Activities: Linking Content to Practice

Allied health care providers must embrace the roots of the profession, develop as professionals, and maintain professionalism and professional ethos. Although a strict understanding of the definitions of these terms is critical, learning activities to evaluate the level of development within these contexts helps preprofessionals make the important connections between theory and practice.

Ethics training and activities have limitations, however. According to Broad and Newstrom,[3] approximately 10% to 13% of what is learned in training is transferred to the job. However, full immersion in self-discovery relative to ethical development in athletic training involves a conscious choice to engage in activities that promote ethical behaviors. The learning activities in this text emphasize individual characteristics, the work environment, and specific parameters for ethical discovery. This intentional organization is intended to promote the transfer of ethics learning to practice. Several studies in social work have shown that previous knowledge, general ability, skill level, motivation level, and sense of efficacy affect how ethics training is incorporated into real-life practice.[2,6] The environment also plays a critical role in ethics training. If a person values—and perceives that others value—ethics training, the likelihood of transferring skills to practical settings increases.[8] Lastly, how learning activities are structured affects the transfer of learning ethics. Four principles govern the design of educational activities relative to ethics training: principle of identical elements, general principles, stimulus variability, and response availability and conditions of practice (Table 2-1).[1,2]

Within any profession, members have responsibilities as professionals, responsibilities to clients, responsibilities to colleagues, responsibilities to the profession as a whole, and responsibilities to society.[6] Activities to promote ethical practice have long been studied in the health care literature; however, a paucity of literature relative to the development of ethical practice exists in athletic training. As approaches to developing as a professional within a chosen profession in a particular professional ethos are examined in this text, several training approaches will be applied. This introductory section presents several learning activities followed by a full section of empirical research to support the learning activities presented in this chapter and subsequent chapters throughout the text.

These activities must be recognized as part of the professional socialization process in the movement toward becoming a professional in athletic training. Students will establish professional relationships and must be able to discern the difference between professional and social implications of these relationships. Discovering your stance on what it means to be a professional enhances your transition into the profession.[19] Self-discovery promotes acculturation into the mores of the profession. While participating in these activities, you must embrace the journey toward becoming an ethical practitioner. Do not be influenced by peer pressure, and take an active role in these learning activities.

Throughout these activities, you will receive feedback from peers and faculty members. Carey and Ness[4] contend that professionalism is facilitated by constant awareness through various modes of feedback.

Table 2-1   TRAINING DESIGN PRINCIPLES

Principles	Definition	Implementation
Identical elements	Transfer of a concept will be facilitated if the training simulates real-life activity.	• Use examples that are similar to actual situations the professional will encounter in the work environment. • Use assessment strategies that closely approximate ethical assessment and decision making that the professional will use in the actual work setting. • Help professionals identify cues that promote recall of training activities related to ethics. • Help learners identify the commonality of each situation to assist in recall of the training strategy.
General principle	Transfer occurs best when general rules and principles underlie the content rather than a specific skill set for each individual situation.	• Make the connections between the general principles and the specific actions but emphasize the general rules. • Promote "mindful abstraction." • Train by using general assessment and decision making strategies that can be used with a variety of ethical dilemmas. • Use parallel processing. • Emphasize metacognitive processing by teaching the student to make connections between the stated code and the resolution of the issue.
Stimulus variability	Transfer of training is best accomplished if a variety of training stimuli are used.	• Maximize examples and learning activities. • Provide examples of ethical and unethical applications of codes of ethics. • Use a variety of examples when using cases to promote the development of broad application of decision making skills.
Response availability and conditions of practice	Transfer of training occurs when strategies promote appropriate responses at appropriate times.	• Allow students the opportunity to solve ethical dilemmas rather than simply discuss options or the dilemma itself. • Practice central ethics skills so they become automatic. • Make connections between the learning and the doing. • Use distributed practice and slowly integrate these skills into real-life situations.

Modified from Baldwin TT, Ford KJ: Transfer of training: a review and directions for future research, *Personnel Psychol* 41:63-105, 1998; and Curry DH: Factors affecting the perceived transfer of leaning of child protection social workers [dissertation], Kent, Ohio, 1996, Kent State University.

Feedback will be formal and informal and should be viewed as constructive. Remember, the ultimate goal in receiving and providing feedback is to promote the advancement of the profession through the enhancement of professionalism. Agreeing to disagree with someone is acceptable, but disagreement should never turn into disrespect. Boundaries within professional conduct exist when persons disagree and no person should feel harassed, disparaged, or intimidated in the process.[4] The demonstration of self-control is a powerful tool and leads to the development of professional behaviors.[10]

Professionals use self-reflection and critical assessment as a means of monitoring professional growth and development.[13,14] The role of reconciling one's personal self with the professional self is a daunting task.[9] While progressing through this text, keep a journal to reflect on the activities you have completed relative to your personal impression of the activity. Express areas in which you felt comfortable, areas that made you feel uncomfortable, and areas about which you still have questions. Try to apply your activities and reflections into practical settings by thinking of one real-life example that highlighted the basic premise of the activity.

At the core of becoming a professional is understanding oneself. Awareness of critical issues in developing as a professional is also critical.[20] The activities in this chapter are designed to encourage personal reflection while reconciling the issues within the profession. The journey toward developing as a professional within the athletic training profession requires traveling along many paths toward discovery and autonomy. Think critically as you progress through these activities to promote raising your level of consciousness relative to professional development.[12]

ACTIVITIES FOR APPLICATION: LINKING CONTENT TO PRACTICE

LEARNING ACTIVITY 1: ETHICAL FOOTBALL

Objectives

1. To familiarize yourself with the NATA Code of Ethics.
2. To provide applications relative to the NATA Code of Ethics.
3. To establish group cohesion and freedom of expression relative to professional ethical considerations.

Description

A football field is set up in the classroom by hanging signs on the walls at equal intervals, marking the end zones as Ethical Hall of Fame and the other as Ethical Hall of Shame.[7] The yard markers (10, 20, 30, 40, 50, 40, 30, 20, 10) are marked on the walls by signs. Students select index cards (see Appendix A). By using the NATA Code of Ethics, the teams (two to three teams) select a representative to move along the field in response to scenarios of compliance and noncompliance provided on the index cards. Other team members stand along the field to provide support to their team member. A team member from the first group randomly selects an ethical scenario card and reads it to the group. Based on the individual response, the group decides how many yards and in which direction the player will move. If no agreement is made on how many yards, move 10 yards. This process is repeated with the remaining cards with the various teams taking turns. The first to reach the Ethical Hall of Fame is the winner.

(Note: You will receive a copy of the standards and scenarios in handout form for future reference.)

Assessment

Using a guided reflective journal entry, provide a written reflection regarding your perceptions of the game and how others' choices affected you. Application of this assignment can be further developed by using the cards to reflect on a real-life scenario that occurred in clinicals that created dissonance.

LEARNING ACTIVITY 2: IS IT ETHICAL?

Objectives

1. To develop a deeper understanding of the NATA Code of Ethics.
2. To facilitate critical thinking and application of the NATA Code of Ethics.
3. To establish group cohesiveness through large-group interaction.

Description

Appendix A provides examples of compliance and noncompliance issues from the NATA Code of Ethics. The coinciding ethical principles are not provided with the examples. Some examples may have practical significance but are not directly linked to a specific principle in the Code of Ethics.[11] Divide your group into teams, discuss the examples, and identify the corresponding principle in the Code of Ethics. If the code does not have a corresponding principle (as with some of the practice examples), identify those as practice issues. Large-group discussion after this activity allows discussion of the principles within the Code of Ethics from a larger scope.

Assessment

Assessment for this activity is accomplished by using the formatted self- and peer assessment tools provided in Appendix B or a personalized self- or peer assessment tool. Identifying the key components is important to assist in gauging your level of participation in group work.

LEARNING ACTIVITY 3: CLASSROOM CODE OF ETHICS

Objectives

1. To establish personal codes of ethics for guiding professional behaviors at each respective level within the program.

2. To enhance the applicability and adaptability of the NATA Code of Ethics to a more personal level and at multiple levels.
3. To establish a student-centered document for addressing professional behaviors within an academic program.
4. To reflect the collective values of each respective class within an academic program.

Description

You will be divided by level within the academic program if not already divided by definition of the class (i.e., freshman, sophomore, junior, senior). After discussing the NATA Code of Ethics and the relevance of codes to all aspects of professional development, you will create your own code of ethics for your particular level.[16]

This code of ethics can be written several ways. First, you may want to write specific principles you would like to see included in the code. These can then be turned in anonymously at a specific location (e.g., box outside the faculty office door) or given to a designated student. The group can then get together to prioritize the submitted principles and develop a working code of ethics.

An alternative option for creating this code is to create a listserv online or within your campus electronic teaching network (e.g., WebCT, Blackboard). Submit your ideas for specified principles to the listserv or discussion group. The group then discusses and decides which principles to include in the working code of ethics. Once the code is established, it can be copied and distributed to each member of the group. It can also be displayed in several key locations such as the academic areas of the building, laboratory spaces, and clinical settings.

(Note: Your instructor also may choose to create a student ethics board to hear complaints or issues relative to the working code for class discussion or redress.)

Assessment

Although this learning activity focuses on a collective product, assessment can occur through individual written work, such as creating a personal document indicating the policies and procedures for reporting violations and including ramifications or sanctions believed appropriate for any breach within the class-

room code of ethics. This project is assessed by using a rubric that highlights key components focusing more on the actual writing and creativity rather than on specific outcomes.

LEARNING ACTIVITY 4: SWOT ANALYSIS

Objectives

1. To encourage critical reflection on the profession and on oneself.
2. To provide a template for designing goals for a specific course or specific clinical assignment.
3. To promote a venue for opening discussion about the direction the profession is headed and how it can be directly related to values.

Description

In any profession, you will be asked to articulate your strengths and weaknesses at some point in your career. Many times these questions are posed as part of an application process or an interview. However, even at the basic levels of an athletic training education program, you should be able to identify and articulate professional strengths and weaknesses. A SWOT analysis is a tool for articulating *s*trengths, *w*eaknesses, *o*pportunities, and *t*hreats that face individuals and the profession as a whole.

CASE SCENARIO

Option A

Perform a SWOT analysis by listing each component as a header down the left side of a piece of paper. Under each heading, identify strengths, weaknesses, opportunities, and threats facing the *athletic training profession.*

CASE SCENARIO

Option B

Perform a SWOT analysis in the same fashion as above; however, this time identify strengths, weaknesses, opportunities, and threats for yourself as *an athletic training professional.*

After this activity, large-group discussion focuses on the analysis of the issues relative to the profession. The individual analysis (which is more personal) will be used by your instructor as a beginning-of-the-year activity followed up by an end-of-the-year written activity that can become part of the personal portfolio. You and your instructor should be able to identify means by which you can maximize your strengths and opportunities and address or limit your weaknesses and threats.

(Note: Because this activity is a wonderful writing activity after discussion of professions, professionals, and professional ethos as it connects the theory to the person, you will likely perform this activity near the beginning of your study of ethics.)

Assessment

Group participation rubrics (see Appendix B) may also be used for the group discussion components. Individual analyses can be assessed as part of the portfolio rubric as they connect to the entire course or clinical assignment. A variety of portfolio evaluation criteria, including clarity and application, may be used to help connect this activity to professional growth.

LEARNING ACTIVITY 5: LINKED LEARNING

Objectives

1. To create a dialogue between you and your peers of various levels within the academic program.
2. To facilitate mentoring within a program.
3. To open lines of communication and initiate discussion about the profession, professionalism, and the professional ethos.

Description

Students are placed in small groups, with a mix of first- and fourth-year students. After a brief introduction, answer the following questions[18]:

1. What is the image of athletic training as a profession?
2. What is your impression of your experiences in athletic training throughout the curriculum?
3. How does the public perceive the profession of athletic training?

After 10 minutes of discussion, you will be given 5 minutes to write a reflective response to the statement: What effect has this activity had on your perspective of the profession of athletic training? Ten minutes of general discussion relative to the written responses follows. First-year students collect the fourth-year student responses, and fourth-year students collect the first-year student responses. Break into groups by year for a larger discussion on the profession, professionalism, and professional ethos. Professional growth and the image of the profession are at the core of this activity.

Assessment

Although this activity involves group discussion, assessment for this activity is best suited to individual reflection. You can provide a written reflection or analysis of the discussion and how your perceptions coincided or conflicted with the other groups' perspectives. Addressing professional implications will help you identify with the profession and how professional development occurs throughout the curriculum. A variety of instruments may be constructed to capture the essence of the nature of the reflection.

LEARNING ACTIVITY 6: THE PROFESSIONAL WILL

Objectives

1. To encourage reflection on personal and professional values and behaviors.
2. To facilitate discussion relative to how personal and professional values and behaviors are perceived by others.
3. To establish a strong understanding of the role of professional image and character.

Description

Create an "ethical will" to leave those who follow you in the profession. The ethical will describes how you want to be remembered.[5] Create a will and connect it to the concepts of profession, professional, professionalism, and professional ethos. This document should describe the legacy you want to leave behind and can be used anonymously in focus groups on the aforementioned concepts. (Note: This activity is an excellent precursor to values activities and will help as you progress into that literature.)

Assessment

Because of the highly personal nature of this activity, feedback focuses on the format and clarity rather than the content. This sensitive activity provides an avenue for you to reflect deeply on who you are and who you want to become.

LEARNING ACTIVITY 7: THREE QUICK QUESTIONS TESTS

Objectives

1. To introduce basic ethical dilemmas.
2. To create dialogue relative to the multiple options for resolving ethical dilemmas.
3. To connect professionalism and the professional ethos into real-life scenarios so you can link professional behaviors and values.

Description

Discuss the following situations[17]:

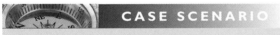

CASE SCENARIO

Scenario A

Supplies are being removed from the athletic training practice areas by fellow athletic training students. Although a rule exists that no supplies can be removed from the athletic training facilities, students are taking the supplies home to practice because they are preparing for their practical examination that determines admission into the program.

CASE SCENARIO

Scenario B

You are asked to assist a faculty member or approved clinical instructor by attending a weekend soccer tournament that was scheduled at the last minute. You have plans to spend the weekend with your friends because one of them is having a twenty-first birthday party.

CASE SCENARIO

Scenario C

You see an upperclassman providing underclassmen with the answers to an online quiz that is part of the introductory course for your program. Students are required to work individually on these quizzes because they are part of the course grade.

After you have completed your discussions, ask the following three questions relative to your responses:

1. Are you following the "golden rule" (treat others as you would want to be treated)?
2. Would you be comfortable having the newspaper report your actions or a television station observe your actions?
3. Would you be at ease having your parents observe your behavior?

Share your solutions to the problems and responses.

Assessment

Group discussion rubrics are an important tool for assessing participation in larger groups. The purpose is not to identify correct or incorrect options but to encourage everyone to think through the options and alternatives. Either the group participation rubric or a self-created rubric may be used. Additional assessment can occur if you create a written document that expresses personal choices compared with group choices and/or identifies areas of dissonance created in the group discussion. Your instructor will choose the most appropriate activity for your class.

LEARNING ACTIVITY 8: USE OF . . .

Objectives

1. To introduce values and the roles they play in professional behaviors.
2. To stimulate thinking about interpretations, policies, procedures, laws, and ethical codes.
3. To increase awareness relative to personal and professional behaviors.

Description

Examine the situations listed below related to the use of certain tools and behaviors in a professional workplace.[21] You are positioned in the middle of the room, and the sides of the room are designated as the "agree side" and the "disagree side." After the instructor poses the questions, move from the middle to one side or the other depending on your position relative to the question. A brief discussion follows each question, limited to 5 minutes. The instructor records how many students moved to each side for discussion. You may address all or only selected numbers of the questions.

QUESTIONS FOR USE OF . . . ACTIVITY	
Use of . . .	**Description**
Time	Cheating on your time at work to keep your job is acceptable (e.g., leaving a few minutes early, stepping outside to smoke, extended lunches).
Telephone and e-mail	Using work computers and time to respond to personal e-mail and telephone calls is acceptable.
Money	Using your employer's money to purchase incidentals and entertainment items while on a business trip is acceptable.
Information	Sharing information about other employees (such as salary, performance evaluations, personal e-mail communications) with other members of the staff is acceptable.
Drugs	Ignoring a colleague who is using illegal substances and/or drinking while on the job (including coming to work with a significant hangover) is acceptable.
Materials	Using company paper for personal invitations or copying and mailing personal items with the company mail meter are acceptable.
Human behavior	Making suggestive remarks to a close co-worker is acceptable.
Work and ideas	Stealing an idea from a co-worker to keep a job and/or take credit for work that was completed by someone else is acceptable.
Environment	Ignoring an environmental hazard, particularly if it will get your superior in trouble, is acceptable.

Assessment

This activity is assessed by having you write a personal interpretation of how the activity went in the larger group by identifying areas of conflict or directly linking the responses (as recorded by the instructor) to the effects they may have on the profession or within the academic program. Evaluation of the written content is based on objective criteria established by the instructor.

LEARNING ACTIVITY 9: LETTER TO A FRIEND

Objectives

1. To encourage you to articulate perceptions in a casual manner.

2. To increase awareness of personal and professional ideas.
3. To assist in processing conflict or agreement on critical topics.

Description

After the introduction to the profession, professional behaviors, and professionalism, students perform an activity that involves informal writing in the form of a letter to a friend who has decided to become an athletic trainer.[15] In this letter, articulate your perceptions of the profession, what it means to be a professional in the field, and why you are pleased the friend has chosen this profession. Another option is to describe what it means to be an athletic trainer to a friend in a letter.

Assessment

Because this is personal reflection, the assignment should evaluate the ability to express oneself clearly and address any possible content errors presented. Expressing your feelings through a personal letter read to the class (volunteers only) may spark group discussion that can lead to group interaction to be assessed by using a group participation rubric.

LEARNING ACTIVITY 10: GOAL RANKING AND MATCHING

Objectives

1. To formulate and rank goals and establish methods for achieving them.
2. To examine the profession and professional development plan.
3. To integrate professionalism throughout the curriculum as you progress toward a career in athletic training.

Description

After discussion on the profession, write several (four to six) learning goals and describe how you plan to achieve those goals. Next, rank the goals in order of importance. These goals should be focused on profes-sional development directly related to the athletic training profession as you progress toward an entry-level career.

Tip: This activity can also be used in a more course-specific manner as part of a portfolio by includ-ing a professional behavior goal or two in each course within the core curriculum. A great culminating activ-ity is to do one of two activities (or both). Compare your goals from the beginning of the year to the end of the year (goals analysis) and/or retain goal state-ments from your early (freshman or sophomore) years and compare them to your senior year goals through a reflective learning activity. This activity reinforces the fluid nature of goals and highlights just how much you have changed throughout the academic program.

Assessment

Goals statements can be assessed by using standard evaluation criteria that include factors such as related-ness to the profession, succinct writing, and depth and breadth of achievement plan. However, goals will not be evaluated as "good" or "bad," because they provide different forms of motivation for each individual. These goals should be referenced throughout the academic curriculum.

REFERENCES

1. Baldwin TT, Ford KJ: Transfer of training: a review and directions for future research, *Personnel Psychol* 41:63-105, 1998.
2. Brittain CR: *The effect of a supportive organizational environment on transfer of training in child welfare organizations* [disserta-tion], Denver, 2000, University of Colorado.
3. Broad ML, Newstrom JW: *Transfer of training: action-packed strategies to ensure high payoff from training investments*, Reading, Mass., 1992, Addison-Wesley.
4. Carey JR, Ness KK: Erosion of professional behaviors in physi-cal therapist students, *J Phys Ther Educ* 15:20-22, 2001.
5. Cornwell L: More people pass on beliefs, values in an ethical will, *The Canton Repository*, March 13:B-10, 2005.
6. Curry DH: *Factors affecting the perceived transfer of learning of child protection social workers* [dissertation], Kent, Ohio, 1996, Kent State University.
7. Curry D, Caplan P: The transfer field: a learning activity, *Child Youth Leader* 7:28-30, 1995.
8. Curry D, Wentz R, Brittain C, et al: *Case scenarios and training implications*, Washington DC, 2004, American Public Human Services Association.
9. Doane G, Pauly B, Brown H, et al: Exploring the heart of ethical nursing practice: implications for ethics education, *Nurs Ethics* 11:241-253, 2004.
10. Emener WG: Consumerism in rehabilitation education and the empowerment of students' personal and professional develop-ment, *Rehabil Educ* 6:265-273, 1992.
11. Feeney S, Freeman NK, Moravcik E: *Teaching the NAEYC code of ethical conduct: activity sourcebook*, Washington DC, 2000, National Association for the Education of Children.
12. Gaylin G: Knowing good and doing good, *Hastings Ctr Rep* 3:36-41, 1994.
13. Heames JT, Service RW: Dichotomies in teaching, application and ethics, *J Educ Bus* November/December:118-122, 2001.
14. Huotari R: A perspective on ethical reflection in multiprofes-sional care, *Reflective Prac* 4:121-138, 2003.

15. McKeachie WJ: *Teaching tips: strategies, research and theory for college and university teachers*, Lexington, Mass., 1994, DC Heath and Company.

16. Schlabach GA: *Classroom code of ethics* [unpublished material], DeKalb, Ill., 2004, Northern Illinois University.

17. Shefrin AP, Harper B: Encouraging ethical excellence, *Appl Clin Trials* 9:52-56, 2000.

18. Smith D, Garteig L: Using a linked learning activity to foster nursing students' professional growth, *J Nurs Educ* 42:227-230, 2003.

19. Teschendorf B, Nemshick M: Faculty roles in professional socialization, *J Phys Ther Educ* 15:4-11, 2001.

20. Triezenberg HL: Beyond the code of ethics: educating physical therapists for their role as moral agents, *J Phys Ther Educ* 14:48-59, 2000.

21. Vincent A, Meche M: Use of ethical dilemmas to contribute to the knowledge and behavior of high school students, *High School J* 84:50-58, 2001.

CHAPTER 3

Ethics Education: Framework for Success

ETHICAL CONCEPTS

Ethics education

Ethical engagement

Values education

Philosophical neutrality

LEARNING OBJECTIVES

After reading this chapter, the student should be able to do the following:

1. Understand the foundation of ethics education.

2. Understand and embrace the importance of studying ethics in athletic training.

3. Appreciate the role of assessing or evaluating progress through the ethical discovery process.

4. Develop a strong understanding of the role of ethics in professional development throughout a career in athletic training.

Being ethical also takes . . . courage. That courage, on occasion, demands resistance; on other occasions, it demands persistence; and on other occasions, it may even demand assertiveness. While fostering courage, however, we have to avoid being self-righteous. Courage must be coupled with the humble acceptance that we will not always make the best decisions or the best choice, but we will keep trying, and we trust our colleagues and clients will help us by providing constructive criticisms (p. 192).[38]

OVERVIEW OF ETHICS EDUCATION

Interest in ethical issues is growing faster than ever.[14] Several formal ethics training programs such as the Kenan Ethics Program—Ethics Across the Curriculum[24] have been established in high schools with attempts of integrating ethics into the academic environment. Medicine, nursing, and physical therapy have looked at ethics education from a professional program perspective. However, athletic training education programs have limited integration of ethics into the curriculum.

Health care professionals deal directly with the health and, oftentimes, lives of the people for whom they are responsible for providing care. The belief that health care providers will provide care and fulfill responsibilities within the scope of trust is often assumed. These professionals, including athletic trainers, must carry out their responsibilities without discriminating for religion, sex, race, nationality, or political or social status.[15] However, the role of ethical development in health care curricula has been controversial. So, how can ethical behaviors be encouraged?

Many educators use established professional codes of ethics as the cornerstone for ethics education. Typically presented in class as a standing document, faculty members have an obligation to take ethics education beyond the presentation of existing documents to encourage critical analysis of the applications of ethics in the athletic training field. Furthermore, ethics education goes far beyond coverage of an established professional code of ethics. This text is designed to immerse readers in the essence of ethics education and place them in conflicting situations to fully develop an ethical framework to guide professional practice. This

process of socialization—in which professional values represented in a code of ethics are internalized—is complex and requires full participation to gain the real benefits of ethics education.[28]

Carr[11] uses the term *ethical engagement* when referencing the different applications of ethics in teaching and learning. "Whereas not all human agents find themselves in the kind of occupational or professional circumstances that might require universally impartial regard for the needs of the sick, or strictly unbiased collection of evidence for legal defense, it should be clear enough that some virtue ethical cultivation of general dispositions to temperance, courage, honesty, justice, and (some measure of wisdom) is a sine qua non of any and all positive moral association" (p. 260).[11] Some professionals may be highly regarded as professionals because of their clinical skills and fidelity to the profession; however, those same people may have less than exemplary moral characteristics. A common conflict that arises in professional educational programs is whose values should be exemplified and how they should be enforced. This illuminates the role of professional socialization and foundational behaviors for professional practice. As young athletic training professionals emerging from your academic programs, you are not only being prepared to challenge (and pass) the Board of Certification examination; you are more importantly being prepared for the profession. Without ethical engagement throughout the curriculum in both the didactic and clinical settings, students will not likely emerge confident enough in personal and professional identity to make sound professional decisions of an ethical nature. That is why this text engages you throughout your academic career to facilitate this transition into the profession.

Although considerable research exists relative to ethics education in the allied health fields, consensus on the philosophy, purpose, and learning strategies has not been reached.[28] This relative state of flux[4] and the uncertainty about ethics education[54] have created a void in many allied health education programs, including athletic training. What the literature does say is that students in professional programs should be able to engage in wise, engaging, imaginative, and life-enhancing conversations rooted contextually in the core curriculum to promote ethical development in a challenging allied health care profession.[11]

The purpose of this section of the text is to present a comprehensive overview of learning strategies related to ethics education, with particular emphasis on the versatility of each strategy. By having a strong theoretic understanding of the techniques used for learning about ethics, students will gain a greater appreciation and understanding of the processes associated with ethical discovery and the ethical decision-making processes.

WHY LEARN ABOUT ETHICS?

The professional needs to develop the skills to see a moral shape, to understand the difference between her own perspective and that of others, and to respond well to what is there to be seen, if she is to become professionally competent (p. 32).[52]

Ethics, or the way a moral person should behave, embodies two concepts: the ability to discern right from wrong and a commitment to do what is good, right, and proper.[45] Being an athletic trainer requires ethical decision making and this, in turn, necessitates an effective learning process. Allied health professionals are faced with increasing challenges as technology and other factors such as medical advances drive change and create more ethical dilemmas and problems.[15] Such changes strengthen the need for ethics education throughout the curriculum at all levels of health care education—undergraduate through continuing education.[20] Ethics education is needed and should continue throughout the educational program in an integrated, real-life setting to prevent deterioration of ethical reasoning as ethical dilemmas are encountered on a daily basis.[13]

Professionals in the field must be able to frame their work in ethically sensitive ways when situations involving ethical dilemmas arise.[41] Beyond a few brief lectures and powerful, often overwhelming, apprenticeships, many allied health care professionals, including athletic trainers, have little training in ethics.[39] Research indicates that increased levels of moral reasoning are associated with ethics education.[8] Ethics education prepares the practitioner to accept the moral responsibilities of clinical practice seen in all allied health care fields. Furthermore, ethics education attempts to restore the human side of health care by focusing on personal and professional values. These are the major reasons for integrating this ethics program throughout a curriculum.

Health care is not the only field that has documented the effectiveness of ethics education. Much can be learned from the business literature that contends that ethics education helps shape leaders and establishes a culture for the organization.[18] Leaders with integrity and social conscience help guide the organization and/or program in good times and bad. Leaders who foster dialogue and dissent also encourage ethical behavior through open communication. Leaders who are willing to reflect on and learn from their actions facilitate ethical behavior by embracing an environment for continuous quality improvement. Establishing a strong leadership foundation encourages ethical behavior by culture of collaboration. Our organizations are beginning to face the same challenges business does and in some cases are taking on similar characteristics and structures of business organizations. This notion of ethics evolving through strong leadership cannot be underestimated.

Athletic training may be assumed to require a high degree of ethical behavior and to hold practitioners to an ethical code, but ethics is not a skill or competency that is typically taught in athletic training education programs. Athletic training students will progress through the academic and clinical programs facing issues wherein wanting to do good—such as acting in the best interest of and showing respect for the patient—is not enough. Conflicting personal values may drive a practitioner to act in a way that creates a sense of ethical discomfort.[49] Understanding why this occurs and how to address this conflict will further shape professionals in the field.

Although business and allied health are rich with support for ethics education, athletic training literature is limited relative to teaching ethics and the development of foundational behaviors for professional practice as a result of ethics education.[12,17,31,33-35,42,52] Nursing and medicine research in ethics education has led the way toward recent advances in ethics education in the physical therapy field. [22,25,27,44,50] Although why athletic training has not yet fully embraced the need for ethics education is unclear, practitioners of practitioners of physical therapy identified the following reasons for the lack of research in ethics education in their field: (1) ethics is not seen as a priority area within the curriculum with the ever-expanding required content areas and (2) the lack of professional expertise on the topic.[5] Athletic training perhaps faces these same issues. However, with the recent transition from affective competencies[36] to the foundational behaviors of professional practice,[37] ethics education must take the forefront to prepare athletic training students for the challenges of professional practice in athletic training.

Ethics education has essentially been confusing because the literature is not clear regarding what the true focus should be. Although required in some allied health and medical programs and in some states by licensure boards, the purpose is often unclear. Ethics education should prepare the student to identify ethical issues, develop moral reasoning and decision-making skills, and improve implementation of ethically rooted decisions. However, the medical literature even acknowledges that simply teaching ethics does not ensure ethical conduct.[19] Therefore some level of ethical discovery needs to be part of the core curriculum in allied health care and medical education. That is why this text involves you directly in the discovery process by encouraging participation in a variety of learning activities to foster your professional journey.

At the core of athletic training ethics education is the development of professional integrity and clinical reasoning.[1] Some literature connects values education with ethics education. Values education is distinctly different, although integrally connected to ethics education. Learning strategies for each are presented.

CONTENT: WHAT IS IT ABOUT? WHAT WILL I LEARN?

Although this may sound odd, the purpose of ethics is not to make people ethical, it is to help people make better decisions.
MARVIN T. BROWN[9]

What do you need to know or want to know about ethics? Barnitt[5] identified a paucity in the litera-ture on what students want to know and an increasing volume of literature identifying recommendations by educators and professional bodies for the content of ethics courses in allied health care. The key concepts relative to ethics education in health care are that it should be taught in a clinically relevant context, involve the development of personal values connected with professional values and codes, and be approached from a process rather than outcome perspective. Teaching how to solve problems a student will potentially face in clinical practice enables confidence when ethical dilemmas and conflicts arise. Students will be provided "opportunities to talk and listen, read, write, and reflect as [you] approach course content through problem-solving exercises, informal small groups, simulations, case studies, role playing, and other activities—all of which require you to apply what you are learning" (p. xi).[32]

Clearly, learning about ethics is not an isolated event that occurs in a vacuum; it is a progressive, integrative journey that leads toward that critical transition from student to professional. Sims and Brinkmann[48] support ethics education throughout the curriculum and across the disciplines to promote a more holistic understanding of ethical dilemmas. Emphasizing moral attitude components such as self-conception, sensitivity, judgment, sharing, motivation, and courage, critical thinking about ethical dilemmas can transcend the entire educational program, including didactic and clinical components. In this model, you should not have to wait until you graduate to apply what you have learned. Developing early opportunities for involvement and communication relative to ethical situations encourages you from the beginning to have a voice in the process of ethical discovery. The tools for ethical discovery will be provided by a variety of approaches across the curriculum.

Fundamental to ethics education is the role of understanding the process as well as the outcome. Essential to professional development, ethics needs to be "uncovered" rather than simply taught by theories. Wiggins and McTighe[53] present filters for understanding that are directly applied to ethics education that serve as a template for content within an ethics education curriculum in any profession. Emphasizing that ethics education should be enduring, at the heart of the discipline, uncovered rather than instructed, and engaging, these filters provide a conceptual structure for the content as ethics educational components are integrated throughout a variety of courses. The conceptual structure centralizes the need for understanding, as depicted in Table 3-1.

A variety of approaches to learning about ethics are documented in ethics education. The *principles* approach identifies four main principles (autonomy, nonmaleficence, beneficence, and justice) that serve as the core of all analysis and judgments.[7] The *ethic of caring* is another content approach for ethics education. This approach emphasizes the relationships and responsibilities associated with providing care for others.[40] *Decision theory* is yet another approach to ethics education. Decision-making models drive this approach as students follow closely prescribed steps to solve ethical problems. Lastly, the topics or issues approach to ethics education is commonly used. This approach emphasizes common topics or issues related to the profession, including codes of ethics, confidentiality, resources allocation, and other issues with ethical implications. Furthermore, models can be applied in the day-to-day activities of an educational or workplace setting to foster ethical behavior (Table 3-2).[45]

Regardless of the approach taken to ethics education, a broad understanding that ethics education is underused in most allied health care programs is imperative. Identification of key concepts to emphasize at each level throughout the curriculum is the approach advocated by the authors. Beginning through advanced students can benefit from ethics education, and the authors are emphatic about the role of ethics education in athletic training curricula. In addition, the integration of ethics in both the didactic and clinical components of the curriculum is essential. This text provides a compass as you journey through this important process.

The goals of ethics education in health care should be to focus on fostering ethical discovery, integrate personal and professional discovery, emphasize rational thinking with subjective experiences, and attend to the complexities of the specified health care field.[16] Literature reflects that bioethics, moral theory, and ethical decision making alone are insufficient to prepare professionals for the challenges of a health care profession.[3,6,26,46] Grounding ethics education into

Table 3-1   FACETS FOR UNDERSTANDING ETHICS

Facet	Definition	Application to Ethics
Explanation	A knowledgeable account of events, actions, or ideas	What is going on here, ethically speaking? What principles, theories, or constructs are at work or in conflict in a given situation?
Interpretation	Meanings that individuals place on events, actions, and experiences	What does this mean? What are the implications? Why is this important, ethically speaking?
Application	Ability to use knowledge in novel situations	How do the principles, theories, or constructs in ethics apply to a specific case? What is helpful in understanding the problem and resolving it? What is not important?
Perspective	Insights and points of view	How would I see this case if I were the patient, spouse, coach, physician? How do values, culture, and other characteristics limit perspective?
Empathy	Ability to perceive the world through the perspective of another	What emotions were evoked in the case? What do emotions tell us about what is important in ethics?
Self-knowledge	Critical self-reflection	Where can I improve? What are my blind spots? How do I know what I know?

Modified from Wiggins G, McTighe J: *Understanding by design,* Alexandria, Va., 1998, Association for Supervision and Curriculum Development, p. 23.

Table 3-2 GOOD PRACTICES FOR FOSTERING ETHICAL BEHAVIOR	
Good Practice Standard	**Practical Example**
Set ethical expectations early in the work or educational relationship	Discuss applicable codes of ethics, policies, and procedures that establish an ethical foundation
Model ethical behavior, and set a good example	Discuss with colleagues and peers regarding their perceptions of your actions; we often see ourselves differently than others see us
Do not look the other way when unethical behavior occurs	Approach the situation through the appropriate chain of command; understand and discuss implications for the entire program and/or facility
See things as they really are and not how you want them to be	Reflect on each situation, and discuss with colleagues and peers regarding the specific incident to ensure your perception is accurate
Foster good communication	Communicate clearly and often, especially in good times so when bad times occur, everyone is comfortable with each other
Pay attention to details	Conduct debriefings (discussion groups) on complex cases so that all the details can be addressed and others' perspectives can lend insight
Ask many questions	Establish a forum (e.g., brown bag lunches, online chats) for encouraging discussion on specific cases (maintaining confidentiality) and/or specific issues

Modified from Shefrin AP, Harper B: Encouraging ethical excellence, *Appl Clin Trials* 9:52-56, 2000.

everyday practice by emphasizing the development as moral agents in a variety of contexts encourages professional behaviors.

Ethics education also should focus on the teamed approach to health care to encourage comfort working as a team member and making joint decisions in the managerial and clinical constraints of potential employment settings.[5] Shulman used the "table of learning" as a framework for organizing how a person learns.[47] Jensen and Richert[23] used this conceptual framework to validate findings in physical therapy students as they develop behaviors for professional practice.[23] This can easily be applied to athletic training. This table of learning has been depicted in several formats, with the most widely accepted model shown in Figure 3-1.

As previously stated, engagement is necessary for learning to occur. Although knowledge is important, the ability to understand is essential to lifelong learning. Students must put into action what they know and understand to perform effectively. Performance and action are two different entities, however, so reflecting

upon actions is critical. Exercising judgment means you can evaluate multiple factors and integrate these factors with existing values and standards to make sound judgments. Connecting with oneself through reflection creates a commitment to an identity—personal and professional.[47] The cyclical representation of this table proposes an alternative look at the same factors (Figure 3-2).

As you journey through these learning activities, you may wonder, "How will I know if I am *getting* it?" A recent study by Lewin et al[29] identifies keys to assessment in medical ethics curricula that could easily be incorporated into athletic training education programs. These authors highlight the use of adult education models in creating rubrics for ethics education. Criteria for the structure of an effective ethics curricula include clear and observable goals and objectives; active learning activities; problem-based relevant content; performance-based evaluation with provisions for individual feedback; and integration of the four components of moral development, including moral sensitivity, moral judgment, moral motivation,

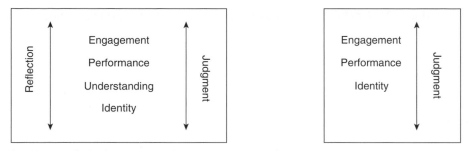

Figure 3-1 ■ "Table of learning." The figure on the *left* represents the table of learning applied to students who engage in a reflective process. The figure on the *right* represents the table of learning applied to students who are overconfident and quick to render judgment in the scenario and who do not appear to engage in a reflective process. *(From Jensen GM, Richert AE: Reflection on the teaching of ethics in physical therapy education: integrating cases, theory, and learning,* J Phys Ther Educ *19:84, 2005.)*

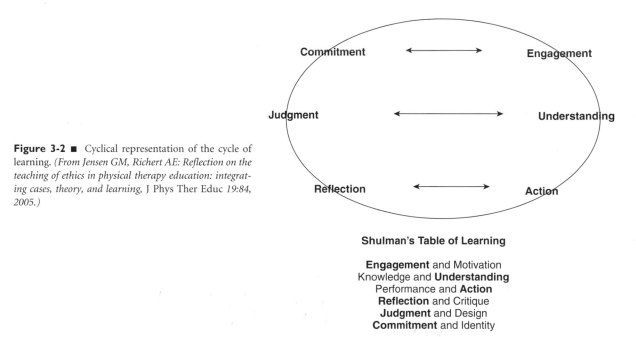

Figure 3-2 ■ Cyclical representation of the cycle of learning. *(From Jensen GM, Richert AE: Reflection on the teaching of ethics in physical therapy education: integrating cases, theory, and learning,* J Phys Ther Educ *19:84, 2005.)*

and moral action. This comprehensive approach to ethics education embraces application within both clinical and didactic education. These factors will permeate the processes by which you will discover yourself and the moral dimensions for the profession.

Many learning activities related to ethics can easily be included in the athletic training curriculum. Small-group activities, moral dilemmas, storytelling, role playing, decision analysis, Socratic questioning, clinical rounds, and case studies have all been used. The authors of this text strongly advocate a multipronged approach to learning strategies, as evidenced in this text.

HOW WILL I BE EVALUATED?

In any course, you are obviously concerned with how you will be evaluated. Because ethics education permeates all aspects of education, it is looked at slightly differently than most assignments or projects. No single way of performing evaluations in ethics education exists; evaluation is more *process* than *outcomes* oriented to encourage discovery of one's self and moral position.

As with all education, the objectives of the activity must be defined. This presents the opportunity to evaluate the degree to which the objectives are achieved.[15] This text provides many activities, each with stated objectives. Objectives help determine what the goals of the activities are and how these objectives can be accomplished. Granted, evaluation in ethics education may appear complex; however, with a clear understanding of the desired outcome (e.g., did you clarify values, or did you follow a prescribed problem-solving strategy?), an objective basis for evaluation can be established without judging the "ethics" because *how* we solve the problems is what matters.

You may also worry that your values and moral compass may not align with those of the instructor or your peers. Emphasizing the role of "philosophical neutrality" is critical in evaluating ethics activities.[51] Philosophical neutrality encourages the student and educator to evaluate each activity from an unbiased perspective. You should strive to obtain neutrality (i.e., not judging others for their perceptions) by evaluating the process by which others came to their conclusions and how they support their position.

Students thrive on constructive and supportive feedback that is individually focused. This feedback is instrumental in both academic and clinical education. With this in mind, feedback should be planned, timely, and nonjudgmental, promoting an optimal learning environment. Most activities in this text are rooted in prompt feedback, sometimes by peers, sometimes by instructors, and sometimes by self-assessment. These variations of feedback will help you through this ethical discovery process by providing a compass by which to gauge your journey. Although complicated by the hectic environment in athletic training education programs, the role of assessment and evaluation, both formative and summative, cannot be underestimated.[30]

In addition, rubrics are often used to provide feedback and input along the way. Evaluation rubrics that emphasize processes rather than outcomes are effective in learning to embrace the activity without fear of getting the "right" answer (see Appendix C for sample evaluation rubrics for ethical decision making). You may even be asked to create your own rubric to evaluate your progress and/or a selected activity, thereby emphasizing the personal nature of ethical discovery.

Many ethical dilemmas typically have multiple answers. Oral and written feedback will be directed with closed- and open-ended questions to guide your work.[5] Because discussion and involvement are critical components in ethical discovery, consideration of involvement and contributions throughout each activity will occur. However, quality of interactions, not necessarily quantity of interactions, promotes ethical discovery. These interactions may be in class or out of class in the form of online discussion boards, other activities, or journal reflections.

Angelo and Cross[2] contend that evaluation in any classroom is characterized by the following principles: it is context sensitive, flexible, likely to make a difference, mutually beneficial to all students, easy to administer, easy to respond to, and educationally valid to reinforce and enhance learning. This is critical in ethics education as well. Ethical discovery requires constant feedback to complete the journey toward professional moral behaviors. Feedback throughout the learning process can either facilitate or hinder the development of moral character. A variety of strategies that encourage self-discovery and dialogue (even debate) without fear of repercussions in an evaluation facilitate moral development. Now that this premise is established, hopefully you will feel more relaxed to enter into the activities involved in this incredibly important journey toward professional development as an athletic trainer.

A map of assessment was created to analyze classroom assessment projects (Figure 3-3).[2] This assessment plan is applicable for designing assessment for the proposed ethics activities in this text. You should understand the focus of the assessment as well as your role in providing input (by way of feedback) to the process. Figure 3-3 depicts an adapted model highlighting key steps that can easily be incorporated into any activity relative to ethics. This 10-step process reflects the cyclical relations among planning, implementing, and responding to activities used in ethical discovery. As you design activities for your own personal use in the future or as an assignment in a selected class, this template can guide your design and implementation.

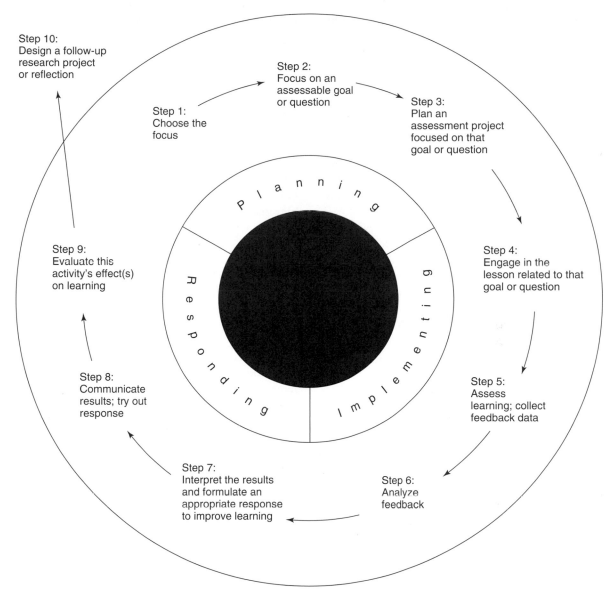

Figure 3-3 ■ Assessment project cycle. *(Modified from Angelo TA, Cross KP:* Classroom assessment techniques: a handbook for college teachers, *San Francisco, 1993, Jossey-Bass, p. 35.)*

Although templates serve as a guide, they are generally nonspecific relative to ethics education. You must understand the generalizability of these instruments and that specific, standardized tests assessing moral sensitivity and moral reasoning exist. Actually, several valid and reliable instruments have been used to evaluate moral sensitivity and moral reasoning. The Defining Issues Test (DIT), a multiple-choice, group-administered, computer-scored test, was developed by Rest[43] to evaluate the degree of moral reasoning of an individual. It is composed of six hypothetical stories, each presenting a moral dilemma. Rooted in Kohlberg's stages, the DIT is the most widely used measurement tool in moral reasoning research.

Although extensively used, little literature supports the use of the DIT in medical and health professions. Challenging the DIT to create a more applicable standardized test for medical professionals, Hebert et al[21] created a Problem Identification Test (PIT) to be used exclusively in the medical field. The use of these standardized instruments is increasing in the allied health care fields as brief and objective measures for evaluating moral sensitivity and moral reasoning affecting subsequent professional behavior. Although limited in their scope, these instruments may be usable in athletic training education programs as part of a comprehensive approach to ethics education.

As a point of emphasis, professional development emerges when the student can *express the process* by which he or she came to that outcome rather than simply the outcome itself. By working together to explore alternative considerations for expressing issues related to ethical behaviors, you can help to connect the personal and professional self with minimal personal conflict.

SUMMARY

Ethics education can appear as an ominous task that requires special training to be effective. However, the key to ethics education in athletic training is integration throughout the curriculum to guide the student along the ethical discovery journey so that ethics will more likely be transferred to real-life professional activities. This approach assists in demonstrating key components while integrating character considerations and shaping potential applications.[10] Additionally, works of virtuous people are interspersed throughout the curriculum. These representations of professionals with strong character traits who have faced ethical dilemmas serve as a constant reference for students. Lastly, reconceptualizing how ethics can be threaded throughout the curriculum may necessitate careful reconsideration of application methods in athletic training courses. This text demonstrates a multifaceted approach to ethical discovery.

Faculty and students alike must be willing to think creatively to facilitate character development and promote professional behaviors. You will be asked throughout this text to perform a variety of activities that will help you on this important journey toward ethical discovery and professionalism. Keep an open mind and participate fully because this is a process that requires reflection and participation. You cannot fully comprehend ethics until you submerge yourself into activities that force you to think about how you think and act.

REFERENCES

1. Akabayashi A, Slingsby BT, Kai I, et al: The development of a brief and objective method for evaluating moral sensitivity and reasoning in medical students, *BMC Medical Ethics* (serial online): www.biomedcentral.com/1472-6939/5/1. Accessed August 27, 2007.
2. Angelo TA, Cross KP: *Classroom assessment techniques: a handbook for college teachers,* San Francisco, 1993, Jossey-Bass Publishers.
3. Bandman EL, Bandman B: *Nursing ethics through the lifespan,* Upper Saddle River, NJ, 2002, Prentice Hall.
4. Barnitt RE: Deeply troubling questions: the teaching of ethics in undergraduate courses, *Br J Occup Ther* 56:401-406, 1993.
5. Barnitt RE: Facilitating ethical reasoning in student physical therapists, *J Phys Ther Educ* 14:35-42, 2000.
6. Beauchamp TL: The role of principles in practical ethics. In Sumner LW, Boyle J, editors: *Philosophical perspectives in bioethics,* Toronto, 1996, University of Toronto.
7. Beauchamp TL, Childress JF: *Principles of biomedical ethics,* New York, 2001, Oxford University.
8. Bebeau MJ, Thoma SJ: The impact of a dental curriculum on moral reasoning, *J Dental Educ* 58:684-692, 1994.
9. Brown MT: *Working ethics: strategies for decision making and organizational responsibility,* San Francisco, 1990, Jossey-Bass.
10. Calabrese R, Roberts B: Character, school leadership, and the brain: learning how to integrate knowledge with behavioral change, *Int J Educ Manag* 16:229-236, 2002.
11. Carr D: Personal and interpersonal relationships in education and teaching: a virtue ethical perspective, *Br J Educ Studies* 53:255-271, 2005.
12. Colston MA: Informed consent: review and implementation, *Athl Ther Today* 9:29-31, 2004.
13. Cotton P, Smith P, Lait M: The ethics of teamwork in an interprofessional undergraduate setting, *Med Educ* 36:1096-1097, 2002.
14. Davis AJ: New developments in international nursing ethics, *Nurs Clin North Am* 24:571-577, 1989.
15. Dinc L, Gorgulu RS: Teaching ethics in nursing, *Nurs Ethics* 9:259-269, 2002.

16. Doane G, Pauly B, Brown H, et al: Exploring the heart of ethical nursing practice: implications for ethics education, *Nurs Ethics* 11:241-253, 2004.

17. Gardiner A: You signed the waiver: NATABOC-exam confidentiality, *Athl Ther Today* 10:54-55, 2005.

18. Gottlieb JZ, Sanzgiri J: Towards an ethical dimension of decision making in organizations, *J Bus Ethics* 15:1275-1285, 1996.

19. Hafferty FW, Franks R: The hidden curriculum, ethics teaching and the structure of medical education, *Acad Med* 69: 861-871, 1994.

20. Hattab AS: Current trends in teaching ethics of healthcare practices, *Developing World Bioethics* 4:160-172, 2004.

21. Hebert P, Meslin EM, Dunn EV, et al: Evaluating ethical sensitivity in medical students: using vignettes as an instrument, *J Med Ethics* 16:141-145, 1990.

22. Hunt G: Right from wrong, *Nurs Times* 89:22, 1993.

23. Jensen GM, Richert AE: Reflection on the teaching of ethics in physical therapy education: integrating cases, theory, and learning, *J Phys Ther Educ* 19:78-85, 2005.

24. Kenan Institute for Ethics: *Ethics across the curriculum,* Durham, NC, 2006, Duke University.

25. Ketefian S: Critical thinking, educational preparation, and development of moral judgment among selected groups of practicing nurses, *Nurs Res* 30:98-103, 1981.

26. Kohlberg L: Moral development. In Sills DL, editor: *International encyclopedia of the social sciences,* New York, 1968, MacMillan.

27. Kramer D, Ber R, Moore M: Impact of workshop on students' and physicians' rejecting behaviours in patient interviews, *J Med Educ* 62:904-905, 1987.

28. Layman E: Ethics education: curricular considerations for the allied health disciplines, *J Allied Health* 25:149-160, 1996.

29. Lewin LO, Olson CA, Goodman KW, et al: UME-21 and teaching ethics: a step in the right direction, *Fam Med* 36:S36-S42, 2004.

30. MacDonald CA, Cox PD, Bartlett DJ, et al: Consensus on methods to foster physical therapy professional behaviors, *J Phys Ther* 16:27-36, 2002.

31. Mensch JM, Mitchell M: Enforcing professional standards or violating personal rights? *Athl Ther Today* 9:28-29, 2004.

32. Meyers C, Jones TB: *Promoting active learning: strategies for the college classroom,* San Francisco, 1993, Jossey-Bass.

33. Miller MA: A clinical quandary, *Athl Ther Today* 8:40-41, 2003.

34. Miller MA: Body art, *Athl Ther Today* 8:52-53, 2003.

35. Mitchell M: From humor to harassment: how context changes everything, *Athl Ther Today* 10:38-39, 2005.

36. National Athletic Trainers' Association: *Athletic training educational competencies,* ed 3, Dallas, 2001, National Athletic Trainers' Association.

37. National Athletic Trainers' Association: *Athletic training educational competencies,* ed 4, Dallas, 2006, National Athletic Trainers' Association.

38. Newman DL, Brown RD: *A framework for making ethical decisions: applied ethics for program evaluation,* Thousand Oaks, Calif., 1996, Sage, p. 192.

39. Nichols B, Gillett G: Doctors' stories, patients' stories: a narrative approach to teaching medical ethics, *J Med Ethics* 23:295-299, 1997.

40. Noddings N: *The challenge to care in schools: an alternative approach to education,* New York, 1992, Teachers College Press.

41. Pew Health Professions Commission: *Critical challenges: revitalizing the health professions for the twenty-first century,* 1995, UCSF Center for Health Professions.

42. Ray R: Ethical practice in athletic training: a thing of the past? *Athl Ther Today* 8:1, 2003.

43. Rest J: The major components of morality. In Kutines WM, Gewrtz JL, editors: *Morality, moral behavior, and moral development,* New York, 1990, John Wiley and Sons, pp. 24-40.

44. Seedhouse D: Health care ethics for medical students, *Med Educ* 25:230-237, 1991.

45. Shefrin AP, Harper B: Encouraging ethical excellence, *Appl Clin Trials* 9:52-56, 2000.

46. Sherblom S, Shipps TB, Sherblom JC: Justice, care, and integrated concerns in the ethical decision making of nurses, *Qualitative Health Res* 3:442-464, 1993.

47. Shulman L: Making differences: a table of learning, *Change* 34:34-36, 2002.

48. Sims RR, Brinkman J: Business ethics curriculum design: suggestions and illustrations, *Teaching Bus Ethics* 7:69-86, 2003.

49. Triezenberg HL: Beyond the code of ethics: educating physical therapists for their role as moral agents, *J Phys Ther Educ* 14:48-59, 2000.

50. Triezenberg HL, McGrath JH: The use of narratives in an applied ethics course for physical therapy students, *J Phys Ther Educ* 15:49-56, 2001.

51. Van Manen M: *The fact of teaching: the meaning of pedagogical thoughtfulness,* Albany, NY, 1991, State University of New York.

52. Verkerk M, Lindemann H, Maeckelberghe E, et al: An interpersonal exercise in ethics education, *Hastings Ctr Rep* 36:31-38, 2004.

53. Wiggins G, McTighe J: *Understanding by design,* Alexandria, Va., 1998, Association for Supervision and Curriculum Development.

54. Wilson BG: Medical ethics for radiography students, *Radiol Technol* 65:313-316, 1994.

Ethical Discovery: Approaches to Learning

LEARNING OBJECTIVES

After reading this chapter, the student should be able to do the following:

1. Appreciate the role of the affective domain in the development of foundational behaviors of professional practice.

2. Understand the multiple ways to approach ethical discovery.

3. Understand the literature related to ethical discovery strategies.

4. Appreciate the processes by which ethics has been studied and embrace the journey toward ethical discovery.

*We cannot avoid the moral dimensions of our lives;
it is always and everywhere present (p. 1).*[33]

The journey toward ethical discovery has many paths. As young professionals, challenges and conflicts encountered along the way are critical elements in the professional development process. Central to integrating the foundational behaviors of professional practice into practice are personal and professional values. "Values reflect our commitments and influence our perceptions. . . . [T]hey guide our behavior even if we do not articulate them to ourselves or others" (p. 84).[3] As early as the 1960s,[42,67] values are believed to be learned, linked to personal experiences, tied to behavior, and evidenced in consistent patterns of behavior (Table 4-1). Clearly, values are both cognitive and affective, requiring careful thought as well as personal feelings.[79]

Since values are directly linked to behaviors, they provide a framework for ethical discovery. Many alternatives will be presented in this chapter to facilitate ethical discovery. Historically rooted in medicine, values education is a cornerstone in the allied health care professions and provides a strong base from which foundational behaviors of professional practice can emerge. However, this does not just happen. Students and, at times, professionals must be immersed in situations—ethical dilemmas—that create dissonance so that ethical discovery can occur, thereby facilitating professional socialization into the athletic training profession. Without this affective skill learning, the cognitive (knowledge) and psychomotor (skills) lack the humanistic factors that demarcate our profession. These affective behaviors reflect attitudes, behaviors, values, beliefs, needs, and emotional responses.[19] The transformation from student to professional and from novice to expert is linked directly to the continual development of the affective domain as well as the cognitive and psychomotor skills.[20]

Ethical discovery in health care has been dominated by principles, codes, and rational models of decision making.[10,54] However, little attention has been given to the best method for learning about ethics. No single way of teaching or learning about ethics exists. Bloom's taxonomy provides a hierarchical framework for learning strategies and provides ways to integrate ethics education into the classroom or clinical setting (see Table 4-1).[9,10,19,42]

The key components of learning strategies in ethics education involve promoting ethical discovery in ways that touch all students and that embrace day-to-day challenges, including competing demands of client needs, ethical principles, ethical and moral dilemmas, personal values, and legal standards.[36] This promotion can occur by starting with simple strategies, as depicted in the upper levels of Bloom's taxonomy, and gradually progressing into the more complex levels. As you progress through this journey, you will understand that simply learning the names of the principles and theories is not enough. What is important is connecting them with what you do on a daily basis and what you will do as a student and professional—evidenced in the latter stages of the taxonomy—that truly cements the role of professionalism. Granted, immersion will become more difficult because analysis, synthesis, and evaluation involve more critical thinking. But these are the vital steps to becoming a professional.

Decision making cannot happen absent of emotion and reason.[22] The process by which a person "discovers" his or her ethical roots is a cognitive as well as emotional journey. Although difficult, this journey is critical for young professionals to discover their personal compass that will guide them throughout their professional careers. Often referred to as *moral reasoning* or *moral responsiveness*, the human side of ethical discovery emphasizes the role of the heart in the process.[45] By understanding the personal, professional, and socially mediated aspects of ethical dis-covery, the young professional can consciously and deliberately navigate the ever-changing professional terrain associated with the athletic training profession.

Personal and professional discovery involves many critical components. Through the management and application of intellect, you will learn to integrate the multiple aspects of this complicated, yet essential, function of professional development. Figure 4-1 reflects the important connection necessary to professional growth.

This figure represents the essential roles that communication, cooperation, self-management,

Table 4-1 **BLOOM'S COGNITIVE TAXONOMY AND KRATHWOHL'S AFFECTIVE TAXONOMY**

BLOOM'S COGNITIVE TAXONOMY		KRATHWOHL'S AFFECTIVE TAXONOMY		COGNITIVE AND AFFECTIVE APPLICATION
Category	*Definition*	*Category*	*Definition*	
Knowledge	Recalling specific facts or general concepts	Receiving	Willingness to attend to a stimulus	Identifying values; differentiating values; appreciating differences
Comprehension	Demonstrating low-level understanding by making use of what is communicated without relating it to other material or applying it to other settings	Responding	Active participation by the student	Understanding values behavior and that behaviors are based on predetermined awareness of chosen and prized values; self awareness and personal values identification; appreciating differences in others' values
Application	Using abstractions in concrete situations by applying principles, ideas, and theories	Valuing	Worth or value that a student attaches to a particular object, phenomenon, or behavior	Exploring values in specific decision making situations related to the profession; Appreciating different approaches to ethical resolution
Analysis	Breaking down the content into specific elements and distinguishing relationships between the content	Organization	Bringing together of different values resolving conflict and beginning the building of an internally consistent value system	Identifying values behaviors in others; appreciating behaviors reflect personal and professional values
Synthesis	Connecting various elements to make a whole that was created independently	Characterization by a value or a value complex	A value system so internalized that it has become a pattern or life style. The behavior is consistent, pervasive, and predictable	Linking values behavior to complex cases and real-life situations; using a variety of ethical discovery techniques to illuminate values behavior; appreciating individual behaviors; acknowledging consistent and inconsistent behaviors
Evaluation	Making judgments about material and methods relative to value for specific purposes			Determining consistency of values behavior in complex settings; critical reflection on value behavior in self and others; acknowledging acceptable and unacceptable behaviors based on personal and professional values system

Modified from Bloom BS: *Taxonomy of education objectives: cognitive domain*, New York, 1956, David McKay; and Bloom BS, Madaus GF, Hastings JT: *Evaluation to improve learning*, New York, 1981, McGraw-Hill; and Davis, CM: Affective education for the health professions: facilitating affective behavior, *Phys Ther*, 61(11),1587-1593: 1981; and Krathwhol D, Bloom B, and Masia B: *Taxonomy of educational objectives: handbook II: affective domain*. New York, 1964, David McKay.

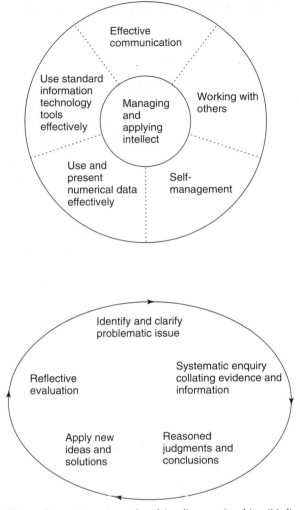

Figure 4-1 ■ Managing and applying discovery in ethics. *(Modified from Rhodes G, Tallantyne F: Assessment of key skills. In Brown S, Glasner A, editors:* Assessment matters in higher education: choosing and using diverse approaches, *Philadelphia, 1999, Open University Press, pp. 107-121.)*

organization, and technology play in the process of discovery. This process highlights the important role that self-management plays because it allows approach to a problem through a controlled, disciplined, and systematic fashion. Additionally, the ability to extract important information and effectively communicate that information in written, oral, or other forms is critical. Lastly, the ability to work collaboratively in a team is an essential function of ethical discovery in athletic training because ethical dilemmas do not occur in isolation and typically affect more than one individual. Acknowledging the connections among each of these elements will assist you in your journey of ethical discovery.

Brown defines ethics as the process of deciding what should be done.[15] This process should allow you to assess the advantages and disadvantages of different courses of action with the ultimate outcome of selecting the appropriate one. It involves consideration of alternative courses of action with opportunities for reflection and communication. This correlates directly with the ability to incorporate each of the above critical elements into the process.

GOOD TO KNOW

Learning is not a spectator sport. This is particularly true of ethics education. "Students do not learn much by just sitting in classes listening to teachers, memorizing pre-packaged assignments, and spitting out answers. They must talk about what they are learning, write about it, relate it to past experiences, apply it to their daily lives. They must make what they learn part of themselves" (p. 5).[16] You must actively engage in the process to successfully discover who you are and what you stand for as a professional in the field and as a person.

The reconciliation of one's personal self with one's professional self is a dynamic and evolving process that is often difficult. You may have found yourself becoming someone other than what you envisioned as an entry-level student. As you progress through an educational program, you will experience educational opportunities that engage you as a professional. These activities are intended to develop your confidence as a moral agent.[22] However, in isolation, without supporting context and education, you may suffer from failure to resolve the personal and professional self, leading to internal conflict. To make sound ethical decisions, you must resolve this conflict. Professionals at all levels must integrate these two worlds to provide a framework for professional behavior and prevent burnout. You must integrate the personal and professional world so that you can seek resolution and effectively deal with the ethical dilemmas you are sure to face as an athletic trainer.

The learning process does not occur in a vacuum.[37] To be productive, you will be given the opportunity to experience the real-world clinical setting to develop skills and knowledge necessary to challenge ethical situations. You will also be provided resources through written and oral interaction that allow discussion and disclosure of concerns and support the clarification of personal self with professional expectations. This vital reciprocity between person, role, context, and moral agent is essential for professional development in health care.[22] Discovering just how central the personal self is to the professional role is the ultimate goal of ethical discovery.

Ethical theory and clinical ethics are intimately related. However, ethics education is seldom viewed from this connected perspective.[18,29,58,61] Some researchers have argued that clinical ethics require a separate educational process other than traditional ethics education.[6,43,68,70] From this perspective, a disconnect occurs between the actual learning process and clinical practice. Medical education models have found that this bridge must be connected to assess resulting changes in student competence.[54] This can only happen with an introduction to cognitive ethical content that can and is applied in the clinical setting. Integration is important in athletic training education programs to facilitate the learning over time of ethical behavior and clinical skills. These two concepts cannot be separated (Figure 4-2). You will be engaged in all aspects of your educational program, including the clinical education components.

VALUES EDUCATION

The role of values in ethics education has been extensively addressed in the allied health care literature.[2,17,34,53,73] Although many programs discuss values, specific learning strategies for developing and discovering values seem to be left to chance.[39] As a person develops as a moral agent, three primary goals evolve that are all rooted in values: (1) promotion of the

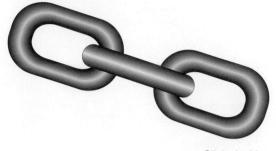

Ethical theory

Clinical ethics

Figure 4-2 ■ Ethical theory and clinical ethics are inextricably linked.

development of moral behavior, (2) promotion of the integration of values and behaviors into the profession, and (3) promotion of the student to have the confidence to engage in ethical discovery through practice.[73] Discovering your values as a critical part of the ethical journey is instrumental to the development of professional and personal consistency.

Although understanding your values is important, you will also encounter situations in which your personal and professional values conflict. Values clarification and value conflicts are at the heart of ethical discovery. Kaufman defines value conflicts as competing moral principles that struggle for primary consideration in a clinical context.[38] Potter contends that when facts in professional practice—contextually defined duties—collide with strongly held personal values, clinicians often struggle to protect their cherished values, resulting in personal dissonance.[66]

You will encounter times of dissonance as you emerge as a professional. Learning about values serves an important process. According to McKeachie,[51] values education serves two important purposes:

> In a multicultural society such as ours, there is a special need for thinking seriously about values—how we differ and what we share. . .we can help students to become more sensitive to values issues, to recognize value implications, to understand others' values, without indoctrination. Even with respect to fundamental values such as honesty, discussion, exploration, and debate about their implications are more useful than simple advo-

cacy. Open consideration of value issues is probably less subversive than disregarding values altogether.

Ethics education clearly should contain some degree of values clarification activities to help you define your position (i.e., your core values) before emphasizing the professional values held in athletic training. Equally important, you will typically have ample opportunities to be placed in situations outside the classroom that gradually expose you to real-life ethical dilemmas that arise within the profession. In a hectic clinical setting, dilemmas arise when immediate discussion of the course of action chosen and the rationale for choosing that particular action is not possible. Therefore these clinical exposures should provide the opportunity to disclose your concerns or perceptions of the dilemma from both a personal and professional perspective to prevent role strain. Willingness to communicate openly regarding ethical dilemmas is essential to development of the foundational behaviors for professional practice. Several learning strategies encouraging disclosure are discussed in greater detail in this text.

LEARNING ABOUT ETHICS

Being a professional requires participation in ethical decision making and this in turn requires an effective teaching-learning process. The involvement and active participation of students in teaching ethics will contribute to the effectiveness of this process (p. 264).[21]

The aim is not to give a protocol that produces moral solutions, but to enhance awareness of the many moral aspects of the daily practice in which professionals operate (p. 38).[77]

The purpose of this portion of the text is to introduce the multiple ways to learn about ethics throughout the athletic training curriculum. Many activities in this text help clarify your moral compass. A brief review of literature is provided to help in understanding the historical evolution of these techniques and the specific merit of each learning strategy. Although you will probably have a favorite by the time you complete your athletic training curriculum, embracing all the techniques is important because as you enter the world

as a professional in the field, you should acknowledge the depth to which ethics affects professional development. You will serve as a role model to many in your professional life, and by having experience with a variety of activities, you can help others clarify their professional roles as they encounter ethical challenges.

Case Analysis or Case Studies

Case studies have a rich history in ethics education and have been found to be an effective method of learning about ethics by facilitating comprehension of theories and encouraging application of material to stimulate the desire to learn.[77] According to Pimple, "case studies are stories, and narrative—the telling of stories—is a fundamental human tool for organizing, understanding and explaining experience."[63] Case studies typically involve the possibility of several alternative solutions or actions and some evaluation of values and costs associated with the different solutions posed.[51] Although not exactly a real-life encounter, a detailed discussion of a case is the closest action to experiencing the ethical dilemma and can help students discern moral from immoral dilemmas involved in the case. Similarly, experiential learning has been found to facilitate the development of skills, knowledge, and behaviors necessary for clinical practice.[66] However, at times you will be unable to develop specific knowledge and skills because of the limitations of clinical exposures. With this in mind, the case study method of learning has been included in the curriculum. If used correctly, case studies serve as a valuable learning tool for students of all levels.

Several formats for case discussions have evolved in the literature. Pimple outlines the format shown in Table 4-2 for the effective use of cases in ethics education.[63]

This common format for case study analysis is useful; however, business professionals also use case analysis and have developed several models that can be used in athletic training. In the following model, two other models were integrated to create a powerful ethics education instrument that can be used in athletic training. In this model, Hosmer[30] synthesizes the philosophical methods emphasizing theory and policy with the practical methods emphasizing strategic and

Table 4-2   EFFECTIVE CASE DISCUSSIONS

Step	Description
Preparation	Define the objectives Define the time allotted Define the assessment tool
Establish ground rules	Define the tone for the activity Emphasize respect for others and openness Clarify the role of opposing opinions
Establish strategies	Is it a position defense activity? Is it a "solve the problem" activity? Is it a role-based activity? Is it a reflective/prospective activity to identify what could have been avoided?
Provide tactics	Identify ethical issues and points of conflict; identify the interested parties; identify the consequences associated with the action; and identify the moral obligation of the protagonist Identify the six factors of the case: facts, interpretations of the facts, consequences, obligations, rights, and virtues
Provide clarification	Distribute the case in written form Read the case aloud; if several characters exist, encourage role play Provide opportunities to ask for points of clarification Provide a few minutes to allow students to record some ideas
Discuss the case	Provide a brief response to the case Record key points on the board or overhead for summary
Close the case	Describe areas of agreement and disagreement Provide the opportunity to express (through written means) any unresolved issues

Modified from Pimple KD: Using case studies in teaching research ethics. *Planning Workshop for a Guide for Teaching Responsible Science,* February, 1997, p. 1.

functional problems into a standardized format for the case analysis of moral issues. Table 4-3 reflects the key components used to analyze cases for moral development.

This integrated model provides a conceptual framework for analyzing cases and can be used as an assessment rubric to track the processes associated with the case analysis. As you consider ethical dilemmas, try to incorporate these steps as you process the information. A template will help you consider all options and alternatives, especially as a novice professional.

The previous models are excellent resources; however, they treat the student as a bystander. The student is provided the information but is not immersed in the case. To fully conceptualize a case, Barnbaum[5] promotes full immersion in case analysis. Rather than viewing the case from "nowhere," Barn-

baum encourages you to remove yourself from the third-person perspective to embrace the case fully. In a similar fashion as role playing, acting out the case in the first person helps the student move beyond the clean, concise ethical principles taught in the classroom. This approach helps demonstrate that the transfer from theory to practice is "messier" when elements of real-life events are considered. This learning strategy has been found to engage observers in the class more actively as well as emphasize the seriousness of the assigned role performed. A resultant appreciation of the complexities associated with moral dilemmas is achieved. "Playing the role" is a rich way to discover all the ethical aspects associated with a particular case.

Although case study and analysis is a widely used and appropriate approach to learning about ethics, this method also has some distinct limitations.

Table 4-3 SUMMARY OF CASE ANALYSIS FOR MORAL DEVELOPMENT

Step	Description
1	Personal moral standards Apparent moral problem • Harm to others • Rights of others • Benefits to others • Wrongs of the case
2	State moral problem
3	Develop other answers List major alternatives Resolve factual issues Acknowledge personal impact Apply ethical principles • Self-interests • Personal virtues • Religious injunctions • Government requirements • Utilitarian benefits • Universal duties • Individual rights • Economic efficiency • Distributive justice • Contributive liberty
4	Research solution Support solution

From Hosmer LT: Standard format for the case analysis of moral problems, *Teaching Bus Ethics* 4:169-180, 2000.

Primarily, empathy is seldom considered in a case analysis because so much of the focus is on solving and analyzing the dilemma.[4] Students often treat each case in a similar fashion by applying the right variables and resolving the case. Students also will likely address cases from a health care provider perspective with little consideration for the patient in the case. Patients tend to become the "other" person, which makes it difficult, particularly for novice students, to empathize with the patient. In this situation, Barnbaum[4] contends that the use of "lottery assignments," in which students are assigned the role of the patient for the entire semester, can be used to facilitate empathy in ethics education.

Reflection

It may be that one of the most important goals of ethics education is facilitating the development of students' reflective capacity as a critical element in their professional formation (p. 84).[35]

Plack and Santasier[65] also support the use of case studies in ethics education; however, they focus more on the reflective processes leading to the development of critical thinking. Through the use of case studies and metaphors, formative and summative reflections can guide ethical development. According to these authors, "reflection is the hallmark of professional practice."[65] In social work, reflective self-awareness has been shown to assist professionals in recognizing their value preferences and alert them to how these values unknowingly affect their approach to ethical dilemmas.[48] Decisions are forged by prejudices brought by the health care provider and influence the process and outcomes of ethical decision making. Taken one step further, Schon[69] contends that reflective practitioners revisit their experiences and coined the terms "reflection in action" and "reflection on action." Characterized by stopping, thinking, and problem solving during actual clinical experience and the thought processes that occur after action, this term has been expanded to "reflection for action."[40] This forward-thinking approach to reflection encourages consideration for improvement of practice combined with retro-reflection relative to what did occur. Integration of reflection in action, reflection on action, and reflection for action can be used as learning tools for linking theory and practice in athletic training education to encourage continuous quality improvement (Figure 4-3).

Several types of reflection are used in ethics education: content reflection, process reflection, premise reflection, reflection in action, reflection on action, and reflection for action. You will be asked to use a variety of these techniques as you journey along the process of ethical discovery. Table 4-4 summarizes the main objectives of each reflective element.

Although reflection seems simple, learning to reflect is a complex task that begins at the personal level and expands to a broader context. Plack and Santasier[65] use the metaphor of an upward spiral to indicate the progressive level of reflective practice (Figure 4-4).

The use of this spiraling approach to professional practice yields several significant outcomes. First, you

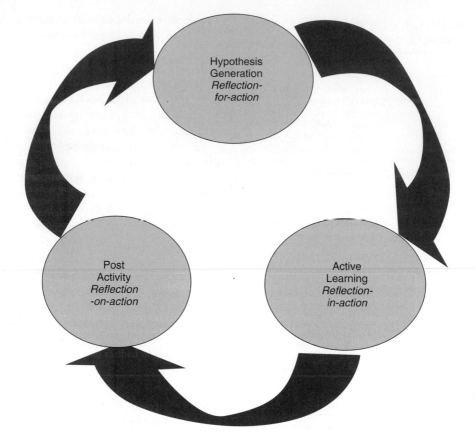

Figure 4-3 ■ Cyclic learning process. *(From Plack MM, Santasier A: Reflective practice: a model for facilitating critical thinking skills within an integrative case study classroom experience,* J Phys Ther Educ *18:4-12, 2004.)*

Table 4-4 TYPES OF REFLECTIVE ACTIVITIES IN ETHICS EDUCATION

Type of Reflection	Goal of Reflective Activity
Content	Identification of the problem, the root of the problem, and potential intervention areas
Process	Exploration of the strategies and processes used to solve the problem and identification of alternate processes that could have been used
Premise	Exploration of existing assumptions such as values and beliefs and how they may have affected the outcome
Reflection in action	Reflection *during* the activity involving analysis of the events AS they unfold
Reflection on action	Reflection *after* the activity regarding actions already taken involving analysis of feelings and outcomes
Reflection for action	Reflection *after* the activity that focuses on future interventions and alternative actions to facilitate outcomes

From Plack MM, Santasier A: Reflective practice: a model for facilitating critical thinking skills within an integrative case study classroom experience, *J Phys Ther Educ* 18:4-12, 2004.

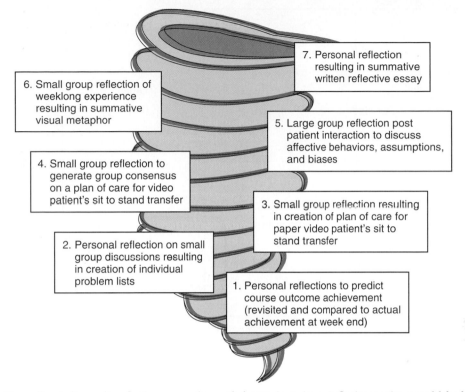

7. Personal reflection resulting in summative written reflective essay

6. Small group reflection of weeklong experience resulting in summative visual metaphor

5. Large group reflection post patient interaction to discuss affective behaviors, assumptions, and biases

4. Small group reflection to generate group consensus on a plan of care for video patient's sit to stand transfer

3. Small group reflection resulting in creation of plan of care for paper video patient's sit to stand transfer

2. Personal reflection on small group discussions resulting in creation of individual problem lists

1. Personal reflections to predict course outcome achievement (revisited and compared to actual achievement at week end)

Figure 4-4 ■ Upwardly spiraling cyclic reflective process. *(From Plack MM, Santasier A: Reflective practice: a model for facilitating critical thinking skills within an integrative case study classroom experience,* J Phys Ther Educ 18:4-12, 2004.)

will learn how to integrate your previous work into the various levels of reflective practice by demonstrating your ability to build and expand upon existing knowledge. This scaffolding connects the information and facilitates understanding. Second, critical thinking skills are developed. As you first process the information individually then collaborate with peers, you develop critical thinking skills while you and your peers consider multiple perspectives associated with resolution of the case. Third, professional values are shaped as you position yourself to interact with others in support of your suggested resolution or in defense of other suggested resolutions. This ability to interact with others (e.g., agreeing to disagree in a professional forum) reinforces the professional values framework through the encouragement of self-awareness.

From a similar perspective, Verkerk et al[77] contends that reflection can be used as a learning tool by focusing on three steps: initial reflection, guided reflection, and mapping responsibilities. Initial reflection is a response or reaction to a case study in the form of a reflection. Guided reflection involves critical examination of the morality of the particular case, and mapping responsibilities involves reconsidering professional actions as they affect daily environment. This text emphasized the critical role of everyday events that spark ethical dilemmas, the deciphering of which helps students transition from the academic to the professional setting. The reflection square shown in Figure 4-5 represents the four dimensions of professionalism: core values and beliefs, actions, social norms, and consequences. Core values and actions are personal, whereas social norms and consequences must be considered as part of the greater environment. Each of these dimensions contributes to the professional identity of the person, which further defines

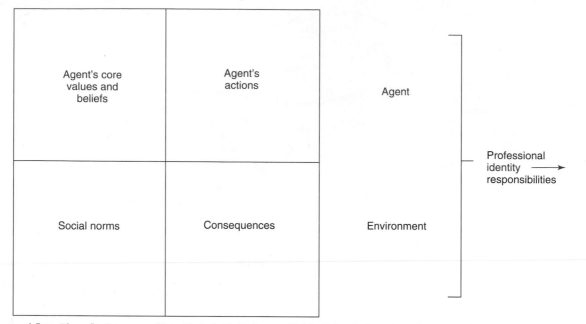

Figure 4-5 ■ The reflection square *(From Verkerk M, Lindemann H, Maeckelberghe E, et al: An interpersonal exercise in ethics education, Hastings Ctr Rep 36:31-38, 2004.)*

responsibilities. This model is used in greater detail in learning activities in future chapters.

Although several specific activities and models have been presented, reflection can be unstructured or structured (guided) or take any form imaginable. The goal of reflective activities is to encourage thinking about events happening to you, around you, and within you during a professional education program. The role of reflection in causing the "stop think process" effect in young professionals is critical. In a hurried clinical program, students often encounter events that cause internal dissonance. Without the opportunity to go back and reflect, a person's professional compass can become slightly skewed. With this in mind, Jensen and Richert suggest the following questions as a guide for student reflection in the health care professions[35]:

- What were the central ethical issues you encountered (in your clinical experience)?
- At the end of the encounter with the situation, why did you choose to resolve the ethical issue the way you did?
- If you were the professional (certified athletic trainer or other allied health care professional), what would you do next?
- What still confuses you about the situation and issue you encountered?
- What did you learn about yourself during this encounter?

These reflections can be used as journal entries or open dialogue to facilitate professional development and disclosure. Reflection from this perspective focuses on personal and professional behaviors and serves as a sounding board. It encourages examination of underlying assumptions and consequences of actions seen in practice as well as personal assumptions relative to political, cultural, and social forces encountered as a young professional. Reflection provides a safe environment for addressing areas of conflict, concern, or discernment.

In another approach to emphasizing the role of reflection in the development of foundational behaviors for professional practice, Mattison[48] created a cycle of reflection that posits the clinician in the center of the reflection and encourages self-awareness (Figure 4-6).[48]

The self-awareness component is critical because it takes the clinician past the "scientific" phase of problem solving and forces the analysis and acceptance of prejudices and prejudgments. This sensitivity enhances the ability to deliberately engage in critical analysis from a personal and professional perspective, especially in light of competing values and loyalties. Active engagement in the cycle of reflection helps an individual constantly reflect on position and its effect on self and others.

In a related context, Huotari[32] emphasizes the role of values in ethical reflection, particularly in multiprofessional care wherein several different professionals must come together to meet the patient's needs.[32] Obviously, athletic training is a multiprofessional care field in which professionals work collaboratively with other allied health care providers to render care. Within multiprofessional environments, the communication and commitment among professionals must be normative. Without a common language, communication is misconstrued and often misinterpreted, leading to less-than-desirable outcomes. Newman and Brown[56] propose the flowchart shown in Table 4-5 to help solve ethical dilemmas involving multiprofessional care providers, which can be quite reflective.[56]

This model does not give predetermined solutions. It allows the integration of personal ethics into the problem-solving approach. It encourages personal reflection and helps the student realize that conflicts may occur. Primarily a cognitive process, ethical decision making evolves by practicing, reading, discussing, and thinking. This model encourages each of these actions by prompting with applicable questions. This model is extremely useful for students and professionals because it helps the individual consider multiple perspectives.

As previously mentioned, reflection is a highly personal process. Although incredibly effective and widely used, reflection requires openness to disclose often personal or concerning issues. Haney[28] encourages students and instructors to consider the dilemmas that may arise as part of reflective work. Anytime you are encouraged to reflect on a potential conflict or concern or are simply provided a safe environment for expressing your voice, sensitive issues, perhaps with ethical implications in and of themselves, likely will emerge. This is an important issue that should be discussed openly, and an established means of addressing these concerns will be outlined to protect both students and faculty. When ethical dilemmas create personal and/or professional dissonance, outside resources can provide another opinion to help discern feelings or concerns. The instructor will provide information about these outside resources, and you may also see them as guest speakers in the classroom. Valuable resources beyond your instructor are available if you have difficulty with some of the challenges relative to personal and professional discovery.

Reflection has been extensively used as a learning tool in ethics education.[24] Described as a process of personal cognitive review of an experience to provide meaningful clarification of the individual experience,[46] reflection serves many purposes and develops multiple components within the context of learning. Specifically, reflection develops skills in self-awareness, description, critical analysis, synthesis, and evaluation. These skills have been found to foster professional behaviors at all levels of the maturity continuum, therefore reinforcing the concept of integrating these activities throughout the curriculum. Many opportunities for reflection are available along the journey of ethical discovery.

Writing Activities

Although reflection is a common writing activity used in ethics education, other forms of writing are also integrated throughout the curriculum to thread ethics education across various courses. Writing provides a valuable tool to process knowledge and apply it to different situations. (See Appendix D for tips on writing about ethical issues.) Although writing is typically seen as a labor-intensive activity, various forms of writing assignments can be instrumental in processing information in ethics education. McKeachie[51] discusses the "letter to a friend" strategy that has the student write an informal letter (two to four paragraphs) to a friend summarizing or reflecting on some issue discussed in class. This writing assignment is informal and has been found to increase comprehension of key concepts. "Minute papers," in which the student has 1 minute at

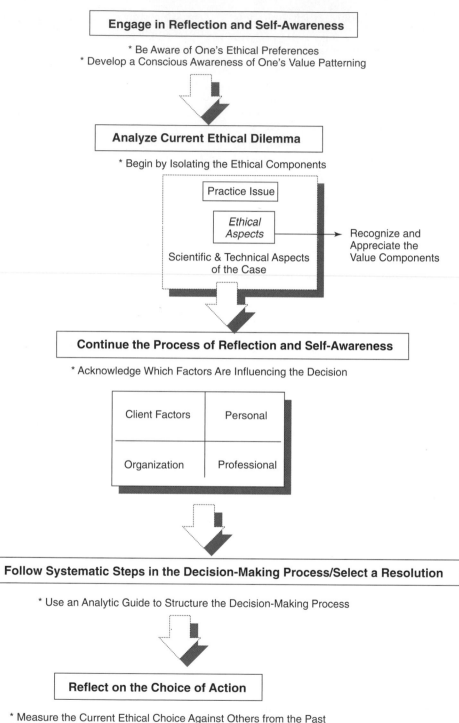

Figure 4-6 ■ Cycle of reflection. *(From Mattison M: Ethical decision making: the person in the process,* Social Work *45:201-212, 2000.)*

Table 4-5   REFLECTIVE DECISION-MAKING FLOW CHART INVOLVING MULTIPLE-CARE PROFESSIONALS

Level	Questions	Decision
Level 1: intuitive sense of potential conflict	Do I respond to my intuitive sense? Do I have time for further analysis?	Stop or pursue concern analysis (move to level 2)
Level 2: rules	What rule, standard, or code applies?	Does a rule, standard, or code apply? (If so, stop or go to level 3) If a rule, standard, or code fits the situation, take action (level 5), move to level 3 for further analysis, or stop
Level 3: principles and theories	Ask questions relative to the principles. What is the relevance of the principles? Do the principles conflict? If so, how can they be balanced?	Stop, consider values (level 4), or take action (level 5)
Level 4: personal values	How do my personal values, visions, and beliefs affect my thinking? What kind of person do I want to be?	Stop or take action (level 5)
Level 5: action	How much stress is involved? What are the risks to me and others? What is my plan? What will my colleagues or organization think? What cultural issues are important to consider?	Stop or implement an action plan Has the plan worked, or must I start again?

From Newman DL, Brown RD: *A framework for making ethical decisions: applied ethics for program evaluation,* Thousand Oaks, Calif., 1996, Sage, pp. 101-119.

the beginning or end of class to summarize either the content coming into or at the conclusion of class, also allow the opportunity to share understanding of the content. Muddiest point activities, in which the student writes about the point or issue most confusing, can also encourage active engagement in learning by allowing the expression of areas that require clarification.

Term papers are another way in which ethics is integrated throughout the curriculum. Obviously a more formal writing project, the research paper enables the student to root his or her writing in the literature. According to McKeachie,[51] research papers provide an opportunity to go beyond conventional course content to become an expert in a specific area and give students opportunities to explore problems of particular relevance to the profession. Frequent feedback (through established deadlines) enables you to stay on track and approach the project in manageable chunks, thereby enhancing motivation. By selecting the topic

for research, you can write about a subject that interests you, which increases motivation. Formal writing in an ethics curriculum is an advanced-level skill that should synthesize theory and practice. Although seen as a difficult task, research can be fun and should be approached with an open mind.

Research papers provide an opportunity to write about a specific topic. However, participating in faculty research can also provide valuable knowledge. This involvement can certainly link to ethics education as research processes can be tied to ethical practice. Discussion of and involvement in the process from the institutional review board application through data analysis and presentation of results can help you understand the importance of ethical behavior throughout the entire process. Linked to professional behaviors and development, this learning activity can provide invaluable insight into many aspects of the athletic training profession. Ask faculty members about the potential to become involved in research projects at your institution.

Peer, Collaborative, and Cooperative Learning

All learning takes place in a societal context. Although individual learning strategies have significant merit, working with others within the various settings has a considerable effect on the student. Peer teaching, in which students teach other students, has been documented in the teaching literature to be extremely effective for a wide range of topics and goals and for students at various levels.[51] Peer teaching is effective because it provides an opportunity for mutual support, stimulation, and elaboration. Students question, explain, express opinions, admit confusion, and reveal misconceptions while listening to peers, responding to questions, questioning their opinions, and sharing information.[51]

Peer teaching can take many forms, including student-led discussions. In these groups, students work together to discuss the content of the course through various methods such as formal presentation and questioning. Student-led groups also allow comparison of ideas and the use of others as a resource, encouraging higher order thinking. Of course, being part of a group involves maturity and cooperation. Conscious efforts must be made by all members to encourage everyone to participate actively at some level and ensure that bias is not perpetuated, which is critically important in an ethics forum.

Peer tutoring can also stimulate a deeper understanding when working through issues related to course content. Research indicates that both the tutor and the tutored benefit from a peer tutoring situation.[44] Clinical education in athletic training is a perfect venue for peer tutoring. The learning cell (or student dyad) is another technique to learn in a cooperative learning environment. In the learning cell, pairs of students alternate asking and answering questions on material presented or read for the content area.[51] Working together with other students to generate thought-provoking questions is an effective means of enhancing learning. Ethical dilemmas typically involve a process for resolution rooted in questioning. The learning cell can tie the theory to the actual practice through a question-and-answer approach.

A variation of peer learning is the syndicate-based peer learning strategy. In this technique, students are divided into groups of four to eight. Each group is given a set of questions to address and then seeks to answer the questions or solve the dilemma. At the conclusion of the class or in class the next day, the "syndicate" reports back to the large group. This technique is a bit different than the dyad in that the content is basically researched (with references) by a small group rather than discussed as questions and each student's perception of the answer.

Linked Learning Activities

Linked learning activities are a student-centered approach to integrating various components of an educational program into related activities. Originally developed to link assignments, linked learning activities have expanded to encourage interaction and dialogue among various groups of people to develop citizenry skills and address multicultural and social issues.[72] This strategy has merit in the athletic training profession. In linked learning activities, students establish an environment of collegiality, share inside perspectives, and envision the profession through others' eyes. Often structured with upper- and lower-level students collaborating, this learning strategy can serve as a type of mentoring program to develop personal and professional skills. Essentially, the structure of this approach is simple; activities are linked across the curriculum to stimulate discussion and interaction, which builds as the students progress through the program. Athletic training education already uses linked learning activities to some degree with peer and approved clinical instructor assessments to facilitate learning over time. However, this approach can be expanded to encompass a wide range of activities such as mentoring programs, combined research projects, case forums, and library club or journal club activities.

The Field Approach: Experiential Learning

Athletic training has long been rooted in experiential learning. Although the shift to the curriculum model has taken some of the focus off the fieldwork associated with athletic training education, clinical experiences remain a critical element in preparation for entering the field. Some students wonder why and how to connect the clinical and the didactic. How do instructors know that students understand the material if they are not in a formal classroom? Most educators would say that "we just know." But ethics education is critical, and it truly needs to be substantiated because the clinical environment is where students will face the real challenges that shape their professional behaviors.

A common practice to substantiate the learning is to use journals or logs. However, other valuable approaches to integrating experiential learning into ethics education include written reports, presentations, and demonstrations to promote long-term learning from the field experiences.

Written reports connected to field experiences may address ethical issues from a "compare and contrast" approach or decision-making approach. Presentations and demonstrations also can create a setting in which real-life situations can be linked to theory. Presentations and demonstrations can lead to group discussions or debates relative to the specific case presentations. An effective method of establishing the problem-solving and decision-making components in health care, experiential learning takes many shapes and is linked to ethics education as how students see and participate in professional practice.

The Principled Approach

The principled approach to ethical discovery has been extensively used in allied health care education programs ranging from medicine to nursing. The Belmont Report was the first publication to address the principled approach to ethical decision making,[55] and subsequent publications provided additional support for this educational framework.[7,23,76] This approach emphasizes the role of ethical theory, principles, concepts, and issues rather than the process of ethical analysis and reasoning.[54] Closely linked to Beauchamp's and Childress' principles of biomedical ethics,[7] this approach has been refined, reviewed, and revised since the late 1970s to result in a more inclusive model that is widely accepted in ethics education.[49]

The principle-based approach to ethics education claims to accomplish three main objectives: (1) iden-

tify that basic principles and the specific actions that guide them are central to decision making in health care; (2) recognize that in any given health care situation, any decision is morally justified if supported by principles, rules, or particular judgments; and (3) support that successful justification is measured by the degree to which it achieves cohesiveness of the entire decision-making process.[49] The common morality that binds all people makes the principled approach to ethics education strong. "The common morality contains moral norms that bind all persons in all places; no norms are more basic in the moral life" (p. 3).[7]

Myser et al[54] contend that this approach enables law to be distinguished from ethics and considers why the law should guide the outcome, especially in the face of conflicting ethical judgments. These authors advocate the principled approach to ethics education because it discourages defensive practice and encourages the processing of conflicting legal-ethical dilemmas. Principlists consider principles to be at the heart of moral life, whereas narrativists view communication as the core.[49] However, from a clinical education perspective, principles can be combined to encourage communication to better integrate these distinct approaches to ethics education.

One method of approaching clinical ethics from a principled approach builds on the previously discussed case analysis model. Typically resulting in a debate format, cases are presented and discussed from a principled perspective and address issues such as justice, beneficence, nonmaleficence, and autonomy. Ethical principles have been simplistically defined: justice is rooted in the fair treatment of others; beneficence involves actions related to the benefit of others; nonmaleficence avoids causing harm to others; and, lastly, autonomy considers the respect for others' views, choices, and actions as central. Legal, social, and ethical issues are at the center of the discussions. Although the weight of the discussion rests on the person assigned the case, other individuals can use templates such as tables, outlines, or concept maps to help identify the key principles and relevant information associated with the particular case.[49] By considering the ethical, legal, and social perspectives separately, courses of action can be distinguished under each category.

The principled approach to ethics education often involves prioritization of the principles. Many situations in athletic training involve more than one principle; therefore establishing a hierarchy of relevance helps resolve the case. This can provide a valuable link to integrating values into the curriculum because students will likely have values conflicts when investigating the implications of principlism in resolving cases. Emphasis on the balance between the two concepts is critical to the success of this approach. Particular focus should continue to be placed on the connection between the principles and how they affect clinical practice.

After prioritization, participants may be asked to disclose their decision regarding the case. By having the opportunity to present the case from one student's perspective (emphasizing the principles involved in the resolution of the case) and giving other students the opportunity to present alternative solutions, ethical principles are reinforced. This progression from individual consideration of options to formal presentation and debate regarding the chosen course of action allows students to reconcile their personal values and posit themselves with strong principled arguments before engaging in a debate with others who may have other options not yet considered (Table 4-6).

Table 4-6   PRINCIPLE-BASED DISCOVERY

Steps for Principle-Based Discovery	Anticipated Outcome
Acquire the facts: medical, social, ethical components through investigating the case	Differentiation of relevant versus irrelevant information in case analysis
Identify the existing and/or anticipated ethical issues	Integration of ethical theory into case review
Distinguish ethical, social, and legal issues	Differentiation of multiple components and categorization of issues
Determine which ethical principles or concepts are relevant in the clinical decision-making process	Definition of ethical principles relative to clinical practice
Identify existing and/or anticipated conflicts between the principle-based obligations	Identification of potentially conflicting processes associated with professional obligations
Provide an explanation why the principle-based obligations clash	Explanation of potential clashes to process multifaceted nature of ethical principles
Clearly state the clinical ethical decision	Decision-making skills
Justify the clinical ethical decision by providing clarification of how the principles were balanced and why, potential objections to the decision, and potential counterarguments to possible objections	Substantiation of decision, personal and professional clarification, and preparation to defend or support decisions made with appropriate reflection on alternatives
Identify relevant laws and how they guide the clinical case	Connect legal and ethical principles to reinforce the strong connection and need to consider both
Examine the relation between the clinical ethical decision and the law	Support why the law supports the ethical action and vice versa
Provide an argument (legal or ethical) for which obligation should guide the case and why. Identify areas of the law that may be perceived as deficient and provide areas that may need to be reformed. Mechanisms for reform may also be addressed (if appropriate).	Critical thinking skills relative to existing knowledge and potential need for change; confidence questioning existing policy and addressing change

Modified from Myser C, Kerridge IH, Mitchell KR: Teaching clinical ethics as a professional skill: bridging the gap between knowledge about ethics and its use in clinical practice, *J Med Ethics* 21:97-104, 1995.

The principled approach to ethics education has several advantages and disadvantages. This method is typically quite systematic and unified. It provides a clear method and vocabulary for identifying concerns and negotiating outcomes on the basis of strong arguments. It provides an ethical framework for addressing emerging issues in health care through a relatively structured process.[7] Additionally, parameters for moral relationships with strangers can easily be defined by this approach.[49] It can be adapted to integrate individual cultural differences for a pluralistic view. The disadvantages of this approach highlight the limitations of using a single-pronged approach to ethics education. This framework has limitations regarding the application of principles, issues with resolving conflicting principles, and the disconnect often encountered when trying to link ethical principles with the complexities of real-life clinical practice.[57] The universal approach to ethical decision making fails to incorporate the critical contexts and relations that influence the dilemma. This approach can be used for introductory through advanced students because it is prescriptive and can be divided into several phases to emphasize one portion of the process more than the others, then later combined into the full model as a culminating experience.

Several key skills are needed to be effective in using the principled approach to ethical dilemmas. According to McCarthy,[49] good principlists need the following:

• Conceptual and analytical skills to identify moral issues and specify principles
• Deductive skills to connect principles to specific health care cases
• Critical skills to assess and weigh arguments and principles
• Reflective skills to generalize from specific cases to general rules

Along with developing these skills, Viafora[78] contends that principlism is critical in clinical ethics. This clinical perspective highlights a systematic approach to using principles to foster ethical discovery through selected questions related to each case. This approach has specific application to athletic training education because it considers multiple perspectives and facili-

tates critical thinking and problem solving. Additionally, it approaches ethical decision making from an experiential as well as principled approach. Table 4-7 provides guiding questions during clinical decision-making situations involving ethical dilemmas.

Problem-Based Learning

Problem-based learning (PBL) has been used as a learning tool in medicine for decades. PBL incorporates any learning environment in which the problem is the stimulus for learning. Found to enhance clinical reasoning skills, retention of learned material, and enhancement of self-directed study, this method of learning provides rich opportunities for ethics education.[1,60] Rooted in the adult learning literature, PBL should involve the following:

1. Resources such as the teacher, other students, and prescribed learning materials should not be imposed to encourage self-directed inquiry.
2. Learning should happen for the sake of learning, which involves self-motivation.
3. Teachers and peers serve as catalysts to encourage inquiry.

For ethics education to emerge in a PBL setting, a brief understanding of the process is necessary. First, learning is most beneficial when it is purposeful and self-directed. This encourages engagement for the sake of learning rather than for a specific outcome. Second, life experiences (and clinical experiences in athletic training) should be considered powerful learning tools. Real-life situations provide a rich ground for evaluating and analyzing processes. Third, motivation is required through this journey of ethical discovery. Therefore the intrinsic and extrinsic motivators must be uncovered and integrated in the process.

Although often combined with the case approach to learning, PBL is a great stand-alone activity that does not necessarily need to be connected to a case. It is diverse enough to integrate basic to complex ideas relative to ethical discovery and should be frequently used throughout the educational process.

Ethics of Care

The ethics of care model typically is framed in the nursing,[25] medical,[13] and feminist[27] literature. Critics

Table 4-7 A PRINCIPLED APPROACH TO CLINICAL PRACTICE	
Major Theme	**Guiding Questions**
Collect clinical data	What are the clinical data relating to the diagnosis and prognosis?
	Do any alternatives exist from a medical or health care perspective?
	What are the constraints that would suggest one alternative is preferred over another?
Assess responsibilities	Was the patient adequately informed about risks and outcomes?
	What are the responsibilities of the individual and the family?
	What are the specific responsibilities of the health care professional?
	Does the intervention suggest consequences that the individual is not likely to assume?
Identify the ethical problem	What are the ethical problems and the values that are involved? Rank them according to context and perceived importance.
Formulate an ethical judgment	What are the proposed solutions and the reasons motivating each solution?
	What are the specific principles that guided the solutions?
	What is the role of experience in guiding the decision?
Elaborate directives from analogous cases	Can the case be reduced to one single ethical issue?
	What are the strategies for preventing a situation like this from occurring again?
	What are the general attitudes and virtues of health care professionals when dealing with cases of this nature?

Modified from Viafora C: Toward a methodology for the ethical analysis of clinical practice, *Med Health Care Philosophy* 2:283-297, 1999.

of this approach contend that it is not an approach but rather a psychological orientation. Focusing on the language associated with this approach, the ethics of care models emphasize the human notion of the developing moral agent as well as a balance between the prevalent existing theories of actions and consequences.[59] Diverting attention away from punishments and obedience may lend a more personal, relational element in allied health care education. "When the rules exert such a priority that humanity is dampened, something has clearly gone awry, and yet the hearts of those around us are the last things considered as we carefully train our students in moral reasoning" (p. 341).[71] In this model, the role of compassion balanced with principles and policies prevents duty-directed compassion and drives a truly caring environment in which to make decisions.

Humanism, another term for care ethics, is defined by Branch et al[13] as "attitudes and actions that demonstrate interest in and respect for the patient and that address the patient's concerns and values" (p. 1067). Although learning methods involving humanistic approaches to values education have undergone scrutiny, several emergent themes have resulted that

facilitate the humanization of ethics education. Furthermore, ethics of care models have been criticized as gender specific. Gilligan[26] contends that women focus more on understanding responsibilities and relationships than do men, which can create a bias. However, this approach to ethics education continues to be extensively used and complements the justice approaches to moral development.

For example, seminal events, role modeling, and active learning skills with an ethics of care focus have been found to facilitate student learning in the medical field in both the didactic and clinical settings.[13] Students are encouraged to be aware of the human aspects of care approach rather than simply the clinical skills being performed. This focus includes attention to social amenities, verbal and nonverbal communication skills, observational skills, humanistic care components, and self-awareness. Strategies for integrating the humanistic approach into ethics education are listed in Table 4-8.

A stepwise approach to incorporating humanism into ethics education also has been defined in the medical education literature. This model emphasizes a practical progression to integrate humanism with

Table 4-8   LEARNING STRATEGIES FOR HUMANISTIC APPROACHES TO ETHICS EDUCATION

Strategy	Objectives	Approaches
Establish a climate of humanism	Treats others with respect Establishes an environment of trust and collaboration Focuses on the human needs of each other	Involve yourself in the process of clarifying the goals, mission, and ground rules for clinical experiences, with an emphasis on humanistic values Encourage presentations that integrate psychosocial and ethical information and strategies Encourage clinical discussions around patients, involving them in the process whenever possible Get to know each other personally and as human beings; perform activities to encourage self-disclosure and self-awareness Promote a cooperative, respectful, and supportive learning environment where mistakes can be made without fear and additional learning assistance is accessible when needed
Recognize and use seminal events	Encourages application to the hidden curriculum associated with health care that shape values and attitudes	When communicating with the patient: • Acknowledge the feelings, concerns, and expectations of each interaction through verbal or written reflection • Focus attention on the use of effective communication skills • Acknowledge the use of insensitive language while providing insight relative to the implications of such language
Role modeling	Encourages active rather than passive role modeling through deliberate mentoring to establish trust and collaboration	Demonstrate desirable skills and behaviors Comment on what you have done and why you did it that way
Actively engage each other	Focuses on doing, discussing, and reflecting throughout the educational process through established learning goals	Involve yourself in tasks that require humanistic skills, such as history taking Ask questions and require reflection on actions and reasons for acting Provide prompt feedback
Be practical and relevant	Creates a connection between real-life situations and theoretical situations to develop an appreciation for the differences	Respect limitations of time and resources Focus on humanistic behaviors that enhance patient outcomes Focus on communication skills that are practical to implement in daily activities
Use ongoing and multiple strategies	Creates a scaffold for each other to relate to the activity in multiple ways from a variety of perspectives, increasing the likelihood of transfer of knowledge	Reinforce and build on existing knowledge and behavior Address differences in individual learning preferences by acknowledging the need for multiple approaches

Modified from Branch WT, Kern D, Haidet P, et al: Teaching the human dimensions of care in clinical settings, *JAMA* 286:1068, 2001.

varied activities throughout the curriculum (Fig. 4-7).

This approach to active learning encourages students who are actively engaged in the educational process to internalize, understand, and remember material. These learning activities are not always staged in a classroom, but instead occur quite naturally in the clinical setting if considered *a priori*.

Although often considered as a single approach, ethics of care models should be balanced with ethics of justice approaches to provide a comprehensive perspective. Ethics of justice focus on fairness, equality, rational decision making based on rules and principles, and autonomous and impartial decision making.[12] Ethics of care models emphasizing caring, need-centered, harmonious relationships are often seen as dichotomous in ethics education. With an integrated approach, young professionals will be able to consider both poles when making ethical decisions, thereby finding a personal and professional balance rather than seeing decisions as an either/or proposition. The benefits of this integrated approach have profound implications in athletic health care.[12]

Narratives

Narrative ethics has evolved over the years as a viable tool for ethics education. Narrative ethics emphasizes the role of communication in the analysis of ethical dilemmas. It involves both telling and knowing and provides a rich medium for discovering the moral nature of health care decisions.[49] Van Manen[75] calls this the *animating ethos*, which enables active engagement in the acquisition of knowledge through animation and interpretation. The central tenets of narrative ethics are provided in Box 4-1.

The narrative approach emphasizes the unique nature of each situation because each story is different.

Box 4-1

CENTRAL THEMES OF NARRATIVE ETHICS

1. Every moral situation is unique. Its meaning cannot be captured by appealing to universal principles.
2. Any decision or action is justified in how it fits with each individual in the situation. Each patient should be considered individually to establish a narrative reflective equilibrium.
3. Opening up discussion and challenging views and norms should be the focus of justification of one's actions in an ethical dilemma.

From McCarthy J: Principlism or narrative ethics: must we choose between them? *J Med Ethics* 29:65-71, 2003.

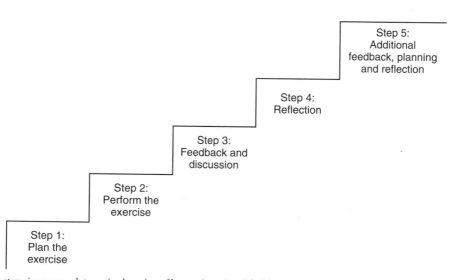

Step 5:
Additional
feedback, planning
and reflection

Step 4:
Reflection

Step 3:
Feedback and
discussion

Step 2:
Perform the
exercise

Step 1:
Plan the
exercise

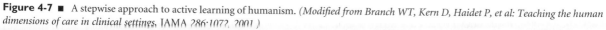

Figure 4-7 ■ A stepwise approach to active learning of humanism. *(Modified from Branch WT, Kern D, Haidet P, et al: Teaching the human dimensions of care in clinical settings, JAMA 286:1072, 2001.)*

The individual life story of each patient should be considered separately in the context of decision making. Brody[14] contends that only a story incorporates the full picture of each ethical dilemma. The story ties together the elements so they are not considered in isolation as disconnected entities. The act of uncoupling a person's actions from the person himself or herself to make the decision fit into specific rules or categories is discouraged.

Moral justification from a narrative approach is rooted in the social embeddedness of the individual rather than his or her ability to make choices and follow rules.[47] The social nature of a person's life shapes decisions he or she makes based on deeply rooted values and conceptions of what is right and what is wrong. The narrative approach is not simply storytelling; however, narratives are tested against criteria such as existing documentary evidence and the stories of others.[49] Other supporting evidence provides a framework for consistency with self-conceptions, thereby expanding the narrative context.

The multiplicity of meanings in each situation encourages different voices to be heard as part of the process. The primary focus of involving as many people as possible in the dialogue to encourage commonly shared perspectives results in the optimal outcome according to narrativists.[31] For example, when a dilemma occurs, considering input from the athlete, coach, physician, athletic trainer, and other health care professionals helps shape the outcome of the dilemma.

The narrative approach has distinct advantages as an educational tool. McCarthy[49] contends that the strength of narrative ethics lies in the ability to interpret and respect unique and personal stories in the decision-making process. This approach emphasizes the personal approach with particular focus on the patient-clinician relationship. It is deeply rooted in personal and professional values and has been found to be an effective way to learn about ethical theory and its application to professional behavior.[74]

McCarthy[49] further supports several key elements to practicing as a successful narrativist:

1. Literary skills and vocabulary that allow the individual to interpret and understand the story
2. Critical skills to tie information in to a larger context of meaning
3. Reflective skills to enable consideration and testing of multiple narratives
4. Communicative skills to negotiate the patient-clinician relationship

Narratives play a critical role in the ethical discovery process. Embracing each story helps discover your position and stance and shapes professional behavior. Narratives are a critical part of what athletic trainers are and what they do and should be used as a learning tool whenever possible.

Role Playing

Role playing has been used in education in a variety of disciplines. Suited well for allied health care and medicine, role playing provides a rich environment to simulate real-life situations to develop professional and interpersonal skills. The goals of role playing are to provide practice in using what has been learned, illustrate principles from course content, develop insight into human relations problems, provide a basis for discussion, maintain interest and motivate, provide a channel for expressing feelings, and develop increased awareness of the feelings of the self and others.[51] This technique frequently is used in health care because it provides a safe environment to test behaviors and decisions in an experimental environment without the risk of negative effects. Role playing is particularly effective when the following components are well defined: time frames, specific roles, objectives, references, and grading criteria. Role playing can easily be dominated by one individual or can become volatile through assertive actions. The instructor should "stage" the role play activities to encourage multiple voices and guide without micromanaging the situation. Much can be learned, particularly relative to cultural competence, in role playing situations that are carefully structured.

Several guidelines apply for successful integration of role playing in ethics education. First, everyone must listen to the others in the role play activity. A calm moderator (who can be a student or a faculty member) facilitates this process to ensure a voice for everyone. Next, the student is given enough information to be able to take the role in the direction necessary. Role play should not be used if a specific script must be followed because it will stifle creativity. Furthermore, role playing should be brief and kept to approximately 6 minutes. This type of activity can help the student evolve in the journey through the assigned role as it is taken in multiple directions.

Role playing likely is followed by a type of reflective activity to help analyze and process what happened. This can be done in a small group, large group, or individually. It can also occur in written or verbal contexts. Often the discussion after the role play has more potential to become volatile than the actual role play itself does, so careful facilitation is needed. Students or faculty can guide the discussion to facilitate the emergence of the professional.

Online Ethics Education

Distance education has recently become a driving force in higher education. As allied health care and medical education programs strive to meet core content areas, ethics education often is addressed nominally in a lecture or two. Athletic training is typically no different. However, online instruction and tools such as WebCT, Blackboard, and Vista can serve as valuable tools for facilitating ethics education. Online discussion can be used to complement an existing ethics education program and provide an environment where the student can be ambiguous and remain anonymous.[80] Remaining anonymous has its advantages, namely self-expression without fear of judgment; however, it also has some disadvantages.

Without being able to identify the individual at the other end of the dialogue, establishing sensitivity to cultural and social differences and legal and ethical issues can be difficult. The structure of online discussions should emphasize regular contributions through the use of deadlines to ensure regular participation.[64] Furthermore, the instructor typically refrains from posting too often and too early so as not to stifle participation. Although this approach lacks the face-to-face interaction of a classroom or clinical setting, online approaches are becoming more popular and have been found to form mutual bonds of trust and support through the establishment of a strong network of peers.[64]

In addition to discussion boards and chat rooms, online resources can provide stimulating case studies and resources for ethics education programs. Phillips[62] discusses the use of chat role playing as a learning strategy that supports Bonk and King's[11] theory of constructivism by scaffolding electronically through learner-centered principles. Through asynchronous discussions, students can resolve issues and cases relative to the athletic training education program (e.g., student grievances, student appeals, injury cases). The Internet can also be used to investigate problems, sort through dilemmas, and challenge commonly held practices. Online resources also provide a breadth of information relative to ethics in athletic training as well as similar health care professions. This information may be used in class projects, discussions, and assignments and will help students connect with other allied health care professionals.

Classroom Discussion

Discussions typically are integrated in ethics education through a variety of strategies. However, effective discussion does not happen naturally. Discussions are used to help you practice thinking about particular subject topics presented in class, learn to take a position and evaluate the logic and evidence for that position, give opportunities to formulate applications of key principles, become aware of problems encountered in readings or lectures, gain acceptance of theories that counter previous beliefs, develop motivation for learning more about a particular topic, and use the members of the group as resources.[51]

Discussion groups are most effective when they start with a common experience. This can occur through a small skit, demonstration, video or movie clip, or brief role-play followed by discussion of the activity that everyone has just seen. Discussions also can start through the presentation of a controversy. Point-counterpoint discussions may evolve, which can stimulate increased interest in the topic.

Questioning is a common means of encouraging discussion; however, asking too many questions does not allow all members in the group to have time to think the problem through to formulate their own thoughts. Questioning should be thoughtful and allow adequate time for members within the group to process the information. Often this may involve addressing questions at the end of a previous class or allowing time to record individual thoughts before the larger group discussion. Questions for stimulating discussion can vary, as reflected in Table 4-9.

Discussion can take on many shapes and should encourage active participation. Discussion can be a valuable tool in ethics education because it helps the student find his or her voice relative to dilemmas that may arise and also provides a strong community for expressing that voice.

Socratic Method

The Socratic method of learning about ethics is rooted in philosophy and mathematics; however, it has strong potential and implications in athletic training education. The Socratic method has a deep, rich history and is based on encouraging students to work through a given problem by using their own intellectual effort without a framework or guidance from an instructor.[8] The Socratic method attempts to teach students to reason toward general principles from specific cases.[51] Emphasizing learning groups, the instructor will serve only to assist with procedures that ensure an open, consensus-oriented discussion.

Governed by specific rules, Socratic group work depends on adherence to preset procedures. First, restraint should be observed to prevent directivity concerning specific questions relevant to the process. Next, participants should remain impartial to protect the members of the group who take longer to contribute. Participants also should be enabled to understand each others' efforts to enhance clarity while holding each other to addressing the specific question. Lastly, group members must work toward a consensus.[8] With this in mind, as part of a Socratic group you must express yourself clearly, make and attempt to understand everyone in the group, use personal experiences as a starting point for discussion, and articulate dissatisfaction or uneasiness if the need arises in the process.

Several rules guide the Socratic method of learning. These rules shape the discussion to encourage consideration of specific cases to link them to a broader application. Often used more as a game rather than an inquisition, specific questions can guide the Socratic discussion (Table 4-10).

The Socratic method of ethics education has a meaningful impact on the professional development of young allied health care providers. This method helps demonstrate that ethical discovery is a process and activity, not a preestablished doctrine. Learning about ethics in small groups (usually five to eight members) encourages fundamental interaction and communication necessary in the health care field. Personal and collaborative thoughts, often highly emotional in nature, can be expressed and considered, which helps the student consider alternative options while maintaining a voice. Furthermore, this method encourages discussion and consideration of concrete cases or irritations experienced by students, thereby encouraging immersion into the ethical discovery

Table 4-9 TYPES OF QUESTIONS TO ENCOURAGE CLASSROOM OR CLINICAL DISCUSSION

Type of Question	Purpose/Outcome
Factual	Check the background knowledge of the group and stimulate problem solving
Application and interpretation	Establish relationships, applications, and analysis relative to content area to broaden the scope of understanding
Problem	Connect to cases—hypothetical or real—to encourage problem solving
Connective and causal effect	Link material and concepts that may not otherwise seem related to deepen understanding and application
Comparative	Compare theories, studies, clinical practices, and treatment protocols to establish commonalities and differences
Evaluative	Establish judgments about the *relative value* or importance of items or concepts compared
Critical	Examine the validity of an argument or discussion presented in a reading or assignment

Modified from McKeachie WJ: *Teaching tips: strategies, research and theory for college and university teachers,* Lexington, Mass., 1994, D.C. Heath and Company, pp. 37-40.

Table 4-10 SOCRATIC METHOD OF LEARNING: GETTING THE DISCUSSION STARTED		
Discussion Starter	**Example**	**Application in Athletic Training**
Ask about a known case	What was the role of the team physician in the recent spine boarding incident at the game on Saturday?	Identifies the role of the team physician relative to the athletic training staff.
Ask for specific factors	Why did the team physician stand back and allow the athletic trainers to command the situation?	Explains specific roles of the health care team. Clarification that the physician needed to be available to treat rather than lift during this situation.
Ask for intermediate factors	Why did the team physician allow the athletic training staff to perform such critical duties?	Identifies the relationships and trust of the health care team. Validation of the education of the athletic trainer.
Ask for prior factors	Why are athletic trainers in command in field evaluation settings?	Identifies the training required to be an athletic trainer. Emphasizes the need to have a standard operating procedure established with the physician.
Ask for insufficient factors	Do all team physicians allow athletic trainers to command the care of an athlete in these situations?	Strengthens the understanding between various venues (e.g., high school vs. collegiate). Fortifies the need for a strong working relationship with the team physician. Identifies various subspecialties of the physicians (e.g., orthopedist versus general medical physician).
Ask for counterexamples	Do you think that the team physicians at all colleges allow the athletic trainers to command the situation?	Establishes an understanding of individual settings and relationships.
Ask for counterexamples if an unnecessary factor is identified	If the counterexample was that the team physician did not like the athletic trainer, then the counterexample could be: How does the personal relationship affect the care that is provide the athlete in this setting?	Establishes a cause and effect relationship. Forces students to address issues that may not be rooted in practice or theory.
Ask for extreme value factors	Does the trust/relationship established by the athletic trainer and team physician have anything to do with the way the athletic trainer performed on the certification examination?	Connects personal and professional values. Facilitates consideration of alternative discussion points that may be of more relevance.
Ask for comparison of two cases	Did the team physician in the video clip (clip of an NFL injury management situation of a potential c-spine injury) act similarly to the team physician at the game here at XYZ university?	Connects behaviors and allows students to contemplate confounding factors that may account for behavioral patterns.
Ask for a prediction for an unknown case	What if the team physician had forced his way into controlling the command position (head) of the spine boarding incident and the athlete ceased breathing?	Facilitates consideration of roles and responsibilities. Engages thoughtful prediction of the "what-ifs" to process the most appropriate alternatives/solutions.

Modified from McKeachie WJ: *Teaching tips: strategies, research and theory for college and university teachers*, Lexington, Mass., 1994, D.C. Heath and Company.

process through real-life experiences. Because the discussions revolve around real situations, motivation for resolution is often heightened. Although not yet documented in athletic training education programs, this method has tremendous potential for serving as a valuable tool in the ethical development of athletic trainers throughout the curriculum.

Storytelling

A rich part of narrative ethics involves storytelling. Often used in medicince[57] and nursing,[41] stories help frame ethical decisions. According to Pimple,[63] stories encourage the audience to interpret and imply causality, intention, and meaning as the story unfolds. According to Triezenberg and McGrath,[74] storytelling promotes moral development by requiring the storyteller to reflect on the actions and consequences taken within the story, thereby providing a rich context. One of the oldest methods of communication, storytelling entertains and creates an environment for addressing cultural sensitivity. Storytelling has much value as a learning and teaching tool (Table 4-11).

Storytelling also is a valuable instrument for addressing diversity within the allied health fields. Faculty members have the responsibility to preserve, collect, and transmit stories of ethical activity to students to demonstrate that good people get into ethical dilemmas in the real world.[50] Stories provide firsthand accounts of situations encountered by students who may have academic or physical disabilities or who are nontraditional students or culturally diverse. Stories from a variety of perspectives serve as learning tools for all health care professionals. These stories (and the underlying messages associated with them) can bring students together as well as prepare them for professional encounters faced in the future. It encourages a deeper understanding of personal and professional issues facing athletic trainers.

Stories are most meaningful when structured to encourage participation and involvement. The content areas of stories have been summarized to include four key areas (Table 4-12): individual values and perspectives, ethical theory, ethical decision making, and professional behaviors and values.

Stories should initially address content from a personal perspective and then progress through stories

Table 4-11 VALUE OF STORYTELLING AS A LEARNING-TEACHING APPROACH

Value	Description
Facilitates thinking	Promotes sequencing, analyzing, and synthesizing information to gain a comprehensive view of the situation
Enhances imagination and visualization	Promotes connections between the story and other similar situations, encouraging transfer of knowledge
Develops appreciation of the beauty and rhythm of allied health language	Assists in the development of a professional language base as new terms are used and as medical terminology is integrated into the story
Supports the review and understanding of athletic training situations	Provides an opportunity to interact to clarify questions that may arise in the storytelling process
Strengthens the creation of caring communities	Provides a venue for clinicians and students to interact as relationships develop and connections are made in the professional environment
Links theory to practice	Encourages sharing among students and professionals to facilitate integration of theoretical concepts into daily practice

Modified from Koening JM, Zorn CR: Using storytelling as an approach to teaching and learning with diverse students, *J Nurs Educ* 41:393-400, 2002.

from current culture to traditional stories to clinical case analysis (Figure 4-8).[74]

Verkerk et al[77] further divides stories into several key categories: stories of identity, stories of relationships, and stories of value, with each having an individual focus. Stories of identity weave together personal issues of the self from one moment to the next and help define who the teller is as a person. These stories often conflict with others' interpretations because they often are biased by personal perceptions. Stories of relationships are important because they define who else is involved in the decisions being made. No ethical decision is exclusively personal; others always are involved. That is why stories of relationships are

Table 4-12 CONTENT AREAS AND PURPOSES FOR NARRATIVES IN ETHICS EDUCATION	
Content Area	**Purpose for the Use of Narrative**
Individual values and perspectives	To introduce a new experience, different moral perspectives, and define personal core values
Ethical theory	To provide a beginning point for ethics conversations, situations in which ethical theory can be tested, and practical applications for ethical theory
Ethical decision making	To develop and refine a personal ethical decision-making model; to provide a safe environment for making ethical decisions and scenarios that will likely be encountered in clinical practice
Professional values and behaviors	To introduce good professional behaviors through clinical stories; to provide time to compare personal values with professional values in the clinical setting and a context for understanding and applying the code of ethics; to facilitate the transition from student to professional

Modified from Triezenberg HL, McGrath JH: The use of narratives in an applied ethics course for physical therapy students, *J Phys Ther Educ* 15:49-56, 2001.

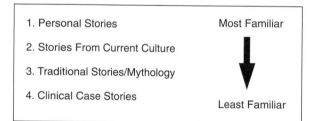

1. Personal Stories   Most Familiar

2. Stories From Current Culture

3. Traditional Stories/Mythology

4. Clinical Case Stories   Least Familiar

Figure 4-8 ■ Storytelling progression. Order of the presentation of different forms of narrative within each content area is based on student familiarity with the type of story. *(From Triezenberg HL, McGrath JH: The use of narratives in an applied ethics course for physical therapy students, J Phys Ther Educ 15:49-56, 2001.)*

important is sorting through ethical dilemmas. Lastly, stories of value involve key elements valued by the teller as well as the profession and are deeply rooted in the terminology of moral meaning. All these stories help make connections with others while negotiating professional responsibilities in the health care arena.

The effectiveness of storytelling in the educational program has been documented in the physical therapy literature.[74] Students reported that using narratives helped provide a framework for understanding the professional role, analyzing ethical issues, developing critical thinking, and clarifying personal values. Narratives also have been found to assist young professionals in considering alternative points of view and clarify cultural differences encountered in the clinical environment. As with all good educational formats, storytelling does have some drawbacks. Some students are not eager to hear others' dilemmas and believe they have an existing model for solving ethical dilemmas. Additionally, sometimes storytelling just does not seem to be formal enough for some students, thereby limiting their participation and input. Despite the negatives, storytelling is an excellent way of introducing and developing an ethical framework into athletic training education programs. After all, ethics education is about transitioning from the student role to the professional role, and stories provide an excellent context for doing so. Storytelling enables the student to be active and engage in the dialogue, which prevents ethics education from becoming a spectator sport; the extra bonus is they are often entertaining as well.

Gaming in Ethics

An interesting approach to considering ethical dilemmas facing the health professions is the gaming approach.[52] Gaming adds to motivation, stimulates learning, reviews course content, and encourages engagement. Gaming also is a more attractive approach than simple lectures when it comes to learning new material.

The gaming approach to ethics education involves presenting an ethical dilemma in a clinical setting after a brief presentation of ethical theory and concepts. Students are then divided into pairs, and each pair is presented a unique dilemma. Students then select any of the ethical decision-making models and apply it to the case. After application of a specific model, each pair must present opposite perspectives on the case to the class, and the class votes on which individual in the pair made the most compelling argument for their case. Scoring consists of a point for each student who

Kent State University Athletic Training Education Program
Professional Course Portfolio Guidelines

The following guidelines are to be utilized for this course in the Athletic Training Education Program (ATEP). This portfolio must be typed and professionally presented. These portfolios will serve as references for you as you progress through the professional phase of this program.

The minimal requirements are listed below; however, the instructor will have the right to add to these requirements:

Section I   **Goals Statements**
Provide short-term (immediate) and long-term (career) goals related to this course. You may use a bulleted list to address each goal followed by an explanation of how THIS course will specifically help you reach these goals professionally.

Personal Strengths and Weaknesses
Address specific strengths and weaknesses related to THIS course content. Address how you plan to maximize your strengths and minimize your weaknesses in this course.

Section II   **Syllabus, Notes, Handouts and other course materials**

Section III Projects, Labs, and Assignments
All written work for this course must be submitted in the portfolio. Completeness of these materials will be evaluated at this time. In this section, also include any references (articles) that you have used as resources for written work (particularly research projects if applicable). Any projects requiring video or CD ROM should have the actual "product" secured in a page protector or similar product.

Section IV   **Professional Journal – Didactic Course (UPPER LEVEL)**
OPTION ONE   For each week that you participate in the classroom assignments, you will be required to write a weekly summary condensing your thoughts. Each week, you will reflect on the following:

***NOTE: THESE ARE TO BE SUBMITTED EACH MONDAY AT THE BEGINNING OF CLASS!!!

a. What area of this week's discussion did you find most helpful/interesting and why?
b. How can this week's information from class assist you in your professional development plan?
c. Identify three scenarios with brief descriptions of situations in which you may find it necessary to incorporate this knowledge/content as you progress in your professional development.

These should be specific—vagueness will not be acceptable.

Section IV   **Clinical Journal – CLINICAL COURSE**
OPTION TWO   For each week that you participate in the clinical assignments for the ATEP, you will be required to write a **weekly summary** condensing your experience. Each week, you will reflect on the following:
a. What did you learn new this week and how does it help shape you professionally?
b. What did you do well this week in the clinicals and why?
c. What did you not do well this week and how do you plan to improve upon your weaknesses?

These should be specific—vagueness will not be acceptable.

Section V   **Reflections**
Provide a separate reflections document on each of the following:
a. Personal Goals Analysis
b. Personal Strengths/Weaknesses Analysis
c. How did you grow conceptually as a result of this course?

Grading will be completed at the end of each semester. It is required that this portfolio be organized in a three-ring binder with appropriate dividers. Portfolios will be held until the third week of the following semester (Fall/Spring). If the portfolio is not retrieved by the deadline, it will be discarded. Grading criteria are based upon the above criteria with additional points for neatness, grammar, professionalism, and creativity.

Figure 4-9 ■ Sample portfolio guidelines. *(Courtesy Kent State University Athletic Training Education Program, Kent, Ohio.)*

votes for him or her. Also, the students who vote for the winning argument also get a point. The student who has the most points at the end of the class session wins. The instructor may use some type of prize (textbooks, pens, t-shirts) to motivate students even further.[52]

The merit of the gaming approach is that it requires active engagement in a process that involves some type of reward for case deliberation and assessment of the merit of other case presentations. This approach teaches analysis of cases from multiple perspectives in a short period. This game can be continued into a writing assignment for personal reflection or deliberation if so desired.

Portfolios

Portfolios are an excellent means of displaying the processes by which ethical dilemmas are resolved and how professional behaviors evolve throughout any given course, semester, or academic program. Although typically time consuming to create, portfolios are a collection of works, projects, reflections, activities, and other artifacts that reflect the application and synthesis of a given time frame of activity.

In athletic training, portfolios can be used to document the development of foundational behaviors of professional practice as they emerge through clinical and didactic assignments. Any number of artifacts supported by explanation of how each activity facilitated ethical discovery creates a comprehensive collection of meaningful work. By articulating goals and performing an assessment of strengths and weaknesses at the beginning of the course or rotation, a reflection at the end of the activity can follow up, with a critical analysis of growth that is supported and linked to artifacts contained in the portfolio. Specifically linking artifacts to the foundational behaviors of professional practice, ethical discovery, and professional growth can be documented. Sample portfolio guidelines are shown in Figure 4-9.

A more specific portfolio may be used in which specific projects and/or activities are all that are included. Creativity is the key, and using a variety of tools to reflect professional growth is a powerful method for learning.

SUMMARY

Athletic trainers are faced with ethical challenges in their daily lives on an increasingly more frequent and complex basis. Formal educational activities that foster engagement in the learning process facilitate a deeper appreciation and respect for the depth and breadth of the ethical dilemmas faced as a professional. By using a variety of approaches to increasing self-awareness on personal and professional levels, athletic training students will be better equipped to address the challenges as young professionals. Ethics education goes beyond learning and reciting the terms, principles, and theories; it requires full immersion into the messiness of what we do, how we act, and how we treat others. This text will help you along this ethical journey by challenging you to look deep within yourself and the profession.

REFERENCES

1. Albanese RS: *Nursing staff development: strategies for success,* St Louis, 1992, Mosby.
2. American Physical Therapy Association: *Professionalism in physical therapy: core values,* 2004, American Physical Therapy Association.
3. Aroskar M: Managed care and nursing values: a reflection, *Trends Health Care Law Ethics* 10:83-86, 1995.
4. Barnbaum DR: Teaching empathy in medical ethics: the use of "lottery assignments," *Teaching Philosophy* 24:63-75, 2001.
5. Barnbaum DR: What I teach my students about. . .moving beyond the view from nowhere in case studies, *BIO Quarterly* 15:9-10, 2004.
6. Beauchamp TL, Childress JF: *Principles of biomedical ethics,* New York, 1989, Oxford University Press.
7. Beauchamp TL, Childress JF: *Principles of biomedical ethics,* ed 2, New York, 2001, Oxford University Press.
8. Birnbacher D: The Socratic method in teaching medical ethics: potentials and limitations, *Med Health Care Philosophy* 2:219-224, 1999.
9. Bloom BS: *Taxonomy of education objectives: cognitive domain,* New York, 1956, David McKay.
10. Bloom BS, Madaus GF, Hastings JT: *Evaluation to improve learning,* New York, 1981, McGraw-Hill.
11. Bonk CJ, King KS: *Computer conference and collaborative writing tools: student dialogue about student dialogue,* Mahwah, NJ, 1995, Lawrence Erlbaum Associates.
12. Botes A: A comparison between the ethics of justice and the ethics of care, *J Adv Nurs* 32:1071-1076, 2000.

13. Branch WT, Kern D, Haidet P, et al: Teaching the human dimensions of care in clinical settings, *JAMA* 286:1067-1074, 2001.

14. Brody H: *Stones of sickness,* New Haven, Conn., 1987, Yale University Press.

15. Brown MT: *Working ethics: strategies for decision making and organizational responsibility,* San Francisco, 1990, Jossey-Bass.

16. Chickering AW, Gamson ZF: *Applying the seven principles for good practice in undergraduate education: new directions for teaching and learning,* San Francisco, 1987, Jossey-Bass.

17. Clark PG: Values and voices in teaching gerontology and geriatrics: case studies as stories, *Gerontology* 42:297-303, 2002.

18. Danner CK, Gert B: A critique of principlism, *J Med Philosophy* 15:219-237, 1990.

19. Davis CM: Affective education for the health professions: facilitating affective behavior, *Phys Ther* 61(11):1587-1593, 1981.

20. DeToit D: A sociological analysis of the extent and influence of professional socialization on the development of a nursing identity among nursing students at two universities in Brisbane, Australia, *J Adv Nurs* 21:164-171, 1995.

21. Dinc L, Gorgulu RS: Teaching ethics in nursing, *Nurs Ethics* 9:259-269, 2002.

22. Doane G, Pauly B, Brown H, et al: Exploring the heart of ethical nursing practice: implications for ethics education, *Nurs Ethics* 11:241-253, 2004.

23. Englehardt HT: *The foundations of bioethics,* New York, 1986, Oxford University Press.

24. Ewing NJ: Teacher education: ethics, power and privilege, *Teacher Educ Special Educ* 24:13-24, 2001.

25. Fry ST: Towards a theory of nursing ethics, *Adv Nurs Sci* 11:9-22, 1989.

26. Gilligan C: *In a different voice,* Cambridge, 1982, Harvard University Press.

27. Glover SH, Bumpus MA, Sharp GF, et al: Gender differences in ethical decision making, *Women Manag Rev* 17:217-227, 2002.

28. Haney MR: Ethical dilemmas associated with self-disclosure in student writing, *Teaching Psychol* 31:167-171, 2004.

29. Hoffmaster B, Freedman B, Fraser G: *Clinical ethics theory and practice,* Scranton, NJ, 1989, Humana Press.

30. Hosmer LT: Standard format for the case analysis of moral problems, *Teaching Bus Ethics* 4:169-180, 2000.

31. Hudson Jones A: The color of the wallpaper: training for narrative ethics, *HEC Forum* 11:58-66, 1999.

32. Huotari R: A perspective on ethical reflection in multiprofessional care, *Reflective Prac* 4:121-138, 2003.

33. Jackson PW, Boostrom RE, Hansen DT: *The moral life in schools,* San Francisco, 1993, Jossey-Bass.

34. Jenson GM, Paschal KA: Habits of mind: student transition toward virtuous practice, *J Phys Ther Educ* 14:42-47, 2000.

35. Jenson GM, Richert AE: Reflection on the teaching of ethics in physical therapy education: integrating cases, theory, and learning, *J Phys Ther Educ* 19:78-85, 2005.

36. Jordan K, Stevens P: Teaching ethics to graduate students: a course model, *Fam J Counseling Ther Couples Families* 9:178-184, 2001.

37. Kansanen P: Pedagogical ethics in educational research, *Educ Res Eval* 9:9-23, 2003.

38. Kaufman SR: Decision-making, responsibility, and advocacy in geriatric medicine: physician dilemmas with elderly in the community, *Gerontologist* 35:481-488, 1995.

39. Kerr DS, Smith LM: Importance of and approaches to incorporating ethics into the accounting classroom, *J Bus Ethics* 14:987-995, 1995.

40. Killion J, Todnem G: A process for personal theory building, *Educ Leadership* 48:14-16, 1991.

41. Koening JM, Zorn CR: Using storytelling as an approach to teaching and learning with diverse students, *J Nurs Educ* 41:393-400, 2002.

42. Krathwhol D, Bloom B, and Masia B: *Taxonomy of educational objectives: handbook II: affective domain,* New York, 1964, David McKay.

43. La Puma J: Clinical ethics, mission and vision: practical wisdom in health care, *Hospital Health Service Administration* 35:257-256, 1990.

44. Lindemann NH: *Damaged identities, narrative repair,* New York, 2001, Cornell University Press.

45. Lovesky DV: Identity development in gifted children: moral sensitivity, *Roeper Review* 20:90-95, 1977.

46. MacDonald CA, Cox PD, Bartlett DJ, et al: Consensus on methods to foster physical therapy professional behaviors, *J Phys Ther* 16:27-36, 2002.

47. Macintyre A: *After virtue: a study in moral theory,* Notre Dame, Ind., 1981, University of Notre Dame.

48. Mattison M: Ethical decision making: the person in the process, *Social Work* 45:201-212, 2000.

49. McCarthy J: Principlism or narrative ethics: must we choose between them? *J Med Ethics* 29:65-71, 2003.

50. McDowell R: *Ethical conduct and the professional's dilemma: choosing between service and success,* New York, 1991, Quorum Books.

51. McKeachie WJ: *Teaching tips: strategies, research and theory for college and university teachers,* Lexington, Mass., 1994, D.C. Heath and Company, p. 375.

52. Metcalf BL, Yankou D: Using gaming to help nursing students understand ethics, *J Nurs Educ* 42:212-215, 2003.

53. Mumford MD, Helton WB, Decker BP, et al: Values and beliefs related to ethical decisions, *Teaching Bus Ethics* 7:139-170, 2003.

54. Myser C, Kerridge IH, Mitchell KR: Teaching clinical ethics as a professional skill: bridging the gap between knowledge about ethics and its use in clinical practice, *J Med Ethics* 21:97-104, 1995.

55. National Commission for the Protection of Human Subjects of Biomedical and Behavioral Research: *Belmont report,* Washington DC, 1979, Government Printing Office. (website): www.ohsr.od.nih.gov/mpa/belmont/php3. Accessed March 17, 2006.

56. Newman DL. Brown RD: *A framework for making ethical decisions: applied ethics for program evaluation,* Thousand Oaks, Calif., 1996, Sage.

57. Nichols B, Gillett G: Doctors' stories, patients' stories: a narrative approach to teaching medical ethics, *J Med Ethics* 23:295-299, 1997.

58. Noble CN: Ethics and experts, *Hastings Ctr Rep* 12:7-9, 1982.

59. Noddings N: *The challenge to care in schools: an alternative approach to education,* New York, 1992, Teachers College Press.

60. Norman GR, Schmidt HG: The psychological basis of problem-based learning: a review of the evidence, *Acad Med* 67:557-565, 1992.

61. Pellegrino ED, Siegler M, Singer PA: Teaching clinical ethics, *J Clin Ethics* 1:175-180, 1990.

62. Phillips JM: Syllabus selections: innovative learning activities. Chat role play as an online learning strategy, *J Nurs Educ* 44: 43-45, 2005.

63. Pimple KD: Using case studies in teaching research ethics, *Planning Workshop for a Guide for Teaching Responsible Science,* February, 1997, p. 1.

64. Pimple KD: Ethics at the interface: a successful online seminar, *Sci Engineering Ethics* 11:495-499, 2005.

65. Plack MM, Santasier A: Reflective practice: a model for facilitating critical thinking skills within an integrative case study classroom experience, *J Phys Ther Educ* 18:4-12, 2004.

66. Potter RB: *War and moral discourse,* Richmond, Va., 1969, John Knox.

67. Raths L, Harmin M, and Simon S: *Values and teaching,* Columbus, OH, 1966, Charles E. Merril Books, Inc.

68. Rodeheffer JK: Practical reasoning in medicine and the rise of clinical ethics, *J Clin Ethics* 1:187-192, 1990.

69. Schon DA: *Educating the reflective practitioner,* San Francisco, 1987, Jossey-Bass.

70. Seigler M, Pellegrino ED, Singer PA: Clinical medical ethics, *J Clin Ethics* 1:5-9, 1990.

71. Shelby CL: Care ethics in education, *Educ Forum* 67:337-342, 2003.

72. Smith D, Garteig L: Using a linked learning activity to foster nursing students' professional growth, *J Nurs Educ* 42:227-230, 2003.

73. Triezenberg HL: Beyond the code of ethics: educating physical therapists for their role as moral agents, *J Phys Ther Educ* 14:48-59, 2000.

74. Triezenberg HL, McGrath JH: The use of narratives in an applied ethics course for physical therapy students, *J Phys Ther Educ* 15:49-56, 2001.

75. Van Manen M: *The fact of teaching: the meaning of pedagogical thoughtfulness,* Albany, NY, 1991, State University of New York.

76. Veatch R: *A theory of medical ethics,* New York, 1981, Basic Books.

77. Verkerk M, Lindemann H, Maeckelberghe E, et al: An interpersonal exercise in ethics education, *Hastings Ctr Rep* 36:31-38, 2004.

78. Viafora C: Toward a methodology for the ethical analysis of clinical practice, *Med Health Care Philosophy* 2:283-297, 1999.

79. Weis D, Schank MJ: Professional values: key to professional development, *J Prof Nurs* 18(5):271-275, 2002.

80. Zembylas M, Vrasidas C: Levinas and the interface: the ethical challenge of online education, *Ethical Theory* 55:61-78, 2005.

Ethical Decision Making

LEARNING OBJECTIVES

After reading this chapter, the student should be able to do the following:

1. Understand the various decision-making models in ethics education.
2. Apply the various decision-making models to athletic training situations.
3. Appreciate the importance of multiple approaches to ethical decision making in the athletic training profession.

The object and reward of learning is continued capacity for growth and that students develop skills and habits of the mind that will enhance their creativity and problem-solving abilities with respect to the issues they are likely to meet (p. 117).[11]

Ethical decision-making models transcend all the allied health care literature. Learning to use ethical decision-making models to make ethical decisions better prepares the student to face the challenges of clinical practice in a rapidly changing environment. Without a strong emphasis on ethical decision making, clinicians could jeopardize "the integrity and the autonomy that the health care professions have worked so hard to achieve."[13] Although each model approaches decision making from a slightly different perspective, each provides a systematic framework for processing complex issues encountered in a profession. Systematic guidelines provide logical approaches to solving ethical dilemmas; however, discretionary judgments also affect the ultimate choice of action.[22] Finding the most appropriate model is a challenge in itself. Students are encouraged to analyze each of the models for its merit and then adapt the one that most suits them and the current dilemma.

Although models provide a framework, competing values or loyalties often complicate an ethical situation (Figure 5-1). Factors such as culture, policy, roles, climate, clinical uncertainty, independence, laws and rules, and professional codes may further complicate the issue. Gender is also known to affect ethical decisions; women are found to have different perceptions and approaches to ethical dilemmas. More critically, the literature indicates that how a person responds to ethical dilemmas depends partially on how he or she has learned to think about ethical issues.[22] Therefore students must be taught to think about ethical issues from multiple perspectives using multiple approaches.

As previously indicated, a certain model may be more useful in a personal values situation, whereas other models may be more applicable in a professional dilemma. The goal is that by exposing a variety of ethical decision-making models, one will become familiar and comfortable enough that you will adopt it as a guide throughout your professional journey. Similarly, with practice in using these models, you perhaps will discover a variation of one of these models that can become your own personal approach to decision making throughout your career.

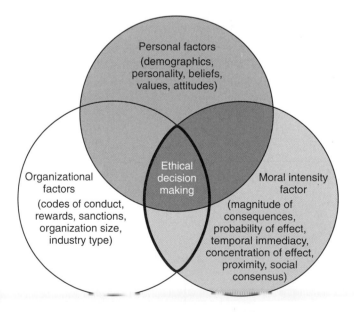

Figure 5-1 ■ Factors affecting ethical decision making. *(Modified from Paolillo JGP, Vitell SJ: An empirical investigation of the influence of selected personal, organizational and moral intensity factors on ethical decision making, J Bus Ethics 35:65-74, 2002.)*

MORAL AND LEGAL TEMPLATE FOR HEALTH CARE PRACTICE

When discussing issues, considering all the critical elements in isolation is difficult. Each decision or action could have legal and moral implications that affect the practitioner or others on a greater scope. Furthermore, others interpret your actions based on their perceptions rather than your intent alone. Geddes et al[17] have developed a conceptual framework for ethical decision making that emphasizes the relation between the morality and legality from individual, group, and societal perspectives (Figure 5-2).

This model demonstrates the complexities of ethical decision making and how issues may pull a person into any of the various quadrants depicted in the model, each having its own implications. This template is not static and does not remain symmetrical; it is always shifting.

VALUES-DRIVEN MODEL

The values-driven model focuses on incorporating the decision maker into the decision-making process by considering the value system and/or preferences of

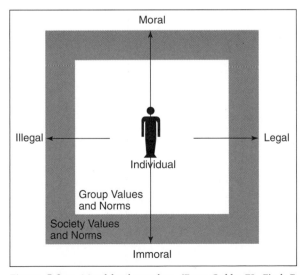

Figure 5-2 ■ Moral legal template. *(From Geddes EL, Finch E, Graham K: Ethical choices: a moral and legal template for health care practice,* Physiother Can *57:117, 2002.)*

that individual.[22] Value tension is at the core of this model. *Value tension* is defined as a no-win situation in which none of the options that resolves the particular dilemma is satisfying because some dissonance in the values emerges throughout the process.

This model is depicted in a triangular graphic (Figure 5-3). In this model, the base of the triangle represents the considerations relative to the case, whereas the personal dimensions of the decision maker become more prevalent as the process progresses. It depends highly on prior socialization and situational factors such as organizational culture, work roles, and attitudes. This model concludes with personal reflection.

After implementation and consideration of the steps in the model, personal reflection is essential to complete the process. After each case is resolved, perform a personal self-evaluation to examine the values that guided the decision. Mattison[22] suggests following the protocol outlined in Table 5-1 for reflection after use of the values-driven model.

This simple self-check will help analyze the effect that value conflicts play in the decision-making process. By acknowledging that these conflicts are present and by addressing them in a personal manner, you can become more cognizant of the various factors that affect professional decisions.

CLINICAL MODEL FOR ETHICAL DECISION MAKING

Bergmann[3] created a model rooted in the resolution of ethical dilemmas that involved real ethical decision making that commences with a presentation of the case followed by fact gathering and definition of the problem, consideration of philosophies and knowledge, alternatives and decisions, and evaluation and generalization. This model leads from the level of specific judgments to a broader level of generality, then finally to the level of ethical theory.[19]

This original model of ethical decision making proved effective for resolving ethical dilemmas; however, application to the allied health care field yielded a modification better suited for athletic training. Han and Ahn[19] created a modification of the Bergmann model that is widely used in nursing and can be

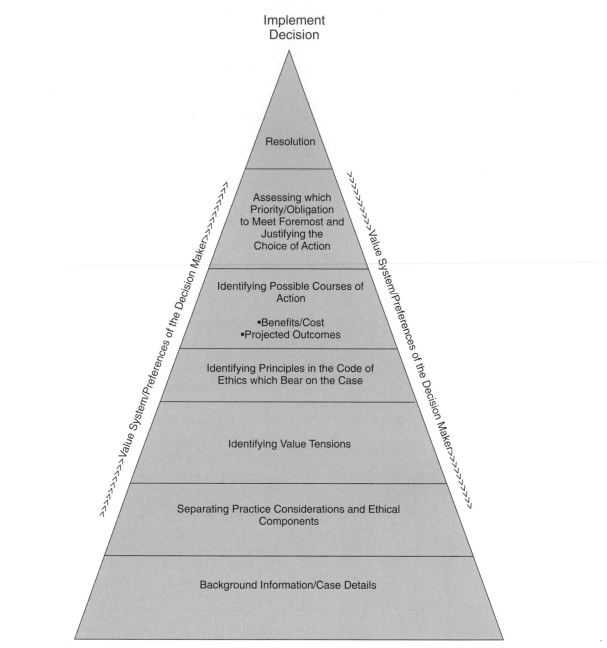

Figure 5-3 ■ Values-driven framework for analyzing ethical dilemmas. *(From Mattison M: Ethical decision making: the person in the process,* Social Work *45:206, 2000.)*

Table 5-1   PERSONAL REFLECTION FOLLOWING VALUES-DRIVEN DECISION MAKING

Question	Option 1	Option 2	Option 3
To what extent did my personal values or philosophies influence the preferred choice of action?	I was aware of my personal bias or preferences and attempted to keep these from unduly influencing the outcome.	I had not considered the extent to which my personal values may have influenced the ultimate decision.	
To what extent did the legal obligation influence my decision in this case?	Not at all	Somewhat	Was a deciding factor in my decision
Was I willing to act outside legal obligations if doing so meant serving the patient's best interest?	My legal obligation took precedence over all other obligations.	If the legal obligation does not serve my patient's best interest, I am not bound to apply the legal rule above other interests.	
To what extent did adhering to organizational policy influence my decision in the case?	Not at all	Somewhat	Was a deciding factor in the decision
If organizational policy conflicted with other obligations to the patient, was I willing to act outside organizational policy?	My first obligation is to the organization.	Organizational policy may not take precedence in all case circumstances.	
To what extent did my role in the agency influence my choice of action? (Do you believe that your choice of action would be different if you were an administrator?)	My choice of action was strongly influenced by my organizational role.	My choice of action was somewhat influenced by my organizational role.	I would have made the same decision regardless of my role in the organization.
If the case involved conflict between patient self-determination and paternalism, which value did I judge to be most essential?	Patient self-determination is the overriding value.	Professional judgment was the overriding value.	
In selecting a choice of action, I viewed as the most important . . .	Evaluating possible costs and benefits for the patient.	Strict adherence to procedural practices (adherence to law and policy).	

easily adapted for the athletic training profession (Figure 5-4).

Several examples are provided for this model (Table 5-2). Specific dilemmas related to the following can be specifically productive by using this approach to decision making, which is useful in clinical practice and educational settings.

As with all models, an effective evaluation tool helps objectify performance and monitor progress.

Several evaluation criteria can be formulated into a rubric for assessing progress through these clinical cases. These rubrics can be helpful in self-reflection or can be used as a peer or faculty assessment instrument in either written or verbal formats. The key evaluation criteria are as follows[7]:

1. Quality of the arguments for moral views
2. Mastery of the theories and principles of ethics

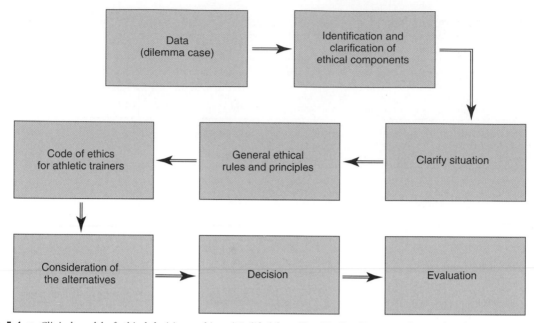

Figure 5-4 ■ Clinical model of ethical decision making. *(Modified from Han SS, Ahn SH: An analysis and evaluation of student nurses' participation in ethical decision making,* Nurs Ethics *7:115, 2000.)*

Table 5-2 SPECIFIC CASES FOR USE WITH CLINICAL MODELS

Dilemma	Examples
Respect for life	• Human experimentation without consent • Abortion
Athletic trainers and clients	• Not telling the truth to the athlete • Failure to maintain confidentiality • Allowing the athlete to decide on treatment without all the facts
Athletic trainers and professional practice	• Practice deviating from principles • Conflicts between athlete's needs and physician orders • Questionable actions by a physician • Allocation of scarce resources • Concealment of a physician's malpractice • Not reporting a medical error • Conflict between athlete's needs and organizational policy • An athlete's distrust of a physician's diagnosis • Insufficient staffing
Athletic trainers and co-workers	• Conflict between athletic trainers • Withholding information about a co-worker's substance abuse • Conflict between physical therapists and athletic trainers

Modified from Han SS, Ahn SH: An analysis and evaluation of student nurses' participation in ethical decision making, *Nurs Ethics* 7:113-123, 2000.

3. Identification of moral issues
4. The ability to argue from both sides of a problem

The following key questions can be used to guide the assessment and evaluate clinical ethical decision making:

1. Were you perceptive in identifying the moral issues?
2. Did you apply the principles and rules of ethics and the code in the ethical decision-making process rationally?
3. Did you have a sense of moral obligation when making the ethical decision?

Written evidence can be evaluated in a similar fashion by using the following questions to guide the review:

1. Do you analyze accurately and participate thoughtfully?
2. Does the written evidence show that sensitivity to ethical issues has increased?
3. Do you make an analysis of a moral dilemma, together with a solution or suitable interpretation?
4. Do you have the ability to adapt and apply something outside the material treated in textbooks while trying to find an ethical interpretation?

Although not exclusive, these questions can be inserted into a rubric to provide substantial feedback relative to your progress in integrating these models while considering ethical dilemmas.

Another clinical ethical decision-making model approaches the resolution of ethical dilemmas from a slightly different perspective.[26] Although the steps appear different, the outcomes are focused on the clinical decision-making processes that athletic trainers face each day. In this model, a broad perspective to each case is gained through careful consideration of options. Table 5-3 reflects the template that summarizes this model.

These clinical models are particularly helpful while you progress through the curriculum and encounter multiple clinical decision-making situations that may create dissonance. Organized approaches to addressing these clinical issues are imperative throughout the academic program to promote acculturation into the profession.

CLINICAL PRAGMATISM PROTOCOL

Ethical cases have been deliberated in allied health care forums for decades. Steinkamp and Gordijn[25] have designed a method of clinical case deliberation rooted in clinical pragmatism that is consensus oriented, analogy based, and democratic (Figure 5-5). With a strong emphasis on ethical reflection, this model approaches ethical dilemmas as conflicts in the context of clinical practice. The steps in clinical pragmatism start with a structural analogy between clinical judgment and the structure of ethical reflection following pragmatism. Although the full model consists of an elaborate list of questions, the basic steps are simple (Table 5-4).

This model has provided considerable guidance in clinical decision making. It encourages a consensus approach when a multidisciplinary team works together. It also encourages deep reflection beyond the written medical record, accounting for the more personal descriptions of the case. As with all allied health care professions, athletic training could gain tremendous insight from the use of this model in clinical decision making.

NIJMEGEN MODEL

Similar to the clinical pragmatism model, the Nijmegen model (Table 5-5) focuses on prospective ethical case deliberation in clinical practice.[27] Typically, a trained ethicist guides a multidisciplinary team through the decision-making processes they encounter in clinical practice. This model is based on the interpretation of clinical reality by assuming that questions are not external to, but intertwined within, the multidisciplinary health care system.[5] This model poses a clear moral question at the beginning of any case deliberation, allowing access to the ethical dimensions to evolve. It is also based on the fact that the health care setting is a complex, multidimensional component that requires considerable understanding of operational procedures in resolving ethical dilemmas; as such, consensus is important but not the most important criterion in ethical decision making. In addition, good facilitation and mediation are essential during case conferences.[25] Although trained ethicists

Table 5-3   CLINICAL ETHICAL DECISION-MAKING MODEL

Step	Goal	Guiding Questions
Collecting clinical data	• Gather information for correct clinical approach implying that the patient is considered whole and unique	• Do any alternatives exist from a medical and health care point of view? • What are the constraints that would suggest, independently of medical indications, a particular course of action over another? • What is the rationale behind the constraint(s)? • Is it the particular organization of work conditions, or the scarcity of resources, the lack of a specific competence, or the internal dynamics of the health care team?
Assessing the responsibilities	• Specific responsibilities of the subjects involved are acknowledged • Patient must be respected and protected • Health care professional responsibilities are legal and deontological	• Was the patient adequately informed? • Are there any reasons to justify inadequacy of the information and responsibility? • What are the responsibilities of the family? • What reasons make their consensus relevant, mandatory, or unreliable? • What are the specific responsibilities of health care professionals involved in the case? • Does the suggested intervention imply consequences that the family cannot reasonably assume? • What kind of support does the family rely on? • Who has the obligation to activate those supporting agencies?
Identifying the ethical problems	• Approach analytically first to investigate values being affected, framed within the clinical context	• Which ethical problems are involved in the case? • Formulate the questions for which each problem might most clearly indicate the possible alternatives for action and the values that are promoted or endangered. • Rank the ethical problems according to their importance and the context in which they are involved.
Formulate ethical judgment	• Evaluate weighing alternative solutions, possible grounds, and choosing course of action promoting values of the ethical paradigm	• What are the proposed solutions for this particular case? • What are the reasons motivating their plausibility of the solution? • Which decision better promotes the values at stake?
Elaborating directives for analogous cases	• Draw indications that may be helpful in dealing with other cases • Morphology of the case, values, principles, and virtues	• Can the case be reduced to a single ethical issue? • Is a kind of typology possible to lay out? • What are the basic strategies for preventing, dealing with, and eventually resolving the most recurring conflicts in similar cases? • What are the virtues and, in general, the fundamental attitudes of health care professionals for dealing with these cases?

Modified from Viafora C: Toward a methodology for the ethical analysis of clinical practice, *Med Health Care Philosophy* 2:283-297, 1999.

are not likely to be present in the athletic training classroom or clinic, this model has considerable application to the profession from a decision-making perspective.

This model highlights the role of the moral dilemma before evaluation of the case facts. By posing a clear-cut moral question, this model taps into the intuitive nature and consciousness of human beings to access everyday moral knowledge balanced with sen-

sitivity. This sets the stage for the discussion of the specific case that is framed in personal experience and connected to common sense and ordinary morality.[25] This model gradually tapers into consideration of the patient from a needs perspective, normative arguments and, finally, a judgment. This inventory process helps evaluate the case from multiple perspectives, considering the multidisciplinary impact of patient care, by combining process and outcome.

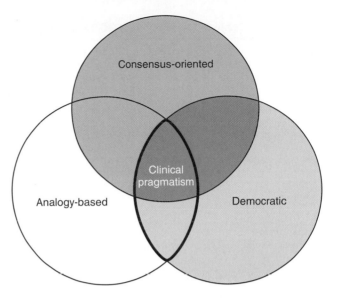

Figure 5-5 ■ Clinical pragmatism in action.

Table 5-4 CLINICAL PRAGMATISM MODEL OF ETHICAL DECISION MAKING

Steps in the Model	Starting Point	Outcome
Assessment of the clinical situation	1. Careful analysis of a clinical situation 2. Medical record is reference point 3. Concentric circles are drawn to reflect contributions of others in the health care team 4. Needs and wishes of the family and patient are added (consider competing interests, issues of power conflicts, and institutional factors)	Wider view of the case from multiple perspectives
Moral diagnosis	1. Identification of the moral dilemma based on how the participants frame the dilemma 2. Narratives, such as moral intuitions and stories, are included 3. Moral considerations are ranked as more or less important and relative to institutional policy, professional ethics, or value agreements 4. Comparison of this case to other similar cases is performed 5. Possible options for solving the dilemma are discussed	Classical casuistry is developing as the case is compared with other similar ones
Goal setting, decision making, and implementation	1. Determine goals of treatment and care 2. Agree on interventions based on the patient's needs 3. Specify goals 4. Decide and implement action plan	Broader consideration of the patient's preferences rather than simply sterile clinical consideration for the case
Evaluation	1. Incidental and continuous evaluation of the outcome is considered 2. Reassessment can occur if other factors arise	Preliminary characteristics of ethical principles are considered; variability of the clinical situation is considered; openness and flexibility in ethical deliberation is encouraged

Modified from Steinkamp N, Gordijn B: Ethical case deliberation on the ward. A comparison of four methods, *Med Health Care Philosophy* 6:235-246, 2003.

Table 5-5 THE NIJMEGEN METHOD OF ETHICAL DECISION-MAKING

Steps	Guiding Concerns	Anticipated Outcomes
What is the moral problem?	• Moral dimensions	• Discovery of moral issues affecting the patient and health care team • Intuitive thoughts expressed before reading the chart
What are the facts?	• Medical dimension • Athletic training dimension • Patient values and social dimension • Organizational dimension	• Discovery of all pertinent information that is factual and documented that contributes to the case
Assessment	• Well-being of the patient • Autonomy of the patient • Responsibility of the health care professional	• Consideration of information in an ethical framework taking into account all aspects of the dilemma
Decision making	• Recapitulation of the moral problem • Unknown details • Arguments • Decision • Evaluation	• Reinforcement of the moral dilemma • Speculation on unknown details that could affect the resolution • Consideration of all components through discussion • Consensus decision • Follow-up and consideration of actions to guide future actions

Modified from Steinkamp N, Gordijn B: Ethical case deliberation on the ward. A comparison of four methods, *Med Health Care Philosophy* 6:240, 2003.

HERMENEUTIC METHOD

The Hermeneutic method is rooted in philosophy and based on understanding and interpretation. The basic tenet of hermeneutics is that anything (e.g., a written document, a morally relevant situation or action) can be best understood when placed in a larger context.[25] By emphasizing the interaction between the actual case and the broader context, athletic trainers are able to frame their decisions on a mutual understanding and explanation of both sides. "A moral problem in clinical practice may be shaped by more general changes in responsibility due to the effects of technical advances in medicine. In turn, in order to comprehend ethical issues in daily clinical practice, a deeper understanding of these effects may prove essential."[1] Hermeneutic dialogue takes into account personal and collective morality and is rooted in tacit reflection on prior experiences (Table 5-6).

Durand suggested a combination method of ethical analysis with the Hermeneutic model approached from a *prospective* rather than *retrospective* perspective (Figure 5-6).[14] It considers multiple alternatives for resolving each clinical case and addresses ethical analysis rather than simply hermeneutic reflection.

This model emphasizes the role of analysis of the narratives presented in any case situation and applying normative reflection to arrive at an interpretation-based conclusion. However, a limitation of this model is that understanding and interpreting the case may be insufficient; athletic trainers usually are required to make decisions. Some users of this model may get so consumed by the interpretation that resolution is never achieved. Action is critical in health care, so this model usually is combined with other models.

SOCRATIC DIALOGUE

As discussed in Chapter 4, the Socratic method of ethical decision making is based on group discussion following a specific plan. The itinerary typically begins with a philosophically relevant everyday question,

Table 5-6 HERMENEUTIC DIALOGUE MODEL		
Steps	**Looking for . . .**	**Outcomes**
Primary intuitions	First impressions of the case	Provide moral intuitions of the health care team
Analysis of the narrative perspectives	Perspective and style of analysis	Provide insight into each person's perspective on the case
Analysis of the narratives	Structure and content	Provide a foundation to build upon embedded intuitions from the case itself to guide toward a more rational understanding of the case
Components of the narrative	Key words Ethical theories	Provide a connection between practice and theory
Significance of considerations for the case	Differences from primary intuitions	Provide multiple perspectives for case resolution

Modified from Steinkamp N, Gordijn B: Ethical case deliberation on the ward. A comparison of four methods, *Med Health Care Philosophy* 6:235-246, 2003.

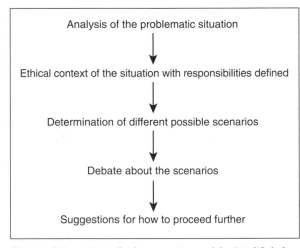

Figure 5-6 ■ Durand's hermeneutic model. *(Modified from Durand G: Introduction to bioethics. In Steinkamp N, Gordijn B: Ethical case deliberation on the ward. A comparison of four methods, Med Health Care Philosophy 6:242, 2003.)*

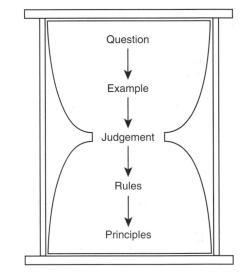

Figure 5-7 ■ Socratic dialogue hourglass analogy. *(Modified from Kessels J: Socratic method. In Steinkamp N, Gordijn B: Ethical case deliberation on the ward. A comparison of four methods, Med Health Care Philosophy 6:244, 2003.)*

Particularly useful in case discussions, this technique focuses on everyday experiences and personal insights. Often referenced as "regressive abstraction,"[2] this strategy brings forth a judgment rooted in reality that is then carefully reflected upon later on an abstract level to gain philosophical insight. An hourglass model illustrates this strategy (Figure 5-7).[21]

Socratic dialogue as a decision-making tool requires careful processes throughout. The facilitator should remain impartial to protect the slowest thinkers, support efforts of all in understanding the different perspectives, constantly pull the group back to the original question, and ultimately drive the group on the direction of consensus.

The Socratic method is useful to the athletic training profession in many ways. Health care providers are constantly placed in situations of moral uneasiness, and experiencing it through this type of activity can spawn confidence. This method also assists young professionals in establishing conceptual clarity to process ethical dilemmas. Each of these components is essential in the development of foundational behaviors of professional practice in the athletic training profession.

A comparison of several specific methods of ethical case deliberation related to various types of moral problems is summarized in Table 5-7. By embracing multiple ways of considering ethical dilemmas, young professionals will develop a strong repertoire for solving complex ethical cases.

FOUR PRINCIPLES MODEL

Although a strong understanding of moral theory is essential in ethics education, many entry-level students are confused by the depth and breadth of applying multiple perspectives in analyzing ethical dilemmas. Therefore a simple, concise model should be established to guide young professionals in decision making. A principle-based approach to ethical decision making proposes 10 sequential steps for solving ethical dilemmas, with emphasis on consideration of the wider framework in which the dilemma exists. The following steps serve as a basic guide to contextualizing ethical dilemmas in health care by using the four principles of beneficence, nonmalfeasance, justice, and autonomy:

1. Ask if the question is an ethical one.
2. List all the people involved.
3. Generate solutions; rule out nothing.
4. Assess the advantages and disadvantages of each solution (using the four principles).
5. Make a decision framed in a basic theory.
6. Discuss the decision with colleagues.
7. Check the precedence (legal, policy and procedure, etc.).
8. Make a final decision.
9. Impart the information to the affected party.
10. Record everything.

Although simplistic, this model provides a useable template for addressing ethical dilemmas from a principles perspective. As you mature as a professional, you will typically need to evolve beyond this simple model and embrace a more comprehensive approach to solving ethical dilemmas. However, the four principles model is extremely useful in the early stages of ethical deliberation.

RATIONAL DECISION-MAKING PROCESS: AN INTEGRATED MODEL

Linked specifically to ethical principles, this multistage model can be used extensively throughout the curriculum. The stages follow a specific sequence and can be used in part or in total for ethical cases (Table 5-8). This model also emphasizes the use of "moderators" to consider while progressing through the decision-making process.

This integrated model carefully considers all perspectives and guides you through multiple layers of analysis. It encourages the decision maker to make

Table 5-7 COMPARISON OF SELECTED METHODS OF ETHICAL DECISION MAKING

Method	Preferred Situation for Use	Perspective	Aim
Clinical pragmatism	Moral conflicts	Prospective	Consensus
Nijmegen method	Moral problem in decision making	Prospective	Justified decision
Hermeneutic method	Moral uneasiness, moral remorse	Retrospective	Comprehension
Socratic dialogue	Conceptual and normative uncertainty	Retrospective	Clarification of basic concepts and principles

Modified from Steinkamp N, Gordijn B: Ethical case deliberation on the ward. A comparison of four methods, *Med Health Care Philosophy* 6:245, 2003.

Table 5-8   TRADITIONAL RATIONAL DECISION-MAKING PROCESS[17,18]

Stage	Description	Questions	Goals
Stage I	Recognition of the ethical dilemma Teleological and deontological	• Does it involve the ends or consequences? • Does it involve the means or duty?	• Peak personal philosophical orientations • Activate background knowledge
Stage II	Generation of alternatives Teleological and deontological	• Alternatives to maximize ends? • Alternatives to maximize means?	• Consideration of alternatives • Conceptualization from multiple perspectives
Stage III	Evaluating alternatives Teleological and deontological	• Which alternative determines the comprehensive alternative? • Which is both good and right?	• Condensing options into a chosen option
Stage IV	Identification of the ideal alternative to solve the problem "Ideal decision"	• Is the proposed choice the best alternative? • Is the synthesis of alternatives to establish the right and good choice correct?	• Reprocessing and reconsideration of alternatives
Stage V	Act on data gathered independent of free will "Existential perspective"	• What is the best end? • What is the best mean? • What creates the most freedom and responsibility?	• Consideration of alternatives from existential viewpoint • Consideration of authentic alternatives
Stage VI	Decision to implement or not implement the ideal decision based on personal intentions "Overt behavior"	• Was the ethical decision comprehensively followed? • If not, why?	• Decision making and analysis of the decision
Stage VII	Evaluate the decision from all perspectives (teleological, deontological, existential) Evaluation of behavior	• Was it good? • Was it right? • Was it authentic?	• Evaluate behavior based on comprehensive ethical behavior • Establish accountability and commitment

Modified from Rest JR: The major components of morality. In Kurtines W, Gerwitz J, editors: *Morality, moral behavior, and moral development,* New York, 1984, Wiley Press; and Nutt PC: Types of organizational decision making, *Administrative Sci Quarterly* 29:414-450, 1984.

authentic choices based on consideration of moderators, including individual moderators (philosophical profile, psychological profile, demographic profile); issue-specific moderators (proximity to the issue, societal consensus, responsibility for results, magnitude of the decision, concentration of the effect, policy, and procedural impact); significant others as moderators (personal, intraorganizational, extraorganizational); situational moderators (organizational ideology, culture, and climate); and external moderators (political, societal, economic, and technological). Each of these factors can influence perceptions of a situation and the direction taken in a decision-making situation. By understanding and recognizing the role each of these

moderators plays along the way to an ethical decision, athletic trainers can fully appreciate the scope of their decisions.

Although sound, this model fails to address critical cultural components that affect ethical decision-making processes. With this limitation in mind, alternative models have been created to expand the potential for cultural sensitivity and cultural competence to evolve.

As previously discussed, this multiple perspective can be interwoven throughout the curriculum. A sample module is presented in Appendix E. This module uses a 12- to 13-week template to incorporate this integrated approach into multiple phases of the curriculum. Your personal development may evolve through a plan similar to this one.

TRANSCULTURAL INTEGRATIVE MODEL

The transcultural integrative model (Table 5-9) is an expanded integrative model that addresses the cultural pieces that many of the prior models have neglected.[16] Combining both values and principles, this model is used extensively in counseling yet has direct application to athletic training. Although a bit more complex than the simple integrative model, this transcultural model is highly sensitive to the cultural needs of both the clinician and patient in the ethical decision-making process.

By identifying personal and cultural bias, athletic trainers can become more sensitive and effective at making ethical decisions in an increasingly diverse world. Documented to be most effective in addressing issues related to informed consent, competence, multicultural counseling, working with minors, dual relationships, sexual orientation, disabilities, and law-ethics interface situations, this model has broad applications in the athletic training profession.

CONSENSUS MODEL

Many ethical decisions are made and serve as critical components in professional lives and practice. As previously mentioned, ethics is about helping people make good decisions to assist in character development. The consensus model considers the less-than-ideal world in which health care providers must make decisions and looks deeply at professional norms and principles, cultural influences, and values (Figure 5-8).[8] This multifaceted approach to ethical decision making highlights the critical role of considering the personal and professional input from all members of the health care team in deciding on the desired action.

Emphasizing the role of consultation with others, this model strives to implement a consultation with others' mentality when facing ethical dilemmas. Health care providers, including athletic trainers, often consult with others because consultation has been proven to stimulate thinking to generate new ideas and options, provide feedback on the ideas already generated relative to quality, increase self-awareness of

personal factors and potential conflicts, support the fact that all options were considered (going the extra mile) in an ethical case, increase confidence and support in the final decision, and reduce legal liability.[4] The advantages of consultation are realized in this model because a collective group is working together to solve the dilemma from multiple perspectives.

This basic model provides a strong framework for solving ethical dilemmas. Although strong, the drawbacks of consensus models are that they are often time consuming and frustrating if a group cannot reach agreement with the proposed courses of action. If this strategy is used in health care, multiple reassessment may be needed to tease out information; however, a decision may need to be made with alternative models if consensus simply cannot be achieved. Obviously, the dialogue will be productive for the decision maker, but the effect of switching from a consensus model to a more directed approach may have considerable effects on those who participated in the consensus model who have now been abandoned. These are all important considerations for the use of this model.

SOCIAL CONSTRUCTIVISM MODEL

Social constructivism approaches ethical decision making from an interactive rather than individual framework. This model involves the following steps (Figure 5-9)[9]:

1. Obtain information from the involved party.
2. Assess the nature of the relationships operating at that specific time.
3. Consult valued colleagues and professional expert opinions (e.g., ethic codes and literature).
4. Negotiate whether agreement or disagreement exists among the sources.
5. Respond in a way that encourages reasonable consensus regarding the outcome.

This model is rooted in the social nature of the health care professions and relies on the processes of negotiating, arbitrating, and consensus building. By being tied to a larger group of professionals, athletic trainers can appreciate the culture that emerges throughout the process. Athletic trainers do not work in isolation. The profession involves a social, collective

Table 5-9 TRANSCULTURAL INTEGRATIVE MODEL FOR ETHICAL DECISION MAKING

Step	Definition	Goal	General Impact	Transcultural Impact
1	Interpreting the situation through awareness and fact finding	Enhancement of sensitivity and awareness	Emotional arousal, cognitive sensitivity and awareness of needs and welfare of all involved	Clinicians' attitudes and emotional reactions aroused; awareness of cultural background; role socialization; acculturation
		Reflection to analyze whether dilemma exists	Consideration of opposing options	Determination of whether proposed actions reflect clinicians' view, patients' view, or both
		Determination of major stakeholders	Identification of legal and ethical relations to all parties	Determination of the impact of the involved parties' cultural values
		Engagement in the fact finding	Reviewing existing information and seeking new information	Gathering cultural information such as family values and community relationships
2	Formulating the ethical decision	Review the dilemma	Determine if dilemma has changed in light of new cultural information gathered	Ensure that all cultural information was considered
		Determine relevant codes, laws, principles, policies, and procedures	Determine the ethics law and practice applicable	Examine whether the code contains diversity clauses, examine discriminatory laws, estimate conflict between laws from various cultural perspectives
		Generate courses of action	List all options	Ensure that all options are culturally sensitive
		Consider positive and negative consequences for each	List all options	Ensure that cultural perspectives are addressed in each consequence
		Consultation	Consult supervisors and other professionals	Ensure consultants have multicultural expertise
		Select preferred course of action	Ensure it is appropriate	Review to make sure that it is consistent with cultural perspectives
3	Weighing competing, nonmoral values and affirming the course of action	Engage in reflective recognition and analysis of personal blind spots	Identify nonmoral values that may interfere with the implementation of the course of action selected	Identify how the clinicians' nonmoral values may be quite different from the patient's
		Consider contextual influences on values selection	Consider context from collegial, professional, institutional, and societal levels	Consider context from multiple cultural perspectives
4	Planning and executing the selected course of action	Develop a reasonable sequence of concrete actions	Divide the action into simple steps	Identify culturally relevant resources and strategies for implementation
		Anticipate personal and contextual barriers	Address the contextual and personal barriers immediately	Anticipate cultural barriers such as biases, discrimination, stereotyping and prejudice; plan for supportive action
		Implement, document, and evaluate the course of action	Evaluate the accuracy of the course of action by gathering information	Identify variables and measures that are culturally specific

Modified from Garcia JG, Cartwright B, Winston SM, et al: A transcultural integrative model for ethical decision making in counseling, *J Counseling Development* 81:268-278, 2003.

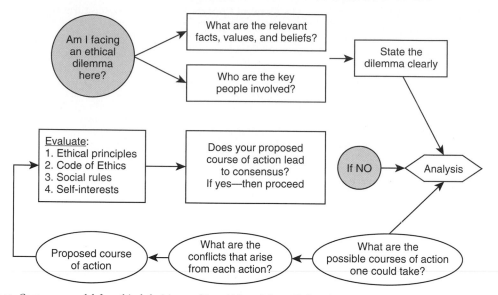

Figure 5-8 ■ Consensus model for ethical decision making. *(Adapted from Chabon SS, Morris JF: Ethics: a consensus model for making ethical decisions in a less-than-ideal world,* The ASHA Leader *9:18-19, 2004.)*

environment and takes advantage of all the resources available. Interactions with others influence and direct the decision-making processes. This model encourages that behavior.

VIRTUE ETHICS MODEL

Virtue ethics is technically defined as *who one is, what one ought to become, and what form of action will bring one from the present to the future.*[15] Rooted in personal characteristics and professional wisdom, the virtue ethics model extends beyond the basic considerations of ethical principles. Because deciding which principle should prevail in most situations is difficult, this model relies heavily on the professional's moral and personal beliefs. Emphasizing the importance of self-responsibility in making ethical judgments, this model focuses on the person making the decision rather than the decision itself. In essence, the action is judged as "right" if it is in sync with what the health care professional believes is correct and reflects how a virtuous health care professional should act. Not defined in steps as many other models are, this approach focuses on reflection, balance, collaboration, and attention to context in the resolution of ethical dilemmas.[16]

COLLABORATIVE MODEL

Although decision making often occurs individually, the collaborative model recognizes the need to obtain a group perspective on ethical dilemmas facing professionals.[11] Based on the values of collaboration, cooperation, and inclusion, this model emphasizes sequential steps to resolving dilemmas (Table 5-10).

This model focuses on the role of multiple perspectives and is favorable in addressing cultural perspectives as they evolve. Because many ethical dilemmas in athletic training involve multiple parties, this model provides a valuable resource for sorting out the key information and input from each of the constituents to try to resolve the problem in a collaborative fashion.

MANAGEMENT MODEL

Much can be learned from the business models when looking at decision making. Although corporate problem solving often involves components unique to such organizations, some overlap is helpful in reviewing moral dilemmas. Rooted in moral reasoning, this particular model is quite similar to the problem-solving models that business managers frequently

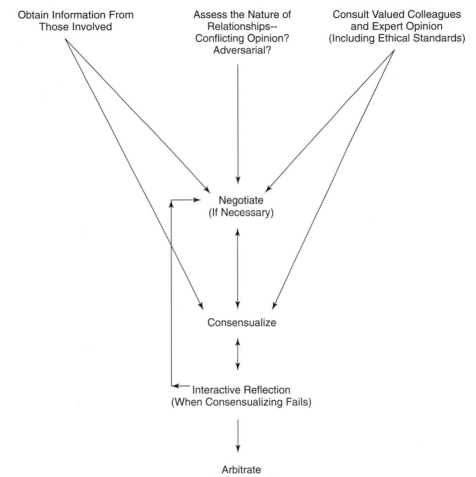

Figure 5-9 ■ Social constructivism model. *(From Cottone RR: A social constructivism model of ethical decision making in counseling,* J Counseling Development *79:43, 2001.)*

Step	Action
	**Table 5-10 COLLABORATIVE MODEL OF ETHICAL DECISION MAKING**

Step	Action
1	Identify the involved parties who are affected by the dilemma
2	Define the multiple viewpoints of each of the parties
3	Develop a solution that is mutually acceptable to all parties based on group work that addresses goals and expectations
4	Identify and implement individual contributions as part of the solution

Modified from Garcia JG, Cartwright B, Winston SM, et al: A transcultural integrative model for ethical decision making in counseling, *J Counseling Development* 81:268-278, 2003.

use.[10] This five-step model is simple and easy to apply to most situations:

Step I: *Analyzing:* Separating the problem of each case into its major components

Step II: *Weighing:* Assessing strengths and weaknesses of alternatives and balancing them against each other

Step III: *Justifying:* Providing compelling and sufficient moral reasoning that appeals to an established moral principle that is consistent with the organizational philosophy

Step IV: *Choosing:* Selecting one or more of the alternatives based on justifications

Step V: *Evaluating:* Reexamining the choices, identifying unanswered questions, and relating discussions to similar cases

This model emphasizes process and content. It is comprehensive in addressing the clinical and administrative dimensions of each situation. A more complex application of a decision-making model is often used in the health care fields.[22] This model is a feedback system that constantly assesses each component to ensure that all factors are being considered (Figure 5-10). By considering personal ethics and organizational structure, this model ties together the larger context in which most dilemmas occur.

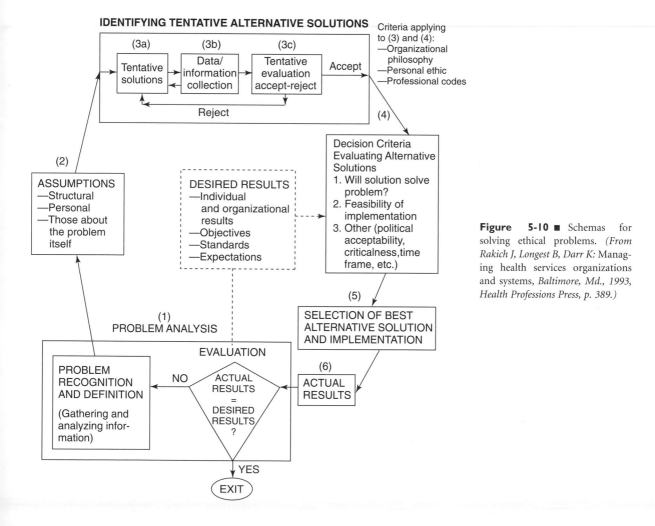

Figure 5-10 ■ Schemas for solving ethical problems. *(From Rakich J, Longest B, Darr K: Managing health services organizations and systems, Baltimore, Md., 1993, Health Professions Press, p. 389.)*

ETHICAL DECISION-MAKING MODEL USED IN NURSING

The nursing profession has been rigorous in ethics education over the past decades. Viewed as a critical element in the educational process, nurses typically complete multiple levels of ethics education throughout their academic program and training. Viewed primarily from a clinical perspective, the proposed ethical decision-making model provides a concise model for entry-level professionals that can easily be applied to athletic training (Table 5-11).[23]

This model moves through sequential steps toward achieving resolution of a case; however, the most important element in this process is the last step. This step is what helps you bridge from a student to a professional. Constant reflection on what you have learned from the process—what could you have done better, what was the impact of your action—is a critical part of becoming a professional in a challenging health care field.

SUMMARY

[Learning about] corporate and professional ethics is fun. It can also be difficult (p. 329).[6]

Ethical decision-making models provide guidance to professionals as they face challenges within their domains. Ethical decisions are made under different circumstances, and professionals rely on a wide variety of strategies to assist them in the process. Value knowledge is essential to the formulation of sound ethical judgment; therefore value education should be integrated into the ethics education framework that permeates the entire athletic training curriculum. Values knowledge reduces confusion and improves the quality and validity of the choices that are made.[18] Additionally, a wide application of various models helps health care providers process the multiple factors that affect these critical decisions. Active learning and extensive use of these models in the clinical and didactic settings will equip the student with the necessary tools to make effective, responsible professional decisions. (See Appendix F for a summary table of selected practice-based ethical decision-making models.)

Interweaving clinical and ethical deliberation provides a strong framework for professionals considering ethical dilemmas because the two are not easily separated.[20] The best way to forge this relationship is to evaluate the ethical dimensions of clinical practice carefully and consistently. By engaging in dialogue with those who hold different values and opinions, you are forced to articulate your position and be open to input from others. This balance provides a strong framework for professional development and growth throughout your career.

Table 5-11 NURSING MODEL FOR ETHICAL DECISION MAKING

Step	Process	Checklist for Data Gathering
1	Gather relevant information and facts	• Clinical indications • Preference of the person • Quality of life • Contextual factors
2	Identify the type of the ethical problem	• Ethical distress • Ethical dilemma • Locus of authority
3	Use theories or approaches to analyze the problems	• Utilitarian • Deontology
4	Explore the practical alternatives	• List each alternative and reasons why
5	Complete the action	• Implement the solution
6	Evaluate the process and outcomes	• Continuous quality improvement • Self-reflection

From Purtilo R: *Ethical dimensions in the health professions*, ed 4, Philadelphia, 2005, Saunders.

REFERENCES

1. Agich G: The question of method in ethics consultation, *Am J Bioethics* 1:31-41, 2001.

2. Badura J: Faculty forum, *Teaching Psychol* 29:136-159, 2002.

3. Bergmann R: Ethics: concepts and practice, *Int Nurs Rev* 20:140-141, 1973.

4. Bowers M, Pipes RB: Influence of consultation on ethical decision making: an analogue study, *Ethics Behavior* 10:65-80, 2000.

5. Brody H, Miller FG: The internal morality of medicine: explications and application to managed care, *J Med Philosophy* 23:384-410, 1998.

6. Cahn S, Pastore J: Decision modeling: an objective approach to moral reasoning, *Teaching Bus Ethics* 7:329-340, 2003.

7. Callahan D, Bok S, editors: *Ethics teaching in higher education,* New York, 1980, Plenum.

8. Chabon SS, Morris JF: A consensus model for making ethical decisions in a less-than-ideal world, *The ASHA Leader* 18-19, 2004.

9. Cottone RR: A social constructivism model of ethical decision making in counseling, *J Counseling Development* 79:39-46, 2001.

10. Darr K: *Ethics in health services management,* Baltimore, Md., 1997, Health Professions Press.

11. Davis M: Developing and using cases to teach practical ethics, *Teaching Philosophy* 20:353-385, 1997.

12. Dewey J: *Democracy and education,* New York, 1916, Macmillan.

13. Dieruf K: Ethical decision making by students in physical and occupational therapy, *J Allied Health* 33:24-30, 2004.

14. Durand G: Introduction to bioethics. In Steinkamp N, Gordijn B: Ethical case deliberation on the ward. A comparison of four methods, *Med Health Care Philosophy* 6:242, 2003.

15. Freeman RE: Business ethics at the millennium, *Bus Ethics Quarterly* 10:169-180, 2000.

16. Garcia JG, Cartwright B, Winston SM, et al: A transcultural integrative model for ethical decision making in counseling, *J Counseling Development* 81:268-278, 2003.

17. Geddes EL, Finch E, Graham K: Ethical choices: a moral and legal template for health care practice, *Physiother Can* 57:113-122, 2002.

18. Grundstein-Amado R: Ethical decision-making processes used by health care providers, *J Adv Nurs* 18:1701-1709, 1993.

19. Han SS, Ahn SH: An analysis and evaluation of student nurses' participation in ethical decision making, *Nurs Ethics* 7:113-123, 2000.

20. Healy TC: Ethical decision making: pressure and uncertainty as complicating factors, *Health Social Work* 28:293-302, 2003.

21. Kessels J: Socratic method. In Steinkamp N, Gordijn B: Ethical case deliberation on the ward. A comparison of four methods, *Med Health Care Philosophy* 6:244, 2003.

22. Mattison M: Ethical decision making: the person in the process, *Social Work* 45:201-212, 2000.

23. Purtilo R: *Ethical dimensions in the health professions,* ed 4, Philadelphia, 2005, Saunders.

24. Rakich J, Longest B, Darr K: *Managing health services organizations and systems,* Baltimore, Md., 1993, Health Professions Press.

25. Steinkamp N, Gordijn B: Ethical case deliberation on the ward. A comparison of four methods, *Med Health Care Philosophy* 6:235-246, 2003.

26. Viafora C: Toward a methodology for the ethical analysis of clinical practice, *Med Health Care Philosophy* 2:283-297, 1999.

27. Wilson Ross J: Case consultation: the committee or the clinical consultant, *HEC Forum* 2:255-264, 1990.

CHAPTER 6

Learning Activities: Linking Content to Practice

Athletic trainers face complex and frequent ethical dilemmas in the fast-paced medical field. While progressing through this academic program, you may have difficulty looking beyond the rules, regulations, and laws that govern practice to the moral choices that guide ethical decisions. Although systematic approaches through various decision-making models provide a strong framework for young professionals, the application of ethical concepts to real-life situations promotes critical thinking and analysis of the multiple components associated with ethical dilemmas.

The activities in this chapter are designed to facilitate the process of ethical discovery through real-life applications to exemplify the cognitive content addressed in earlier chapters. Each activity includes three factors: (1) the key learning objectives, which identify the focus of the activity; (2) the description, which details the activity and serves as instruction for completion; and (3) assessment ideas regarding how the completed activity is evaluated (to provide the criteria for assessment and/or serve as a self-check or assessment tool). Assessment is often broad, and the activities typically look at the process rather that elicit one specific answer. As such, be candid and reflective in your work.

Although each learning activity is designed according to selective content, these strategies are versatile and can be applied to different situations. They are designed to help the student process information from multiple perspectives. These activities can be used as study guides and professional development activities even if they are not assigned for this course.

ACTIVITIES FOR APPLICATION: LINKING CONTENT TO PRACTICE

LEARNING ACTIVITY 1: ETHICAL LEGAL GRID

Objectives

1. To encourage insight beyond rules and norms in ethical decision making
2. To acknowledge the complexity of ethical situations facing athletic trainers
3. To integrate morality (the sense of right and wrong) and law from personal, professional, and societal perspectives

Description

Use the moral-legal template shown in Figure 6-1, which depicts dichotomous components of morality and legality with the individual centered among group values and norms and society values and norms.[2] This static and symmetric depiction of the model reflects balance between the inner square (individual moral stance), middle square (moral and legal stance of groups to which the individual belongs), and the outer square (moral and legal stance of society as a whole).

After a brief explanation of the roles of morality and legality in the decision-making process, analyze a case and shift the individual toward the appropriate quadrant based on his or her perception of the proposed dilemma. The shift in the individual reflects the emphasis placed on the case by the student or group of students. The goal is to change the template dynamically based on scenarios provided for consideration.

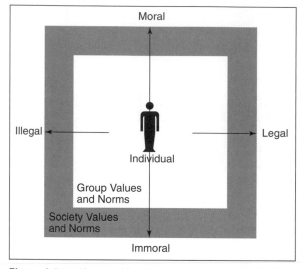

Figure 6-1 ■ The moral-legal template. *(From Geddes EL, Finch E, Graham K: Ethical choices: a moral and legal template for health care practice,* Physiother Can *57:113-122, 2002.)*

A head athletic trainer is asked to join a search committee to hire a new assistant athletic trainer. Many candidates have applied for this position, but the university will allow only three interviews. The search committee (composed of the head athletic trainer, the assistant athletic director, various coaches, and a student-athlete) reviews the files and selects the top three candidates to interview. After receiving the selections from the committee, the athletic director notices that the three candidates are all white and male. The athletic director instructs the committee to review the files again carefully to ensure that a diverse pool is provided for interviews. The head athletic trainer then takes this information to the committee members, who are offended but agree to allow the head athletic trainer to replace one of the candidates with a lesser qualified minority candidate to satisfy the request of the athletic director.

Discussion

Discuss the outcome of this case and shift the individual in the moral-legal template to reflect the discussion. Be prepared to discuss why you chose to shift the model in the way that you did. Also be prepared to discuss alternative ways in which the case could have evolved and how that would have affected the moral-legal template.

Assessment

Assessment of this activity can be multidimensional. If group discussion is used, the group discussion rubric is a good option for providing feedback. Furthermore, if this activity is used as an individual assignment, either in class or as a take-home activity, objective criteria can be used to assess the level of understanding of the morality and legality of each situation. This activity can also be used as a reflective class assignment after any case discussion.

Tip: This case can also be used as part of a clinical assignment by creating a summary of a specific case and applying the template to the case with a rationale for each dimension: individual, group, and society.

LEARNING ACTIVITY 2: DEFINING FEATURES MATRIX

Objectives

1. To help develop an understanding of the various components of ethical decision-making models or learning strategies
2. To encourage critical thinking about how each of the models and strategies is designed
3. To reinforce the key elements of each model to promote student learning

Description

Use the matrix provided (or create your own) to identify features of the models you have learned about in class.[1] Create a summary sheet by noting a defining feature by a plus sign and a feature not prevalent in the model by a minus sign. This assignment can be used as a self-assessment tool, an individual assignment, or a group activity. Several examples are provided for review; however, this template can be used for any model or learning strategy to help process the elements with key concepts.

COMPARISON OF SELECTED DECISION-MAKING MODELS

Feature	Hermeneutic Decision Making	Social Constructivist Decision Making
Emphasizes first impressions and intuition		
Interactive rather than individual perspective		
Seeks expert opinions as consultants		
Focuses on interpretation		
Relies on negotiation, arbitration, and consensus		
Emphasizes the larger context of all situations		
Rooted in philosophical theory		
Collective morality is a central consideration		
Involves dialogue and debate relative to the best solution		
Appropriate model for consensus decision making		

COMPARISON OF SELECTED LEARNING STRATEGIES

Feature	Case Analysis	Role Playing
Encourages active participation by all students		
Allows students to evaluate multiple options for any dilemma		
Encourages dialogue		
Is based on facts		
Can be linked to real-life scenarios		
Is more scientific		
Can be continued as an out-of-class activity		
Helps students clarify personal and professional values		

Assessment

Assessment will likely involve quantifying the number of correct responses identified as features under each model. Additionally, these matrixes can be shared with the group for open discussion, which can turn into a debatelike situation. Evaluation tools that emphasize participation and engagement are most appropriate.

This activity can also involve creating a matrix with plus and minus signs that can be assessed for accuracy and serve as a study tool.

Tip: Create these matrixes and share them with classmates to serve as a study guide. Encourage your instructor to select some of the student-created matrixes on a written examination.

LEARNING ACTIVITY 3: EMPTY OUTLINES

Objectives

1. To provide a template for gaining cognitive understanding of key concepts and principles related to ethics.
2. To encourage active engagement in cognitive material presented to facilitate comprehension.
3. To challenge critical thinking about the connections between selected content to minimize rote memorization.

Description

Use the empty outline to guide note taking.[1] This outline provides various levels of guidance to use in class or as a study guide.

Ethical Decision-Making Models

A. Clinical Pragmatism Model
  1. Assessment of the Situation
    a. Starting Points
      i.
      ii.
      iii.
      iv.
    b. Outcome
      i.
  2. Moral Diagnosis
    a. Starting Points
      i.
      ii.
      iii.
      iv.
      v.
    b. Outcome
      i.
  3. Goal Setting, Decision Making, and Implementation
    a. Starting Points
      i.
      ii.
      iii.
      iv.
    b. Outcome
      i.
  4. Evaluation
    a. Starting Points
      i.
      ii.
    b. Outcome
      i.
B. Application

Create a real-life scenario that illustrates the clinical pragmatism model of ethical decision making used in clinical assignments. Did it follow these steps exactly? How can this model be modified to better fit your process of decision making?

Assessment

If used as a before-class assignment, this activity can be graded by simply checking correct responses and providing feedback. It can also be used as a study guide if the instructor provides a jumbled list of headings and subheadings and has students organize them in a sequential order or by providing main headings and having students fill in subheadings. Additionally, creating your own outline or collaborating to create the outline reinforces social relationships and group dynamics. Lastly, critiquing completed outlines created by peers reinforces the content and encourages students to look critically at the content. An appropriate rubric that emphasizes group work or peer evaluation is essential.

LEARNING ACTIVITY 4: MEMORY MATRIX

Objectives

1. To promote recall of critically related items in a particular unit
2. To relate given information to information that must be recalled
3. To identify key elements in a unit

Description

By using the following matrix, complete the cells under the appropriate categories by recalling information from previous knowledge.[1]

MEMORY MATRIX FOR REFLECTIVE ACTIVITIES IN ETHICS EDUCATION		
Type of Reflection	Goal of the Reflective Activity	Applications to Clinical Practice
Content reflection		
Process reflection		
Reflection in action		
Reflection on action		
Reflection for action		

Assessment

This activity can be an individual, class, or take-home assignment. Evaluation is essential, considering the appropriate selection of material presented. Because this activity promotes recall, accuracy in responses is critical. This activity can become a peer-designed learning tool by creating matrixes and having a peer complete them. Evaluating each other's work is helpful to reinforce recall from the two perspectives of design and evaluation.

LEARNING ACTIVITY 5: PRO/CON LIST

Objectives

1. To differentiate potential advantages and disadvantages of selected actions
2. To examine the multiple influences that affect an ethical decision
3. To formulate a decision based on critical thinking

Description

After a situation is presented, create a pro/con list to analyze the advantages and disadvantages of the decision being made.[1] Often completed on a sheet of paper folded in half with pros on one side and cons listed on the other, this is a visual way to evaluate potential choices before the final decision is made. Create a pro/con list based on the following scenario.

CASE SCENARIO

An athletic training student is asked to cover a field hockey game so that the certified athletic trainer does not have to attend this contest on a Sunday. The team physician will be in attendance at the game, and the athletic training student is instructed to call the certified athletic trainer if any problems arise.

The athletic training student is contemplating reporting this situation to the athletic training education program director because the policy and procedures manual states that an athletic training student should not perform clinical duties in the absence of the approved clinical instructor.

Pros	Cons

After completing a pro/con list, discuss as a larger group some of the issues that were identified and how they affected the decision. This activity can lead to a debate or formal presentation with justification for selection of pros/cons on the list.

Assessment

Depending on whether the activity is performed individually or as a group, assessment should be tailored to identify the process by which you considered options. Furthermore, a debate evaluation rubric and/or group discussion rubric can provide meaningful feedback.

LEARNING ACTIVITY 6: PROBLEM RECOGNITION

Objectives

1. To connect related problems with the appropriate problem-solving strategy
2. To examine the relatedness of selected concepts
3. To practice problem-solving strategies based on applied cases

Description

Match the following problems to the appropriate problem-solving approach.[1] These problems are rooted in ethical dilemmas and encourage problem solving from multiple perspectives. Explain why you selected each approach.

Problem 1

Jeff works for a private clinic as an athletic trainer. He is certified and works on a team with a physical therapist. At a recent staff meeting, the supervisor tells all the physical therapists and athletic trainers that they must begin billing according to the codes that provide the highest reimbursement for each patient's insurance carrier. In essence, if XYZ Insurance Company reimburses ultrasound at a higher rate than electrical stimulation, then the clinician should select ultrasound over electrical stimulation in the treatment protocol. Jeff has some disagreement with this directive and wants to speak to the supervisor.

Problem 2

Suzy is a certified athletic trainer who has been consulted by a student-athlete regarding a potential problem on her team. The student-athlete suspects that several of her teammates are using ephedrine-based medications for stimulation during practice and games. She is uncertain regarding whether to tell the coach or confront the teammates because she wants everyone to like her. She is concerned about their health status.

Problem 3

Louise is a certified athletic trainer currently employed by a Division I NCAA school. She has primary responsibilities with the women's basketball team. She has disclosed to you, as her co-worker and friend, that she is looking at another position out of state that begins just before basketball season. She has not told anyone else that she is looking for another job and has stated that she will have to leave immediately to fill her new position, thereby leaving without providing 2 weeks' notice. You are confused regarding what you should do in this situation.

Problem-Solving Approaches

A. Principlism
B. Ethics of care
C. Virtue ethics

Assessment

This activity can be performed in pairs or in small groups. Use appropriate rubrics to evaluate the ability to apply the content of each of the problem-solving strategies to the cases. Further evaluation can occur based on a formal presentation of the justification of each selection relative to clarity, thoroughness, and professionalism.

LEARNING ACTIVITY 7: HOROSCOPE

Objectives

1. To assist in articulating a vision or futuristic perspective
2. To relate professionalism to personal goals
3. To examine the perspective from which you approach the profession

Description

You are charged with the task of writing your own horoscope relative to the profession of athletic training. This horoscope should be brief (maximum of three sentences) and should be done individually.

Assessment

The personal nature of this activity makes assessment difficult. The most effective assessment is to provide feedback in the form of nonjudgmental comments to acknowledge the direction of the horoscope. You can also peer review these documents and make comments or pose questions that may arise from reviewing the documents of other students.

LEARNING ACTIVITY 8: APPROXIMATE ANALOGY

Objectives

1. To identify relations between selected concepts
2. To demonstrate an understanding of key concepts
3. To illustrate the complex nature of conceptual issues

Description

Complete the following analogies.[1]

1. *Storytelling* is to *narrative ethics* as *consensus* is to _____.

2. *Moral uneasiness* is to *hermeneutics* as *moral conflict* is to _____.

3. *Moderator* is to *rational model* as *culture* is to _____.

4. *Beneficence* is to *"doing right"* as _____ is to *"doing no harm."*

Assessment

Evaluation of the appropriate responses is the most efficient way to assess the analogies. However, using this tool as a writing activity in a journal entry is another way to evaluate the level of understanding and relations present. Group discussion also serves as a valuable means of reinforcing the connections being fostered. Group discussion rubrics are applicable here.

REFERENCES

1. Angelo TA, Cross KP: *Classroom assessment techniques: a handbook for college teachers,* San Francisco, 1993, Jossey-Bass.

2. Geddes EL, Finch E, Graham K: Ethical choices: a moral and legal template for health care practice, *Physiother Can* 57:113-122, 2002.

Level II: Professional Enculturation

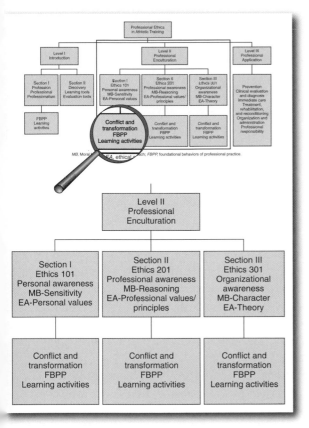

In order to gain a full appreciation of ethical behavior and the complexity of ethical inquiry in athletic training, Level II is called *Professional Enculturation*, which is the process of transitioning from a novice to a professional by learning and internalizing norms, values, beliefs, and corresponding behavior in a profession such as athletic training. It is divided into three sections (Sections I, II, III) that parallel your maturation beginning with entrance into the Athletic Training Education Program (ATEP) and ending with employment in an organization. Section I corresponds to the new student's commencement in the ATEP. At this stage in the academic program, clinical experiences are well-supervised. The newly admitted pre-professional is dependent on the faculty and clinical instructors to guide him or her through a variety of learning experiences. In fact, faculty and clinical instructors direct the new student's behavior by outlining rules and regulations in ATEP policies and procedures manual and modeling appropriate professional behaviors. This section encourages introspection and introduces the pre-professional to moral sensitivity, the first step of moral behavior. Also, Section I promotes active participation by encouraging you to identify and examine your personal values that shape your ethical norms, attitudes, and beliefs and influence your behaviors. Finally, this section will prompt you to think critically about *foundational behaviors of professional practice* and circumst-ances using reflective paradigms to resolve conflict and formulate acceptable judgments relative to right conduct.

Section II builds upon Section I and mirrors the student's second year in the ATEP. The student examines his or her professional identity, the *professional therapeutic relationship,* and the second step of moral behavior, called *moral reasoning.* Furthermore, universal health care principles are considered as well. During this stage of matriculation in the ATEP, the student becomes semi-autonomous. In other words, the student has a mix of dependent (directly supervised) and independent (first aide) learning opportunities. Active learning strategies encourage the student to process professional conflict and ethical inquiry by considering a variety of approaches: professional values, Code of Ethics, and health care principles. Lastly, the promising student learns the importance of reflection that serves to facilitate understand and guide *foundational behaviors of professional practice.*

Section II prompts you to examine the athletic training profession from the perspective of the *professional therapeutic relationship,* in other words, to see yourself in relation to a patient/athlete in the athletic training practice setting. Not only is it important to *get in touch* with yourself as a person, it is equally important to *get in touch* with yourself as a professional. Section I stressed the importance of self-awareness. Similarly, Section II stresses the importance of professional-awareness, specifically in the establishment of a healthy *professional therapeutic relationship.* Thus, to facilitate insight and professional-awareness, you will be introduced to inherent attributes of the certified athletic trainer that are foundational to the professional identity. Furthermore, ancillary understandings relative to trust, which underpins the *professional therapeutic relationship,* will be examined.

Enculturation is a transitional process that is advanced by learning and internalization. Furthermore, it encourages the emergence of the athletic training professional identity. Early interactions with athletic training faculty, clinical staff, and patient/athlete in the classroom and clinical setting facilitate professional enculturation. As you develop into a competent professional, you will continue to cultivate the *professional therapeutic relationship,* as well as other appropriate interpersonal relationships with health care professionals and patient/athletes. You will develop these relationships using an ethical approach, which is integrated in the *foundational behaviors of professional practice.*

In the backdrop of the professional identity awareness, insights into ethical standards of professional practice will be examined through the perspectives of professional values, moral reasoning, and the principled approach to ethical challenges. Remember from Section I that moral reasoning builds on moral sensitivity in the three-step process of moral behavior development. The appreciation of moral reasoning and the principled approach to ethical challenges guide how certified athletic trainers *ought to treat the patient/athlete* in the *professional therapeutic relationship.*

Finally, Section III builds upon Sections I and II and emulates your entrance into the real world as a young professional. Autonomy describes the professional's practice. The final step of moral behavior—moral character—is introduced. It is here that you learn about organizational climate and culture and potential challenges that threaten your professional integrity. You will be prompted to examine organizational conflict and ethical inquiry by means of philosophical theories and other approaches (e.g., professional values, Code of Ethics, health care principles) previously learned in Sections I and II, which guide *foundational behaviors of professional practice.*

Thus collectively, Sections I, II, and III are segments that sequentially build upon each other in an ethical journey that presents considerations and insights as you strive to do good and do right on your journey toward becoming a professional in athletic training. Professional values, health care principles, and moral theory are ethical approaches that will serve as a professional compass and encourage appropriate *foundational behaviors of professional practice.* As an important postscript, it is imperative to be mindful that although you, the professional-in-training, will not be involved with complex ethical health care issues, such as right-to-life and/or the morning after pill, you will engage in subtle ethical issues that arise on a day-to-day basis. The ethical issues that you may face encompass interactions with the patient/athlete or other professionals involving team approach to practice, legal practice, advancing knowledge, cultural competence, and professionalism *(the foundational behaviors of professional practice).*

As you journey along the emerging professional pathway in Sections I, II, and III, you must be ever vigilant to the ideals of the professional practice from which the real standards of practice emerge into a singular professional identity.

CASE NARRATIVE

You are introduced into Level II, professional enculturation, through the eyes of Maria, a prospective athletic training student.

Maria spent the better part of her second semester in college going through the application process for the university's athletic training program. She was required to submit an application form that included several essays, her academic transcripts from high school and college, and three letters of recommendation—one of which had to be written by one of the health care professionals with whom she interned during her *Introduction to Health Professions* course. The most nerve-racking part of the process was the interview. Maria had to be interviewed by both the athletic training program director and the university's head athletic trainer. Competition for admission was stiff with only about 25% of qualified applicants earning a spot in the program. About a month after the interviews, Maria received the letter informing her that she would be admitted to the program effective with the beginning of her sophomore year. Both Maria and her parents were thrilled by the news.

Maria received a copy of the athletic training student manual in the mail during the summer before she began the program. The manual was filled with policies and procedures related to the operation of the university's athletic training room, rules for student behavior, and information on required courses and clinical experiences. A letter from the program director that accompanied the manual informed Maria that she would be tested on its contents during the first ten days of the semester. Maria spent the rest of the summer reading and re-reading the manual so that she would know it well once school began in the fall. This proved to be

Continued

(Case narrative continued)

a challenge since Maria had to hold down two jobs to earn money for the portion of her tuition not covered by her scholarship. She would get up before the sun six days per week and get home after her parents and sisters had finished dinner. She would then spend an hour or so poring over her athletic training manual before falling exhausted into bed. Sundays were for family and church, though she tried to steal a couple of hours for the manual as well. She never thought summers without classes would be more difficult than the school year!

Maria reported to school 2 weeks before the beginning of the semester to take part in preseason practice and to go through the orientation program for new athletic training students. Even though she knew most of the staff and students, Maria was very nervous. She had spent the last 2 years of her life contemplating and preparing for this moment. She didn't want to screw it up! The clinical coordinator met her at the door of the athletic training room and welcomed her to the program. He handed her a binder that contained a schedule for the orientation program. Each element on the schedule was cross referenced with a number of policies and procedures from the athletic training student manual. The first item on the agenda was a tour of the facilities. Maria and the ten other new students were instructed to bring a pen and notebook and make notes as they followed Tom, a senior student, around the various on-and off-campus facilities used to support the athletic training program. One of the first stops was the office of the head athletic trainer in the university's main athletic training room. In addition to providing work space for this very busy professional, the office also contained private examination space for the team physician, a medical records room, and a locked cabinet. Tom walked over to the head athletic trainer's desk where a key hung from a hook on the wall and unlocked the cabinet. "This is where Dr. Ingram keeps all of the medicine he needs to treat athletes when he comes to the athletic training room for his clinics," said

Tom. "We're not allowed to go into this cabinet without permission," Tom said as he reset the lock and placed the key back on its hook.

After dinner the clinical coordinator met with all the new students. "We're going to go through an exercise designed to get you thinking about the professional behaviors that are most important to you. This is important for a couple of reasons. First, I want you to know about the behaviors that most people agree serve as the foundation for professional practice in athletic training. Second, and perhaps more important, I want you to think about these behaviors enough so that when two or more of them conflict with each other—which they will— you'll be able to make a good decision about the course of action. The clinical coordinator then passed out a sheet that contained the *Foundational Behaviors of Professional Practice* as contained in the fourth edition of the NATA's *Athletic Training Educational Competencies*:

- Primacy of the patient
- Teamed approach to practice
- Legal practice
- Ethical practice
- Advancing knowledge
- Cultural competence
- Professionalism

The clinical coordinator asked students to take turns explaining to the group what they thought each of these concepts meant. Then Maria was paired with another student and instructed to develop short case studies that emphasized each of the behaviors. After sharing all of the cases, the students were asked to identify their most important behavior. Maria thought for awhile, raised her hand, and announced "I think all of these behaviors are very important. It's really hard to have to pick just one. But I guess if I could only act on one of these for some reason I would choose 'legal practice.' I mean, if you're doing something as an athletic trainer that's not legal, then nothing else would really matter. I

(Case narrative continued)

could be outstanding in all the other areas, but if I'm guilty of doing something that breaks the law, then nobody will give me credit for the other things I do well."

Maria got back to her dorm at the end of her first day in the athletic training program excited but very tired. It had been a long day. As she lay in bed, she thought about everything she had seen and heard that day. She felt good about the fact that everyone she had met seemed nice, and she thought she'd be able to handle the responsibilities she'd have. Only one thing bothered her—the medication locker in the head athletic trainer's office. She thought she remembered a reference in her athletic training student manual that led her to a website that talked about the laws governing the storage and dispensing of prescription medicines. If what she remembered from that website was correct, the way that the head athletic trainer kept prescription medicines in the athletic training room might not be legal. She made a mental note to ask one of the older students about it the next day as she drifted off to sleep.

CHAPTER 7

Introduction to Ethics

ETHICAL CONCEPTS

Administrative law

Constitutional law

Descriptive ethics

Ethics

Judicial law

Morality

Metaethics

Nonnormative ethics

Normative ethics

Professional enculturation

Professional ethics

Statutory law

LEARNING OBJECTIVES

After reading this chapter, the student should be able to do the following:

1. Define ethics.

2. Define morality and describe how it plays out in everyday life.

3. List important Greek philosophers who studied and wrote about ethics.

4. List important Western philosophers who studied and wrote about ethics.

5. Describe nonnormative and normative ethics.

6. Define professional ethics.

7. Describe law and the types that play out in everyday life.

8. Describe real or fictitious stories that contain (1) both an ethical action and an illegal action, (2) both an unethical action and a legal action, and (3) both an unethical action and an illegal action.

9. List the foundational behaviors of professional practice.

Unfortunately, professionals, precisely as professionals, are confronted with serious conflicts of duty and conflicts between duty and self-interest. The stakes are high for both the integrity of the professional and the welfare of others (p. 13).

JOHN KULTGEN[7]

Changes in technology, managed care, and reimbursement expose athletic trainers to the perils of the professional world by placing increased moral and legal responsibilities on them in patient/athlete care decisions. Maintaining balance on the moral, high road of professional life requires an understanding of ethics.

NORMATIVE AND NONNORMATIVE ETHICS

"Ethics is a systematic reflection on morality (p. 15)."[11]

Ethics, a branch of philosophy, is a systematic inquiry and judgment about the moral dimensions of human conduct or morality. *Morality* refers to values, principles, and judgments made in relation to right or wrong conduct and based on cultural, religious, and philosophical concepts.[11]

The Greeks, and later the Romans, were the first to study ethics seriously and analytically. Well-recognized ethicists from early societies include Socrates, Aristotle, and Plato. Modern Western philosophy began with the work of eminent ethicists such as Thomas Hobbes, David Hume, and Immanuel Kant. Their work was followed up by the utilitarians Jeremy Bentham and John Stuart Mill.

Ethics can be divided into two broad categories: nonnormative and normative (Box 7-1). Nonnormative ethics is composed of two major subcategories: descriptive ethics and metaethics. Descriptive ethics describes what people actually do and how people think or have thought about morality. As Box 7-1 outlines, descriptive ethics is essentially a neutral description about what "is" as it relates to values and moral conduct in a society. It compares morality between and among cultures without bias. Metaethics seeks to understand the meaning of moral language, such as good and bad. Thus this approach studies the nature of the ethical statement.

Normative ethics examines issues and behaviors relating good and bad and right and wrong. It identi-

fies principles and appraises how people *ought* to act on them. Also, normative ethics studies how people make moral choices and how rules apply to the individual. Take the Golden Rule, for example: "Do unto others as you would have them do unto you." Thus this approach is about standards of morality or moral codes and rules.[4,15]

To consider how these two distinct ethical categories may work in the athletic training setting, a simple case scenario helps emphasize the differences in ethical examination.

Box 7-1

ETHICAL CLASSIFICATIONS

Nonnormative Ethics

Descriptive ethics: descriptive (what *is* done)

- What do people claim to be their moral norms?
- How do people behave when dealing with moral issues?

Metaethics: analytical (the nature of moral rightness)

- What does normative ethics mean by *good* and *right*?
- Can moral judgments be proved? How?

Normative Ethics

Action guided or prescriptive (what *ought to be* done)

- What is one's moral obligation?
  - What is right?
  - What is wrong?
- What is the moral value?
  - What is good?
  - What is evil?

CASE SCENARIO

XYZ Athletic Training Education Program (ATEP) requires the athletic training student to record accurately the clinical hours accrued at the end of the week. The policies and procedures manual of XYZ ATEP states that the student should attain a minimum of 12 clinical hours per week. Ann accrued only 10 hours but recorded 12 hours.

How would this brief case be examined by non-normative ethics (descriptive and metaethics) and normative ethics?

A descriptive ethical style might observe that athletic training students at XYZ ATEP typically record clinical hours accurately and honestly. A metaethical approach would be interested in what is meant by "right," and how does a "right" behavior compare to a "wrong" behavior when recording clinical hours. On the other hand, a normative ethical response would be concerned with reasons of "right and wrong," and how "right or wrong" behavior relates to the XYZ ATEP policies and procedures manual or the National Athletic Trainers' Association (NATA) Code of Ethics.

Another example relative to the distinction of normative ethics and nonnormative ethics is considered in the following scenario.

CASE SCENARIO

XYZ university just received a large shipment of 40 ankle braces for the men's basketball team at no cost from their sponsoring corporation, Nike. The head athletic trainer asked Tony, an athletic training student, to stock the braces in the storage room. Tony was amazed by the number of ankle braces, given that the men's basketball team had only 11 active players. In fact, he did not think they would miss a package of braces. So he placed a package of braces in his backpack and zipped it up. Later that evening, Tony was playing intramural basketball with other athletic training students. Lenny noticed Tony's new ankle braces and said, "Hey, Tony, those are nice braces; where did you get them?" Tony said, "Don't say anything, but I got them out of the athletic training storage room." Lenny chuckled and said, "Don't worry, dude, I'm cool; I'm not going to snitch."

How would this case be examined by nonnormative ethics (descriptive and metaethics) and normative ethics? A descriptive ethical style might note that, relative to Tony's actions, athletic training students at XYZ university typically stock supplies in the storage room,

and it is understood that no one takes anything from the athletic training room. Furthermore, this ethical style might depict Lenny's behavior by expressing that all students at XYZ university are expected to report misconduct. The second nonnormative approach, metaethics, would be interested in what is meant by "right" and how a "right" versus a "wrong" behavior expresses itself while stocking equipment in the storage room. Additionally, what is meant by "right," and how does a "right" compare to a "wrong" behavior appear relative to reporting misconduct? In comparison, a normative ethical response would be concerned with reasons of right and wrong—how "right and wrong" behavior relates to stocking the storage room, and how "right and wrong" behavior relates to reporting misconduct at XYZ university on examination of all policies and procedures manual (university and athletic training) or the NATA Code of Ethics.

A final example of how normative and nonnormative ethics are viewed is a case involving a head athletic trainer who chooses to buy a particular sports drink for his athletic teams from a vendor in exchange for a golf bag and a set of clubs.

How would this case be examined by nonnormative ethics (descriptive and metaethics) and normative ethics? A descriptive ethical style might observe that the giving or receiving of gifts, other than those of nominal value, to or from any person doing business with the university typically is prohibited. Metaethics focuses on what is meant by "right" and how a "right" compared to a "wrong" behavior expresses itself while purchasing sports drinks for the athletic teams. Normative ethics would ask how "right and wrong" behavior relates to purchasing sports drinks, and how "right and wrong" behavior relates to the policies and procedures manual (university and athletic training) or the NATA Code of Ethics.

Professional Ethics

Live in such a way that you would not be ashamed to sell your parrot to the town gossip.
—WILL ROGERS

When morality is viewed through a philosophical lens, the notion of ethics emerges. Taking that concept one step further, when morality is viewed though a professional lens, the notion of *professional, applied,* or *practical* ethics surfaces. Thus when a professional group draws on ethical standards to examine specific professional actions, professional, applied, or practical ethics are put to use.[4] The importance of morality in health care professions was underscored by the Hastings Center Report of the Commissions on the Teaching of Bioethics, which reported that future health care professionals need to receive preparation in ethics because of the increased moral and legal liability.[2]

Originally, professional ethics got its start from delving into controversial moral issues in the field of medicine such as euthanasia, abortion, and animal rights. For an issue to be thought of as a professional ethical issue, two aspects need to be apparent: (1) it must be so controversial that a critical mass for and against the issue is evident, and (2) it must be a distinctly moral issue, one in which the focus is on universal obligatory practices. The duty to do no harm is not restricted to one professional group. Today professional ethics has been divided into a broad variety of fields, such as medical/health care ethics and business ethics, which serves to address unique moral issues of a particular profession.[3,4,9]

Thus professional ethics aims to develop or evaluate moral standards in a well-defined group. Important philosophical and theological works provide insights and cognitive frameworks with which to explore the morality of real-world professional circumstances. Because of unique health care roles and relationships, universal principles have specific rules that serve to guide the moral conduct of specific professional groups.[9] Take, for example, the universal principle of respect of autonomy, self-determination. Specific health care rules, such as informed consent and confidentiality, pertain to this universal principle and serve to direct the actions of the health care professional.[1,14] Relative to athletic training, professional ethics, a component of normative ethics, serves to guide the conduct of athletic trainers by means of the NATA Code of Ethics and the Board of Certification Standards of Professional Practice.

Ethics and Law

Laws are rules and regulations by which a society is governed; failure to abide by laws leads to legal consequences and sanctions.

Box 7-2
TYPES OF LAW
Constitutional Statutory Administrative Judicial

Several types of laws are listed in Box 7-2. Constitutional law contains the essential principles of a nation or society (e.g., the Bill of Rights). Statutory law is typically created by elected officers of the legislative branch of government and includes civil law (contract law) and criminal law (penal law). Administrative law refers to the authority of administrative agencies to regulate practice. For example, state boards regulate the practice of athletic training. Finally, judicial law is decisional in nature and is represented by courts (trial, appellate, supreme) that interpret and wrangle over legal issues.[5,6,16]

The practice of athletic training is not perfect; in fact, the practice can fall into one of four quadrants: legal and ethical, legal and unethical, illegal and ethical, and illegal and unethical. Figure 7-1 illustrates this concept.[12,13]

Certified athletic trainers should strive to keep their practice within legal and ethical boundaries. Occasionally, ethics and law conflict. Law is standardized, bureaucratic, and impersonal, whereas ethics is humanistic, personal, and dependent on conscience.

Failure to abide by the law may result in a felony (a serious crime) or a misdemeanor (a lesser crime). Being professionally unethical is a judgment made by a group of peers; if a professional's actions are deemed unethical, sanctions will apply. Box 7-3 outlines sanctions that can apply to an unethical NATA member.

In the examination of the "rightness" of a particular act, ethics is not precise and, in fact, encourages serious reflection through a number of moral lenses before arriving at a moral decision and/or action. Law, on the other hand, is fairly straightforward; a judgment relative to a legal or illegal act is rendered on the basis of interpretation of the law.

Consider the following case scenario.

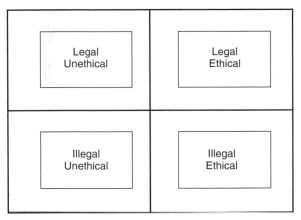

Legal Unethical	Legal Ethical
Illegal Unethical	Illegal Ethical

Figure 7-1 ■ Actions relative to professional practice may be described in one of four quadrants.

Box 7-3

NATA MEMBERSHIP SANCTIONS FOR UNETHICAL CONDUCT

Denial of membership eligibility
Cancellation of membership
Nonrenewal and suspension of membership
Public censure
Private reprimand

CASE SCENARIO

Speeding Through a School Zone
The characters: Kathy, an experienced high school certified athletic trainer, and Randy, a high school baseball pitcher.

The Spartan High School baseball team practices 4 miles off school grounds in Mr. Dudson's farm field. During one practice, Randy, Spartan High School's best pitcher, was hit on the temple by a high-velocity line drive. Randy immediately fell unconscious to the ground. Kathy, the school's certified athletic trainer, immediately went onto the field. She pulled her cell phone off her belt to make a phone call to the hospital. Much to her dismay, the batteries were dead and no one else had a cell phone at the practice field. Kathy stabilized Randy's head and neck and asked the coach and players to help transport the athlete to her sport utility vehicle. After stabilizing the athlete in the vehicle, Kathy drove to the hospital, which was not too far away. Given that Randy has a history of head trauma, Kathy realized that time was of the essence. Kathy drove a constant speed of 55 mph along mostly county roads. When she came to the elementary school crossing she slowed to 45 mph, although the posted speed was 25 mph. A police officer caught her on radar, and he followed Kathy with his lights on trying to encourage her to pull over. She arrived at the emergency room in 18 minutes. After the neurosurgeon evaluated Randy, he said to Kathy, "It is a good thing you got him to the hospital as quickly as you did."

Which quadrant did Kathy's actions fall into? Do any legal issues apply? What about ethical issues? What should the police officer do? What should Kathy do?

FOUNDATIONAL BEHAVIORS OF PROFESSIONAL PRACTICE AND ATHLETIC TRAINING EDUCATION

The origin of athletic training education is in competency-based education. Over time, these competencies have evolved into the fourth edition of the *NATA Edu-cational Competencies*. Many of the affective domain competencies have been folded into the foundational behaviors of professional practice, more specifically: (1) primacy of the patient, (2) teamed approach to practice, (3) legal practice, (4) ethical practice, (5) advancing knowledge, (6) cultural competence, and (7) professionalism.[8] In short, these foundational behaviors relate to principles of right conduct. The need to infuse these behaviors in all aspects (e.g., classroom, laboratory, clinic) of the athletic training education program is monumental. The first step in developing ethical professional behavior is cognitive understanding because cognitive competence informs appropriate professional behaviors. Ethics education can advance the understanding of ethical professional behavior by incorporating activities that encourage ethical discovery and decision making into the curriculum.[10]

REFERENCES

1. Beauchamp TL, Childress JF: *Principles of biomedical ethics,* New York, 2001, Oxford University Press.
2. Dieruf K: Ethical decision-making by students in physical and occupational therapy, *J Allied Health,* 33:24-31, 2004.
3. Edge RS, Groves JR: *The ethics of health care,* Albany, NY, 1994, Delmar.
4. Gabard DL, Martin MW: *Physical therapy ethics,* Philadelphia, 2003, F.A. Davis.
5. Jacobson PD: Health law 2005: an agenda, *J Law Med Ethics* 33:725-739, 2005.
6. Krause JH, Saver RS: Ethics in the practice of health law, *J Law Med Ethics* 32:766-770, 2004.
7. Kultgen JH: *Ethics and professionalism,* Philadelphia, 1988, University of Pennsylvania.
8. National Athletic Trainers' Association: *Athletic training educational competencies,* ed 4, Dallas, 2006, National Athletic Trainers' Association.
9. Peer KS, Rakich J: Ethical decision making in healthcare management, *Hospital Topics* 77:7-14, 1999.
10. Peer KS, Schlabach GA: Ethics education: the cornerstone of foundational behaviors of professional practice, *Athl Ther Today* 12:34-37, 2007.
11. Purtilo R: *Ethical dimensions in the health care setting,* ed 4, Philadelphia, 2005, Saunders.
12. Scott R: *Professional ethics: a guide for rehabilitation professionals,* St Louis, 1998, Mosby.
13. Scott R: Supporting professional development: understanding the interplay between health law and professional ethics, *J Phys Ther Educ* 14:17-20, 2000.
14. Snyder L, Leffler C: Ethics manual: ed 5, *Ann Int Med* 142:560-583, 2005.
15. Tschudin V: *Ethics in nursing,* ed 3, St Louis, 2003, Butterworth Heinemann.
16. Wacker GG: *Legal and ethical issues in nursing,* ed 4, Upper Saddle River, NJ, 2006, Prentice Hall.

CHAPTER 8

Self-Awareness and Cultivation of Personal Identity

LEARNING OBJECTIVES

After reading this chapter, the student should be able to do the following:

1. Name three well-known Greek philosophers who described insights about self-awareness, and describe those insights.

2. Describe existentialism, phenomenology, and humanism.

3. Explain the importance of self-awareness in athletic training.

Even before the new student entered the athletic training education program (ATEP), he or she has endured a long journey. First, the journey consisted of deciding which ATEP to attend. Then the new student discovered the application timelines and procedures in place to be considered as a viable applicant into the program. As part of the limited admission's process, he or she may have submitted formal transcripts, letters of recommendation, clinical observation hours, and essays. The applicant also had a physical examination, all the necessary immunizations, and obtained signed a technical standards form. The applicant may have been invited to the academic department to be interviewed by the athletic training faculty, students, and/or others on the limited admission's committee.

Just when the newly admitted athletic training student (ATS) thinks the process is over, he or she learns that liability insurance and a criminal background check are required before clinical coursework. Additionally, the new student must have cardiopulmonary resuscitation and automated external defibrillator training. Finally, the new student is given a thick ATEP policies and procedures manual that contains preprofessional expectations relating to dress, conduct, health, academics, and profession.

The new preprofessional has been swiftly ushered into the professional culture of athletic training. The student will discover the importance of personal and professional values and trustworthiness, which are conveyed in foundational behaviors of professional practice. Thus one goal of the ATEP is to develop a cultural orientation toward acceptable professional values leading to appropriate practices and behaviors that impart professional distinctiveness. In Section I of this text, the focus is on the promising student. In the following chapters, the student engages in self-discovery and gains an understanding about moral development and the first step of moral behavior—namely, moral sensitivity.

SELF-AWARENESS

The easiest thing in the world is to be you. The most difficult thing to be is what other people want you to be. Don't let them put you in that position.
—LEO BUSCAGLIA

Healthy relationships begin first and foremost with self-awareness that is initiated with introspection and honest discoveries about one's values, beliefs, prejudices, and motives. Although this type of activity can be humbling, these important understandings can assist the preprofessional when dealing with all types of relationships (e.g., faculty, peer, clinical instructor, student-athlete). To know and understand another human being means to know and understand oneself.

Values give rise to beliefs, feelings, and prejudices, which motivate behaviors. In turn, these behaviors may be conveyed in subtle or obvious ways. For example, subtle behaviors, such as passive-aggressive actions, may be revealed in animated, nonverbal mannerisms such as slamming a door. Self-centeredness and insecurity may be conveyed in animated posturing and facial expressions. Aggressive behaviors are overt, such as shouting or loud profanity. The preprofessional must be aware that his or her values shape beliefs, feelings, and prejudices and serve to motivate the corresponding behaviors.[1]

The importance of self-awareness was described as early as the fifth century BC. The notion of self-awareness has evolved over time, and contemporary philosophy views it through three major lenses: existentialism, phenomenology, and humanism.

GREEK PHILOSOPHY

An unexamined life is not worth living.
—SOCRATES

The quote above is one of the earliest acknowledgments emphasizing the importance of self-awareness. Socrates (Figure 8-1, *A*), a Greek philosopher, is thought to be the father of moral philosophy, or ethics. This great Greek philosopher, along with Plato and Aristotle, distinguished himself as a scholar of the minds contemplating the mind, the seat of self-awareness.[2]

Although Socrates left no writings, he is known through the dialogues of Plato (Figure 8-1, *B*), his most prominent student. His contribution to philosophy was that knowledge could be approached through the soul, which was the origin for the waking con-

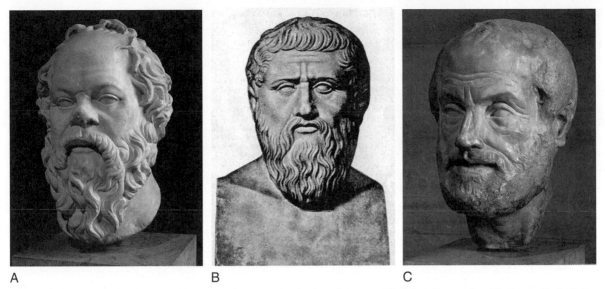

Figure 8-1 ■ Greek philosophers. **A,** Socrates; **B,** Plato; **C,** Aristotle. *(A and C, From Eric Gaba, photographer, The Louvre, Paris. **B,** From Baumeister:* Denkmäler des klassischen Altertums [Monuments of Classical Antiquity], *volume III, 1888, p. 1335.)*

sciousness as well as moral character. Socrates' conviction was that all virtues merge into one, which is the good or the knowledge of one's authentic self. He professed that holding virtue and having knowledge were indistinguishable; thus no one can act wrongly with proper knowledge of virtue. Accordingly, to know honesty means to be honest. Moreover, wrongdoing is a result of ignorance of virtue.[2,4,5]

Plato added to the concept of self-awareness by identifying its location in the mind (i.e., psyche). Motivation, will, and knowing were said to be located in the psyche, sometimes referred to as the soul. He surmised that a fixed amount of motivation and psyche was inherited.[3] However, Plato's well-recognized student, Aristotle (Figure 8-1, *C*), considered the soul as having unlimited potential for development. He also considered the soul to be divided into two spheres, a rational sphere (mind) and an irrational sphere, which give rise to self-awareness. Furthermore, Aristotle contended that morality emerged as a result of conflict between the rational and irrational spheres. Finally, he believed that truth surfaced from the rational sphere and guided behavior.[2-4]

CONTEMPORARY PHILOSOPHY

Know thyself.
—Plato

Self-awareness continued to evolve through philosophical writings in the areas of existentialism, phenomenology, and humanism. Existentialism asks, "Who am I?" and is concerned with the examination of the "authentic" and "inauthentic" self in human life. The authentic self genuinely accepts the values created for it through decisions that have been made, and human beings are willing to bear the consequences of those decisions. The inauthentic self has not considered its own values, beliefs, or behaviors and lives thoughtlessly or distractedly.[5]

Phenomenology literally means "the science of the phenomena" and describes structures the way they appear to the conscience without reference to theory, deductive reasoning, or assumptions. Edmund Husserl, the founder of phenomenology and a twentieth-century German philosopher, introduced the concept of intentionality, which supposes that thoughts, feelings, and behaviors are interconnected when directed at others or objects. In contrast to existentialism, which encourages full engagement in the human experience, he advocated detachment as a method to better understand that experience.[4,5]

Important components of existentialism and phenomenology were distilled into the basic principles of psychology and include premises such as self, self-actualization, being, becoming, individuality, and meaning. Self-examination and open and honest relationships are underscored in humanistic psychology.[4,5]

Lastly, humanism and the importance of self-awareness were brought to the health care field through the nursing profession. Humanism is a philosophical theory that affirms the dignity of all people.[1,6]

SELF-AWARENESS AND ATHLETIC TRAINING

People of the world don't look at themselves, and so they blame one another.
                                                    —RUMI

Before newly admitted preprofessionals engage in a health care relationship with a patient or athlete, clinical instructor, faculty member, or another preprofessional, they must have an authentic understanding of their own ethical standards (values and corresponding behaviors) that are expressed in overt and covert behaviors and are essential in developing healthy relationships. Personal values are shaped by cultural, ethnic, familial, environmental, and educational experiences and are important in athletic training because they guide and inform foundational behaviors of professional practice. Personal values are further discussed in Chapter 9.

Prejudices are unfounded, preformed opinions based on inadequate information and inaccurate stereotypes. They tend to have judgmental overtones. Athletic trainers must be cognizant of their prejudices and at times suspend judgment to attend to the needs of the patient or athlete. The following clinical scenario illustrates this point.

CASE SCENARIO

Cindy plays for the Chicago Lakers amateur softball team. Off the field, she is known to be a lesbian. One day after popping a ball deep into right field, she rounded first base and slid into second. Her pant leg rolled up, and she sustained a significant abrasion to her lower leg. Josh, the team's athletic trainer, grew up in a family espousing conservative values and beliefs. Josh does not agree with or support homosexual relationships. But when he noticed that Cindy was hurt, he promptly ran out to the field, quickly evaluated the situation, helped Cindy off the field, and cleaned and bandaged her abrasion. Cindy was grateful for Josh's professional assistance and was able to reenter the lineup.

Josh's actions reflect a mature, professional athletic trainer. This case scenario pointed out that although personally Josh takes issue with Cindy's homosexuality, he was able to ignore his prejudices and carry out his professional responsibilities.

Motivation, the incentive to act in a particular way, to be an athletic trainer should be examined as well. Healthy motivations in the profession of athletic training surface from the desire and enjoyment of caring for a patient-athlete. They evolve from moral values. Sometimes detrimental motivations, originating from nonmoral values, emerge from a selfish need to belong, feel important, or increase self-esteem. Wholesome motivations emerge from the intention of giving, not receiving.

SUMMARY

Clearly the concept of self-examination is not new. The realization that self-awareness crystallizes an authentic personal identity is valuable to the athletic training student. Insights into motivations, prejudices, and values yield a unique perspective. Knowledge of that perspective, and how it may or may not shape a relationship with the patient, is foundational.

REFERENCES

1. Eckroth-Bucher M: Philosophical basis and practice of self-awareness in psychiatric nursing, *J Psychosocial Nurs Mental Health Services* 30:32-40, 2001.

2. Kurtz P: *Sidney Hook: philosopher of democracy and humanism,* Buffalo, NY, 1983, Prometheus Books.

3. Stumpf SE: *Philosophy: history and problems,* New York, 1994, McGraw-Hill.

4. Tymieniecka AT: *Phenomenology and science in contemporary European thought,* New York, 1962, Farrar, Straus and Cudahy.

5. Warnock M: *Existentialism,* Oxford, UK, 1970, Oxford University Press.

6. Westphal EA: *The activity of philosophy,* Englewood Cliffs, NJ, 1969, Prentice Hall.

CHAPTER 9

Development of Moral Behavior: Step 1—Moral Sensitivity

ETHICAL CONCEPTS

Cultural competence
Cultural responsiveness
Moral behavior
Moral character
Moral motivation
Moral reasoning
Moral sensitivity
Preprofessional behavior
Values
Values clarification
Values conflict

LEARNING OBJECTIVES

After reading this chapter, the student should be able to do the following:

1. List the components of moral behavior. Describe the frameworks of moral behavior developed by Andre, Rest, and Triezenberg and Davis.
2. Explain a personal value system.
3. List the seven criteria of values clarification, and distinguish between a value and a value indicator.
4. Discuss moral motivation and its relation to values clarification.
5. Explain how cultural competence can help develop moral sensitivity.
6. Describe why awareness of one's personal value system is important regarding the issue of moral sensitivity.
7. Discuss how personal values shape foundational behaviors of professional practice.

The basis of foundational behaviors of professional practice in athletic training is ultimately distilled from ethical standards. One of the first objectives of an athletic training education program (ATEP) is to introduce the preprofessional to an awareness of moral behaviors in the professional setting. Table 9-1 identifies three frameworks of moral behavior: (1) Andre's components of moral appreciation,[1] (2) Rest's components of moral behavior,[12] and (3) Triezenberg and Davis's components of moral behavior.[16] The most notable distinction between Rest's and Triezenberg and Davis's components of moral behavior is that Triezenberg and Davis believe that moral motivation is integrated into moral behavior through the development of moral sensitivity.[16] For the preprofessional to elevate to a level of professional autonomy, he or she must move sequentially through the stages of moral behavior.

Given that knowledge has the ability to inform behavior, three important elements of moral behavior should be examined: moral sensitivity, moral reasoning, and moral character. An examination of the framework of moral behavior developed by Triezenberg and Davis[16] provides important information for the promising athletic training student. This three-step module representation of moral behavior relates adequately to athletic training and can be folded into the ATEP. As Table 9-1 illustrates, the first component is moral sensitivity, which is the ability to recognize and identify ethical issues (more specifically, how a person's actions affect others). The second component is moral reasoning and prompts a person to distinguish right from wrong and interpret, judge, and make a decision. The third component is moral character, which reflects the strength of an individual's temperament to persevere against adversity.[16]

STEP 1: MORAL SENSITIVITY

Figure 9-1 shows that moral sensitivity is the first of three steps in the overall concept of moral behavior. Moral sensitivity involves an awareness of and atten-

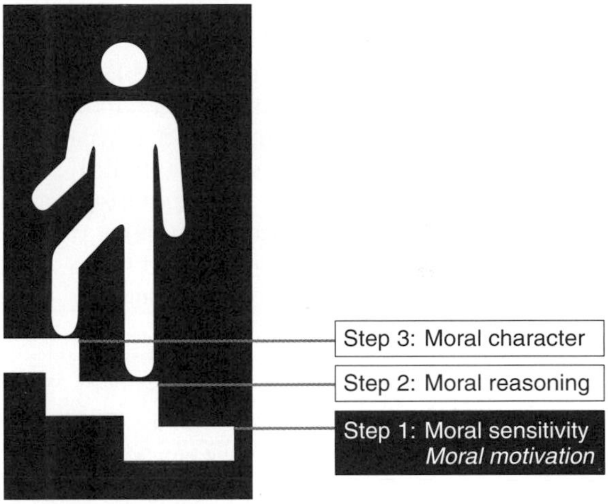

Step 3: Moral character
Step 2: Moral reasoning
Step 1: Moral sensitivity
Moral motivation

Figure 9-1 ■ Triezenberg and Davis's model of moral behavior has three steps, beginning with moral sensitivity.

Table 9-1   STAGES OF MORAL BEHAVIOR

Stage	Moral Appreciation (Andre)	Moral Behavior (Rest)	Moral Behavior (Triezenberg and Davis)
1	Helpful relationships: understanding how to help and care for others	Moral sensitivity	Moral sensitivity
2	Socialization structures: understanding how social structures cause good and bad	Moral judgment	—
3	Thinking fruitfully: moral reasoning	Moral motivation	Moral reasoning
4	Moral strength, traits, and skills to be able to act	Moral character	Moral character

Adapted from Andre J: Beyond moral reasoning: a wider view of the professional ethics course, *Teaching Philosophy* 14:359-373, 1991; Rest JR: Background: theory and research. In Rest JR, Narvaez D, editors: *Moral development in the professions: psychology and applied ethics*, Hillsdale, NJ, 1994, Lawrence Erlbaum, pp. 1-27; and Triezenberg HL, Davis CM: Beyond the code of ethics: educating physical therapists for their role as moral agents, *J Phys Ther Educ* 14:48-59, 2000.

tion to relationships.[1,12,16] Moral sensitivity requires the preprofessional to interpret a situation and judge whether a moral transgression has occurred relative to how an individual's actions may affect others. Research in moral sensitivity suggests that well-educated women seem to have an edge in demonstrating insight in recognizing ethical components.[7] This chapter focuses on moral sensitivity and how personal values, cultural diversity, and foundational behaviors of professional practice sharpen a person's awareness.

Personal Values

Try not to become a man of success, but rather a man of value.
—Einstein

Chapter 8 discussed values in relation to self-awareness. Personal values define who a person is and what he or she holds most meaningful in life. A personal value system is one of several major value systems. Other major value systems include professional and organizational value systems, which are discussed in later chapters. A personal value system includes values that were chosen after serious consideration and helps a person lead a "good" life.[10] In addi-

tion, within each major value system, values can be bundled into exclusive subsets. For example, a personal value system may have value subsets that describe spirituality, esthetics, prestige, and corporeal, pragmatic, and economic values.

Those in touch with their personal values see themselves as authentic individuals, appreciate others, and interpret the world in general with remarkable clarity and focus. Continuing with the analogy of a train from Chapter 1, values could be comparable to directional switches in a railroad track. When a switch is activated, the train takes the triggered tracks in a precise direction. Similarly, values guide an individual's behaviors and influence attitudes, motives, and beliefs. Moreover, personal values are transparent for the world to see because they are evident in written, verbal, and nonverbal communication and behaviors.[15,18]

Personal values, regardless of value subset and moral orientation, are viewpoints about what is perceived as worthy. Values are learned, arise from personal experiences, and form a basis for behavior that becomes transparent and consistent (Figure 9-2).[9,18]

Moral Motivation

In Triezenberg's and Davis's three-step model of moral behavior, moral motivation is incorporated into moral sensitivity. Motivation is the process of prioritizing moral action (behavior) when confronted with conflicting values.[7] Keeping in mind that many types of value systems exist, moral motivation requires a person to ignore other value systems and focus on the moral value system as well as prioritize one moral value above other competing values.[1,12,16] An individual may

Personal values

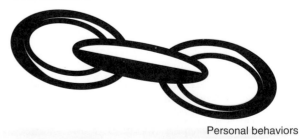

Personal behaviors

Figure 9-2 ■ Personal values inform personal behaviors.

Table 9-2 VALUES CLARIFICATION PROCESS AND SEVEN CRITERIA

Value Process Phases	Value Process Criteria
Choosing	1. Choosing freely 2. Choosing from alternatives 3. Choosing after thought consideration of the consequences of each alternative
Prizing	4. Cherishing—being happy with the choice 5. Affirming the choice to others
Acting	6. Doing something with the choice 7. Acting repeatedly in some pattern of life

Adapted from Raths LE, Harmin M, Simon SB: *Values and teaching,* Columbus, Ohio, 1978, Merrill Publishing Company.

be tempted to act in nonmoral ways because he or she may be motivated by nonmoral values (e.g., self-interest, pleasure, financial advantage, or institutional loyalty). Values clarification helps the student identify and prioritize moral values.[11]

Values Clarification

Introspection may not be easy for everyone. To assist in self-discovery, Raths et al[11] identified a three-stage process containing two or three criteria, within phases, to help a person discover his or her personal values. Table 9-2 illustrates sequential phases in value processing, which include choosing, prizing, and acting. Raths et al attest that a value must meet all seven criteria outlined in Table 9-2, which help distinguish true values from more immature needs, wants, and aspirations. Elements that almost, but not completely, satisfy all seven criteria are identified as value indicators, such as a belief or an attitude.[4] Because value processing requires thoughtful reflection, value development has both a cognitive and affective component.

Values clarification is rooted in John Dewey's work and is thought to help people integrate values into their own lives. When values become internalized, they are conveyed in foundational behaviors of professional practice. Internalized values direct consistent patterns of verbal and nonverbal professional behaviors. Raths et al[11] agree and maintain that values arise from personal experiences and are learned and integrated into *consistent patterns* of behavior.

The following case scenario presents some dilemmas and reinforces the notion of values and the influence of moral motivation.

CASE SCENARIO

The characters: Skippie, a young, inexperienced assistant athletic trainer whose ultimate value is respect; Peggy, an experienced associate athletic trainer whose ultimate value is truth and honesty; and Camden, an experienced head athletic trainer whose ultimate value is loyalty.

Skippie prides himself in being a respectful person. Skippie works with Peggy and Camden, who do not share the same philosophy regarding athletic care, which has created tension between these two individuals. Camden is frustrated that Peggy does not agree with his philosophy regarding athletic care and believes she is not loyal to him. He would like nothing more than to release Peggy from his staff. Through several experiences, Skippie has learned that if he is disrespectful to Peggy, he gets rewarded by Camden. In fact, Camden encourages Skippie to be mean spirited toward Peggy in hopes that she will become irritated by the situation and look for another job. Skippie privately obliges Camden.

Is the value of respect truly Skippie's top value? Is Skippie morally motivated? Is the value of loyalty truly Camden's ultimate value? Is Camden morally motivated?

Now consider the following case scenario.

CASE SCENARIO

The characters: Kim, a graduate assistant athletic trainer whose top professional value is care; the head athletic trainer, whose top value is promise keeping.

Kim's assistantship is at a midsize university with 17 intercollegiate sports. The athletic training staff consists of the head and assistant athletic trainer and two graduate assistants. Without a doubt, the staff is tired and exhausted as they try to provide coverage to all the teams. The university requires that graduate assistants should not work more than 20 hours a week. Kim already has put in 57 hours while covering women's soccer, and it is only Friday. Fed up with how overworked his staff is, the head athletic trainer sent Kim home before Friday's practice. Privately, the head athletic trainer hopes to send a message to the athletic department that athletic training is understaffed. Kim knew there would not be another athletic trainer to cover her sport. Kim left the athletic training room and managed to sneak on the soccer field to provide coverage. When the head athletic trainer found out that Kim went out to cover soccer practice, he was furious and suspended her for 3 weeks without pay.

This case scenario prompts several questions. Is the value of care truly Kim's top value? Is Kim morally motivated? Is the value of promise keeping truly the head athletic trainer's top value? Is the head athletic trainer morally motivated?

Consider the next case scenario.

CASE SCENARIO

The characters: Adam, a senior athletic training student whose top value is excellence; Jane, a senior athletic training student whose ultimate value is integrity.

Adam is by all appearances a promising young professional. He is consistently well groomed and attends class in a suit and tie, is prepared and respectfully attentive in class as exhibited by his copious notes, arrives punctually at his clinical site dressed in a pressed polo and khakis, and communicates respectfully to his peers, teachers, and clinical instructors. Jane is also a promising young professional. She and Adam were running for presidency of the student council. Jane won by a small margin; publicly Adam took the loss gracefully but privately revealed to a close friend that he was devastated.

The ATEP faculty asked Jane to chair a student committee to help the program get ready for continuing accreditation. The faculty emphasized that student committee members would not have clinical responsibilities for the following 2 weeks so they would have the necessary time to work on the project. Jane has always been impressed with Adam's work ethic and asked him to be a member of the student group, and Adam agreed. Jane met with the student group, divided the workload evenly, and was available to anyone who needed assistance. Jane distributed committee minutes via e-mail. Adam's committee assignment required time and attention. Adam e-mailed Jane to seek clarification of his assignment, and Jane replied promptly in an e-mail with detail. Adam was privately frustrated with his assignment because he recently learned that the football team at his clinical site was going to the state playoffs. The opportunity to work the state playoffs would give Adam the public recognition that he privately needed. He decided that he would help provide football coverage and try to put something together for his assignment. The student committee met 1 week before their assignment was due to the faculty. All committee members had their assignments completed except Adam. As Jane was adjourning the committee meeting, she asked Adam if he could have his assignment in by the next day. Adam's face turned red, deadpan, and drawn, and he blurted, "Jeez, Jane, you never asked me to do that." Jane remained calm but was privately stunned by Adam's reaction and dishonesty. Jane adjourned the meeting. Adam shoveled his papers into his backpack and marched to the door, opened it, and slammed it on his way out.

Is the value of excellence truly one of Adam's top values? Is Adam morally motivated? Is the value of integrity truly one of Jane's values? Is Jane morally motivated?

Cultural Diversity

Cultural diversity illustrates different value systems. Moral sensitivity draws attention to different value systems and encourages mindfulness when interacting with others following a different system.

History reveals diversity in athletic training. In 1950, when the profession of athletic training was established, the professional membership was entirely male. With the passage of Title IX, the Educational Amendment Act of 1972, athletic training rooms in higher education opened their doors to allow female athletes. This landmark federal legislation bans sex discrimination in education and athletics. The *Journal of Athletic Training* took note, and Holly Wilson, athletic trainer at Indiana State University wrote a column, "Not for Men Only."[5] Her first column noted the change in the athletic training culture:

> The entry of women into the field of athletic training is a long overdue necessity, for we, too, have a moral obligation to our sports programs. Although presently there are few jobs available for women athletic trainers, the need definitely exists, and it will certainly be a growing field as it becomes increasingly accepted and understood. . . . The great rise in women's competition will certainly warrant the need for trained professional athletic trainers to properly care for the athletes (p. 67).[5]

Although the professional membership was nearly an equal blend of the sexes by the year 2000, the number of ethnic and racial minorities remained significantly low. In fact, in 1998, of the nearly 15,000 certified members, 1% were black, 2% were Hispanic, 1.5% were Asian Pacific Islander, and 0.5% were American Indian. Jack Rockwell, 1977 NATA Hall of Fame inductee, commented in the winter 1968 *Journal of Athletic Training,*

> Why should an athletic trainer be differentiated by skin color? This is where understanding is needed; the black athlete should not, cannot, and must not be treated in any way differently from the white athlete. . . . As individual athletic trainers who all have pride in your work, and display the integrity and character needed to perform your tasks, I sincerely hope you will all show the greatest concern and understanding in this situation that prevails in our country today.[5]

These 1968 thoughts were well intentioned and sincere in that *every* athlete should be treated with the exceptional competence. Today, however, the need exists to provide competent treatment equally to all athletes as well as to respect, examine, and be aware of cultural differences by transitioning from a singular to a multifaceted perspective in the delivery of health care services to athletes and patients. In fact, *Healthy People 2010,* the agenda for disease prevention and health promotion in the United States, has two central points: to (1) increase quality and years of healthy life and (2) eliminate health disparities, which include gender, race and ethnicity, education and income, disability, geographic location, and sexual orientation.[17] Moral

CULTURAL COMPETENCE

Cultural competence is the willingness and ability of a system to value the importance of culture in the delivery of services to all segments of the population. It is the use of a systems perspective that values differences and is responsive to diversity at all levels of an organization: policy, governance, administrative, workforce, provider, and consumer/client. Cultural competence is developmental, community focused, and family oriented. In particular, it is the promotion of quality services to underserved racial or ethnic groups through the valuing of differences and integration of cultural attitudes, beliefs, and practices into diagnostic and treatment methods, and throughout the system to support the delivery of culturally relevant and competent care. It is also the development and continued promotion of skills and practices important in clinical practice, cross-cultural interactions, and systems practices among providers and staff to ensure that services are delivered in a culturally competent manner.

Cultural competence activities include the development of skills through training, use of self-assessment for providers and systems, and implementation of objectives to ensure that governance, administrative policies and practices, and clinical skills and practices are responsive to the culture and diversity within the populations served. It is a process of continuous quality improvement.

From *CEO services: cultural competence online*, www.culturalcompetence2.com. Accessed August 15, 2005.

GOOD TO KNOW

The fourth edition of *Athletic Training Educational Competencies* states that cultural competence is one of the foundational behaviors of professional practice threading its way through the ATEP. Cultural competency in health care refers to the awareness of the cultural differences in racial and ethnic groups and applying that knowledge to health care practices.

Many culturally determined and equally appropriate value systems exist.[13] The literature emphasizes that the first step in becoming morally sensitive and culturally competent begins with self-awareness of one's personal values and beliefs, including styles of communication and body language; in other words, one's ethical standards.[13,16] The understanding of one's cultural identity provides the consistent framework and perspective to understand, appreciate, and respect customs and traditions of diverse populations. Many excellent online resources are available for health care professionals (Box 9-2).

GOOD TO KNOW

Ethnocentrism is the belief that one's culture is the best. Human beings have a tendency to believe that everyone in every culture believes as we do, and when that does not happen others are judged on the basis of what we think is right in our culture. In fact, a culture can be viewed in many ways: religious, spiritual, historical, political, and societal. To avert ethnocentrism, consider the following:

1. Be aware of and examine your own beliefs and values.
2. Learn as much as you can about different cultures' beliefs, health care, language, customs, and values.
3. Be aware of nonverbal communications: personal space, clothing, food, and medicine.

sensitivity, the first step in moral behavior, and cultural competence, the first step toward cultural responsiveness, requires conscientiousness and attentiveness to ethical standards, such as values, beliefs, attitudes, and behaviors of oneself and others (Box 9-1). Cultural responsiveness, then, requires taking that knowledge and applying it to practice. This requires the athletic trainer to be clinically flexible by respecting and adapting to the unique and diverse patient-athlete population.

Box 9-2

A SAMPLE OF ONLINE HEALTH CARE RESOURCES RELATING TO CULTURAL HEALTH

NATA Ethnic Diversity Advisory Committee: www.edacweb.org

NATA International Committee: www.nata.org/international/index.htm

athealth.com: www.athealth.com

The Cross Cultural Health Care Program: www.xculture.org

U.S. Department of Health and Human Services, Agency for Healthcare Research and Quality: www.ahrq.gov/research/minorix.htm

Diversity RX: www.diversityrx.org/HTML/ESLANG.htm

National Institutes of Health, National Center for Complimentary and Alternative Medicine: nccam.nih.gov

Global Health Council: www.ncih.org

Foundational Behaviors of Professional Practice

Professionals acting professionally do not just "do" things, they are called to "be" something, to serve in a certain way that reflects moral consciousness and conscience.[16]

The athletic training student enters the education program with personal values motivated by moral and nonmoral beliefs. An individual's values and belief system usually are biased and emerge from the family, are learned, and are evident in consistent patterns of behavior.[11] Before entering the ATEP, students have well-developed behaviors that reflect their personal values. Because the students' behaviors have become automatic over the years, they give little thought to how they act out. Those values-based behaviors are so instilled in their repertoire that they remain in the unconscious regions of their minds.

Consciousness-raising activities are purposeful in bringing issues to the forefront and shedding light on important moral concerns. Moreover, such endeavors help the student recognize how his or her behaviors affect others and therefore serve to reinforce the notion of moral sensitivity.

CASE SCENARIO

One such example of a consciousness-raising activity includes asking male athletic trainers what behavior, if any, they found offensive about female athletic trainers. The male athletic trainers reported that they found it irritating when female athletic trainers huddled in a group and whispered and giggled. The women had no clue that this was offensive, but this consciousness-raising activity brought the behavior to the forefront, and now the female athletic trainers refrain from such activity.

Through consciousness-raising activities, students can examine and accept alternative values and the behaviors associated with them. Repetitive positive reinforcement of specific value-laden behaviors may help beginning students develop instinctive patterns of behavior reflective of the foundational behaviors of professional practice.[16]

Because newly admitted students have little professional insight regarding appropriate practice behaviors of athletic trainers, institutions develop rules and regulations to help guide new preprofessionals. The student begins to learn that the ATEP partners with many institutions that have distinctive institutional policies and procedures. Each institution and profession honors and emphasizes particular values that reflect institutional significance and the clientele whom they serve and operates to direct professional behaviors. Table 9-3 outlines general professional behaviors in the health care professions of nursing, occupational therapy, and physical therapy.

Students often operate under several policy and procedures manuals (e.g., institution, department, ATEP, intercollegiate athletics, high school). These differing manuals may not be uniform in the expectations of student conduct. When two or more organizations' policies and procedure manuals differ regarding a particular issue, the general principle of conduct is to adhere to the most conventional and explicit guidelines.

Consider the following examples relating to dress.

Table 9-3   PROFESSIONAL BEHAVIORS IN HEALTH CARE

Author	Identified Behaviors
Chickering	Developing competence Managing emotions Moving through autonomy to independence Developing mature interpersonal relationships Establishing identity Developing purpose Developing integrity
Kasar and Muscari (occupational therapy)	Dependability Professional presentation Initiative Empathy Cooperation Organization Clinical reasoning Supervisory process Verbal communication Written communication
Koenig, Johnson, Morano, and Ducette (occupational therapy)	Time management Organization Fieldwork experience Self-directed learning Reasoning and problem solving Written communication Initiative Observation skills Supervisory process Verbal communication and interpersonal skills Professional and personal boundaries Use of professional terminology
Macdonald, Cox, Bartlett, and Houghton (physical therapy)	Communication Adherence to legal and ethical codes of practice Respect Empathy and sensitive practice Best evidence-based practice Lifelong learning Client-centered practice Critical thinking Accountability
Miller, Abbott, and Bell (nursing)	Higher education Autonomy Code of ethics Continuing education and competency Communication, publication Professional organizations Community service Research involvement

Adapted from Chickering AW: *Education and identity*, San Francisco, 1993, Jossey-Bass; Kasar J, Muscari ME: A conceptual model for the development of professional behaviours in occupational therapists, *Can J Occup Ther* 67(1):42-51, 2000; Koenig K, Johnson C, Morano CK, et al: Development and validation of a professional behavior assessment, *J Allied Health* 32(2):86, 2003; MacDonald CA, Cox PD, Bartlett DJ, et al: Consensus on methods to foster physical therapy professional behaviors, *J Phys Ther Educ* 16(1):27, 2002; Miller BK, Adams D, Beck L: A behavioral inventory of professionalism in nursing, *J Prof Nurs* 9:290-295, 1993.

CASE SCENARIO

ATEP of Mid-American University
The characters: Jenny, a first-year athletic training student, and Paul, a third-year athletic training student.

As part of the orientation to the program, four policies and procedures manuals were reviewed: (1) Midwestern University, (2) the ATEP, (3) Intercollegiate Athletics, and (4) St. Mary's Downtown High School, where Jenny and Paul will engage in their first clinicals.

1) Mid-American University policies and procedures manual states the following:

- All students should dress appropriately and not attract amusing or degrading attention to themselves through their dress selection.

2) The ATEP policies and procedures manual states:

- Dress like a licensed health care professional at all times in the athletic training room and at all practices and events.
- A neat, clean, professional appearance is expected.

3) The Intercollegiate Athletics policies procedures manual states:

- Khaki pants or shorts and wind pants are acceptable at all times; shorts must be at least mid-thigh length. No jeans are allowed while working as an athletic trainer.
- Polo shirts provided by intercollegiate athletics must be worn. All shirts must be tucked into the pants.
- When attending outside events, athletic training students are encouraged to wear intercollegiate jackets, coats, sweatshirts, or hats.

4) St. Mary's Downtown High School's policies procedures manual states:

- Shirts: assigned practice or game shirts. Must be tucked in at all times.
- Shorts or pants: short length should be no shorter than 1 inch above the top of the kneecap. Color should be black or khaki.
- Shoes: white or black tennis shoes are required. Mudders are acceptable when weather conditions warrant them. Absolutely no sandals, flip-flops, or other open-toed shoes should be worn.

Can Paul wear mid-thigh shorts at Midwestern University? In the ATEP? At St. Mary's Downtown High School? At Intercollegiate Athletics?

Can Jenny wear a midriff belly-shirt at Midwestern University? In the ATEP? At St. Mary's Downtown High School? At Intercollegiate Athletics?

Given that the new athletic training student has limited insight regarding the ethical standards and values that influence attitudes, beliefs, and practices of the profession, he or she will not appreciate what constitutes appropriate foundational behaviors of professional practice. Therefore the preprofessional is inundated with rules and policies from both the ATEP and assigned clinical sites. These rules and regulations often are bound into policies and procedures manuals and help the emerging professional behave in ways that reflect the ethical standards, attitudes, values, beliefs, and practice of the profession of athletic training (Figure 9-3).

The policies and procedures manuals of the ATEP and the clinical site provide a sense of the organization's mission, values, vision, and operating rules and principles. Policies are statements that articulate the nonnegotiable standards of the program and define

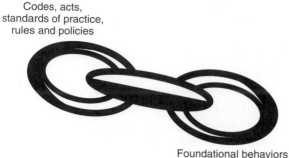

Figure 9-3 ■ Foundational behaviors of professional practice are guided by state practice acts, the NATA code of ethics, BOC standards of practice, and ATEP/institutional rules and policies.

what is acceptable to ensure program success. Procedures illustrate in detail the steps needed to be taken to show *how* a specific function is to be carried out in the program.[8]

Overall, policies and procedures manuals identify ethical, legal, and program professional obligations and are expressed as program rules. NATA's Code of Ethics describes principles and rules of acceptable behaviors for professionals. Similarly, the Board of Certification (BOC) standards of professional practice provide statements of expectations that define structures and procedures that must be in place to enhance the quality of care. Thus ATEP policy and procedure manuals should be congruent with the ethical and legal expectations of the NATA Code of Ethics and the BOC Standards of Professional Practice.

GOOD TO KNOW

NATA Code of Ethics

Principle 4.5: Whenever possible, members are encouraged to participate and support others in the conduct and communication of research and educational activities that may contribute knowledge for improved patient care, patient or student education, and the growth of the athletic training as a profession.

PERSONAL CONFLICT AND TRANSFORMATION

The metaphor of the reflective practitioner has been proposed for one who develops an appreciation for those gray areas of clinical practice where value conflicts and moral dilemmas are encountered and where the true artistry of professional practice is evident.[2]

Moral values are aspects of affective behavior associated with the way people *ought* to be treated. The interconnectedness of values and moral behavior is complex and entwined in the ethical framework of professional ethics. Moral behavior is the culmination of moral sensitivity, moral reasoning, and moral character, which fuse to yield moral conduct that is ultimately conveyed in foundational behaviors of professional practice.

Personal values conflict is good and an important stressor that assists the emerging professional to disembark at the next ascending step of the moral behavior staircase, moral reasoning (see Figure 9-1).

The ultimate consequence in the development of moral behavior is ethical fitness. It can be analogous to physical fitness in that the body needs appropriate levels of stress to acquire intended and healthy results. Thus personal values conflict strengthens ethical fitness and facilitates an automatic and effortless response to challenging situations.

The inner struggle to shed light on contradictory values and resulting behaviors defines personal conflict. A conflict or dilemma in chosen values indicates a readiness for learning and the readiness to develop ethical fitness.

Given that ethics is about morality, right versus wrong and good versus bad, what might constitute an ethical value conflict? Reflect on the following case scenarios.

CASE SCENARIO

Conflicting Values
The Character: Betsy, a first-year athletic training student

Betsy is a new student in the ATEP and was excited to get money from her grandmother to go to the university because her family could not afford it. During the second week of the semester, Betsy learned that her grandmother had died, and although Betsy had enough money to attend school for the next 4 years, she did not have enough money to buy the new car she had been longing for.

Betsy enjoyed her classes and was learning so much. In her Introduction to Athletic Training class, Betsy learned that her top moral value was accountability. She believed that accountability described her because that word suggested reliability and responsibility. All Betsy's preprofessional behaviors consistently implied her chosen value, and she was well received by both the football players and coaches. Betsy was excited when she learned that she was assigned the local high school, Barbs High School, to gain clinical athletic training experience. Betsy's approved clinical instructor emphasized accountability and talked about its importance almost every day in the athletic training room. The Barbs football team was performing quite well that fall, and of course Betsy was thrilled to be part of a successful team.

Meanwhile, an alum of the ATEP, a certified athletic trainer working for the National Football League (NFL), posted a position note about a job for an athletic training student that involved performing menial, boring chores each Sunday for $200.00 per day. Betsy learned that the Barbs team would not practice on Sundays, meaning that the NFL position would not interfere with her clinical experience. She immediately applied for the position as a way to buy the car that she wanted. Much to her relief, she got the job.

Betsy's family was planning a big family Thanksgiving in honor of her grandmother. Betsy thought long and hard about her financial situation and her Thanksgiving weekend and asked the NFL athletic trainer if she could take that Sunday off even though she knew that she would be giving up $200. The NFL athletic trainer said taking that Sunday off would not be a problem as long as she found a substitute. Sally, a friend of Betsy's, volunteered to help and earn some extra Christmas money.

The month of October was grueling for Betsy; she spent 4 to 5 hours a day (Monday through Saturday) providing coverage for the Barbs football team. She was proud of "her team" and "her players," and everyone could see how much Betsy was appreciated by the team. November was proving to be just as grueling. The team survived demanding regional and then sectional playoffs. The state playoffs were scheduled for the first Sunday in December, which meant everyone was looking forward to Thanksgiving break. It also meant that Betsy had to make another difficult decision.

Betsy deliberated for hours and made a decision whether to commit to travel downstate on the Sunday after Thanksgiving. The ATEP program director indicated that traveling downstate with the team was voluntary. Although Betsy felt tremendous anxiety, she decided that she needed to work in the NFL locker room on that Sunday.

Was this a dilemma or moral dilemma? In the ethical framework regarding the way we ought to treat others, did Betsy make the appropriate moral decision? Why or why not?

CASE SCENARIO

Conflicting Values

The characters: Lisa, a third-year student whose primary value is truth; Joey, the head athletic trainer, whose top value is loyalty; and Susie, a first-year athletic training student.

Because of her advanced cognitive and clinical skills, Lisa, a student in the ATEP, was given a large amount of responsibility by Joey, the head athletic trainer for Kaneland University. When Joey talked to the five new students and staff, he would refer to them as "my staff," "my rules," and "my athletic training room," which reinforced his position of authority. Susie, a first-year student, had always done well in school and wanted to do well in her first clinical athletic training class. After Joey's first meeting with students and staff, she felt a bit flustered and admitted to Lisa that she did not know how to please Joey with her clinical performance. Lisa, in her matter-of-fact way, said to just do what he asks.

One Friday afternoon, Joey was joking and having fun with the new athletic training students. The students finished cleaning the athletic training room and invited Joey and Lisa to the local bar for happy hour. Joey and Lisa stayed behind after the new students left to take care of some insurance matters. They planned to stop by the bar for a short time to say hi to the new students. The new students were having fun and playing a card game. Joey and Lisa sat down and had a beer or two and played cards with the new students. Joey teased Susie about her long blonde hair, and Susie showed signs of embarrassment and left the card game to go to the women's room. Joey left the card game as well to get another beer at the bar.

A few minutes later Lisa said goodbye to her younger classmates and headed to the door, where she saw Joey and Susie. Joey appeared to have drawn Susie close to him, and Susie seemed to be squirming with embarrassment. Lisa quickened her pace to the door and left.

On Monday morning Joey found out that the athletic director was asking questions about him and the incident Friday night. Joey said to Lisa, "Hey, I know you are loyal to me—tell the athletic director that nothing happened." When the athletic director questioned Lisa, she said that she observed Joey grasping Susie.

Was this a dilemma or moral dilemma? In the ethical framework regarding the way others ought to be treated, was Lisa morally motivated? Why or why not?

Personal values have a sense of fluidity. Because of their relative and interactive nature, an ordered, hierarchical value system results. When a person's behavior is guided by values, conduct becomes predictable and consistent over time. In fact, science has identified the mind-body connection (Box 9-3). Personal values tend to be relatively stable over time. The tendency to maximize specific values when faced with an ethical dilemma is expected; however, personal values may presuppose a temporal and circumstantial moment in time, meaning that an individual may defend another important value depending on the circumstances.

Moreover, regular reflection in relation to value conflict and ethical dilemmas may encourage an individual to reorder his or her personal value system on occasion.

SUMMARY

The focus of Section I of this text was on the athletic training student. Self-discovery is the first step in building healthy, moral, professional relationships with the patient-athlete. Moral sensitivity encourages examination of how behaviors affect others.

Furthermore, given that values guide behaviors, dedicated reflection of values, prejudices, and motivations facilitates an understanding about behavior and why human beings do the things they do. Cultural

Box 9-3

THE MIND-BODY CONNECTION

The mind and body are connected. The reticular activating system (RAS) is a group of cells near the top of the brainstem. The RAS processes sensory information and compares data. For example, it examines an incoming stimulus with accepted values, positive and negative (threats) thoughts, and beliefs stored in memory.

The results of RAS processing and comparison are communicated to the amygdala near the mid-brain. It is part of the limbic system and plays a role in intense positive or negative emotions, such as anger, fear, and joy. The amygdala produces neurochemicals that cause emotions consistent with the nature of and proportional to the match between environment and values. The neurochemicals initiate the chemical processes needed for the action (behavior) to be taken. If the emotions produced are strong enough, the perceived information is blocked from reaching the logical, rational, and conscious executive center of the brain, resulting behavior will be automatic and completely in accordance with the person's strongest held values and/or identity.

Thus a person's beliefs about chosen values determine his or her response to the stimuli received from the environment. These beliefs are stored in the subconscious mind, are subject to change by the conscious mind, and have a powerful influence on foundational behaviors of professional practice.

sensitivity broadens perspective and helps people realize that everyone is different; this awareness helps the student care for the patient-athlete and not simply the injury or illness. This insight about oneself and others is critically important before entering a health care relationship with a patient-athlete.

REFERENCES

1. Andre J: Beyond moral reasoning: a wider view of the professional ethics course, *Teaching Philosophy* 14:359-373, 1991.
2. Clark P: Values in health care professional socialization: implications for geriatric education in interdisciplinary teamwork, *Gerontologist* 37:441-452, 1997.
3. *Cultural competence online.* Available at www.culturalcompetence2.com. Accessed July 15, 2006.
4. Davis CM: Affective education for the health care professions, *Phys Ther* 61:1587-1593, 1981.
5. Ebel RG: *Far beyond the shoe box,* New York, 1999, Forbes.
6. Grundstein-Amado R: Values education: a new direction for medical education, *J Med Ethics* 21:174-179, 1995.
7. Killen AR: Morality in perioperative nurses, *AORN J* 75:532-541, 2002.
8. Konin JE: *Developing an athletic training program policy and procedure manual,* 1996 (website): www.nataec.org/documents/articles/pp_manual.html. Accessed October 21, 2005.
9. Lumpkin A, Stoll SK, Beller JM: *Sport ethics applications for fair play,* St Louis, 1994, Mosby.
10. Purtilo R: *Ethical dimensions in the health professions,* ed 4, Philadelphia, 2005, Saunders.
11. Raths LE, Harmin M, Simon S: *Values and teaching,* Columbus, Ohio, 1978, Charles E. Merrill.
12. Rest JR: Background: theory and research. In Rest JR, Narvaez D, editors: *Moral development in the professions: psychology and applied ethics,* Hillsdale, NJ, 1994, Lawrence Erlbaum, pp. 1-27.
13. Shaw-Taylor Y, Benesch B: Workforce diversity and cultural competence in healthcare, *J Cultural Diversity* 5:138-147, 1998.
14. Sisola S: Moral reasoning as a predictor of clinical practice: the development of physical therapy students across the professional curriculum, *J Phys Ther Educ* 14(3):26, 2000.
15. Stern DT: The development of professional character in medical students, *Hastings Ctr Rep* 30:S26-30, 2000.
16. Triezenberg HL, Davis CM: Beyond the code of ethics: educating physical therapists for their role as moral agents, *J Phys Ther Educ* 14:48-59, 2000.
17. U.S. Department of Health and Human Services: *Healthy people 2010,* Washington DC, 2000, U.S. Government Printing Office (website): www.healthypeople.gov/document. Accessed August 15, 2005.
18. Weis D, Schank MJ: An instrument to measure professional nursing values, *J Nurs Scholarship* 32:201-205, 2000.

CHAPTER 10

Learning Activities: Linking Content to Practice

The tools of ethical decision making include developing "habits of thought" for reflection on complex, changing situations that are part of everyday practice. Facilitating reflective habits of the mind is a necessary but difficult task in a professional education environment (p. 79).[6]

Learning activities that emphasize personal behavior and values often elicit a strong response in young people. These activities are designed to help the student think about *how* he or she thinks and *why* he or she thinks that way. Much human behavior is guided by the values that people hold personally while trying to make them "fit" within professional situations. Remember, each person comes to this profession with a different background that affects how he or she acts.

Personal discovery facilitates professional development through the ability to reflect on how a person has acted and provide rationale for why he or she acted in that particular way. By practicing these behaviors in a variety of settings, the student will be in a position to address any situation that may arise professionally. Understanding what you stand for is essential as you journey toward a career in the athletic training profession. While moving through the activities in this chapter, the specific objectives will help you move toward personal discovery and professional growth. Information about how you may be assessed will help you focus on the purpose of these activities as you complete them.

ACTIVITIES FOR APPLICATION: LINKING CONTENT TO PRACTICE

LEARNING ACTIVITY 1: VIDEO AND AUDIO TAPE ANALYSIS

Objectives

1. To examine professional behaviors during group activities
2. To encourage communication during group activities
3. To facilitate cultural sensitivity in group problem-solving activities

Description

Review the following case scenario. You will be videotaped as you work together to solve the case or perform a procedure.[1]

Respond in the fashion related to the facts of the case by using communication skills discussed in class. Feel free to elaborate on each case and take it in the direction that it evolves throughout the interaction (i.e., go with the flow). Try to stay in character. Think out arguments before the taping begins; you will have a minimum of 10 minutes of tape time with active dialogue between you. Take approximately 15 minutes to prepare your arguments or rationale. Only prepare your rebuttals; do not work collaboratively to create the scenario. The purpose is to see how you will respond as an individual as the "rebuttals" arise.

CASE SCENARIO

Character A: You were recently appointed program director of an athletic training education program at a large division I institution. You work with a head athletic trainer who is extremely conservative and does not permit women to travel as health care providers with the football team. You are in a meeting with this individual to provide rationale for why female students should be able to serve as health care providers for the football team at away games and the importance for men and women alike of serving the team on away trips as part of the clinical education process.

Character B: You are a "silent generation" (that is, quiet, hard working for long hours, strong work ethic) head ATC who has worked at a large university for 27 years. You have had a successful program thus far, but now the new curriculum director states you have to allow women to travel with the football team. In the past, a female athletic training student (ATS) traveled with the football team and an inappropriate act occurred. Since then, no women have been permitted to travel with the team. You do not believe the argument that the accreditation board requires that this take place and think that the standard is being met by allowing them home experience.

Assessment

Assessment can occur in several ways in a videotaped presentation. Self-evaluation by using a reflective assignment will help you articulate what you could have done differently in a private manner. Peer assessment, with the persons playing the roles critiquing each others' arguments and communication style, can be done by using a strengths/weaknesses evaluative tool. Larger group evaluation of the respective videotapes may be helpful, but they should be balanced with pros and cons of the performance. Ideally, the evaluation should focus on the professional behaviors and content arguments provided. Evaluating the written assignment (preparatory work) is another avenue for assessment.

LEARNING ACTIVITY 2: CLASS OPINION POLL

Objectives

1. To encourage critical thinking about issues of particular relevance to the athletic training profession
2. To demonstrate personal differences in the face of ethical challenges
3. To promote confidence in presenting differing opinions and supporting opinions by using content knowledge among peers

Description

After the presentation of selected controversial topics, an opinion poll will be collected from the class in response to each topic.[1] This opinion poll is typically performed by a show of hands but can also be performed by physically moving to one side of the room or another to reflect choice.

Several selected scenarios are provided for consideration. Feel free to create your own scenarios by using examples from previous classes, clinical experiences, or professional activities.

CASE SCENARIO

A head athletic trainer (male) and an assistant athletic trainer (female) are talking in their office after a hard day of work. The door is open and the two are joking with each other, and one of the jokes has a sexual connotation. An athletic training graduate assistant (female) happens to hear the joke and is greatly offended by the content. She intends to pursue sexual harassment charges against the two professionals.[9]

- Can a private conversation exist in a work environment such as an athletic training facility?
- Are professionals in a work setting obliged to ensure that no one can hear if they are having a personal conversation?
- Were the two athletic trainers unprofessional in their behavior?
- Are athletic trainers socialized into the "locker room" mentality in which sexually explicit jokes are acceptable?

CASE SCENARIO

An athletic training education program requires that athletic training students be free of facial hair to participate in clinical activities. An incoming student with impeccable grades disputes this policy and argues that facial hair has nothing to do with performing athletic training services.

- Is the policy regarding facial hair fair?
- Should athletic training education programs have dress codes for students?

CASE SCENARIO

As an athletic training student, you are preparing for the Board of Certification (BOC) examination. You approach a fellow athletic training student who recently successfully completed the examination for assistance. The athletic training student, a close friend, assists you by answering questions relative to general content but not specific questions that she encountered on the board examination.[4]

- Is this athletic training student in violation of the BOC examination confidentiality waiver?
- If you were a program director and you overheard this conversation, would you report this athletic training student to the BOC?
- Is the athletic training student asking the question guilty as well?

CASE SCENARIO

An athletic training education program has a student in the program who works as an exotic dancer in a gentlemen's club in town. She is a good student and performs successfully in clinical assignments. She is set to graduate and take the board examination in a few months. Conversations around the athletic training room and from athletes on several teams indicate that many people know of her employment, although she has never disclosed it to the athletic training program director or her clinical supervisor. Her clinical supervisors ask that she be given an ultimatum: quit the club or complete her education. The clinical supervisors indicate that her job is interfering with athletic health care because the athletes are talking about it.[7]

- Should the student be required to quit her job to complete the program?
- Is it appropriate for the clinical instructor to consider this in her year-end evaluation?
- Is the student in violation of the NATA Code of Ethics?

CASE SCENARIO

An athlete reports to the athletic training room with a brand that he received on induction into a local fraternity. The athlete is in considerable pain and asks the athletic trainer to help him care for the wound. The athletic trainer refuses to treat the athlete, stating that it is not an athletic injury and that he self-inflicted the wound so he deserves to be in pain. The athletic trainer does, however, provide the athlete with the opportunity to use supplies (adhesive bandages, ointments) from the athletic training room and gives the athlete the phone number of the team physician.[8]

- Should the athletic trainer have provided treatment for the branded area?
- Is the team physician responsible for caring for this injury?

CASE SCENARIO

An athletic training student reports to the athletic training program director that a clinical supervisor at an affiliate site has inquired about the next student who is assigned to that high school. While standing on the sidelines of football practice, this affiliate site supervisor inquires about the personality, clinical skills, and sexual orientation of the incoming student in an informal manner.

- Should the athletic training student disclose to the athletic training education program director the questions she was asked by the clinical supervisor?
- Should the clinical supervisor ask a fellow athletic training student about another student to better prepare for the incoming student?
- Should the athletic training education program director contact the clinical supervisor to discuss the issue?
- Should the athletic training education program director withdraw the current student and remove the affiliate site as a clinical venue for the program?

Assessment

Participation in the group activity is the simplest way to evaluate this activity. A group participation rubric that evaluates level of participation and ability to articulate the argument is preferred. This activity can also be given as a take-home assignment in which you must argue your position on each scenario, evaluated as a written assignment or used as a precursor to an in-class debate. After the group activities, you may also be assigned a written assignment of justifying the opposite stance.

Tip: Create questions by yourself or in small groups for the polls, and collect the data to share with the class after collecting the information from peers, supervisors, or faculty members.

LEARNING ACTIVITY 3: DIRECTED PARAPHRASING

Objectives

1. To enhance communication skills
2. To facilitate interpersonal skills, including nonverbal communication
3. To demonstrate cultural sensitivity in allied health communication

Description

Read the following scenarios, which include highly specific information that must be communicated to selected populations.[1] This activity is designed to help students decipher detailed medical information and break it down into understandable knowledge for patients.

CASE SCENARIO

Communicate the following information to a parent of a high school athlete:

A 16-year-old female gymnast fell off the balance beam and dislocated her left ankle. Radiographs of the ankle reflect a displaced fracture to the lateral malleolus; ruptures of the anterior talo fibular, calcaneo fibular, and posterior talofibular ligaments; a talar dome compression fracture; and partial rupture of the deltoid ligament. Damage to the posterior tibial artery has resulting in occlusion. The patient requires immediate surgery. The physician anticipates significant damage that will affect her ability to perform gymnastics in the future.

CASE SCENARIO

Communicate the following information to a collegiate basketball player:

A diagnosis of type 2 diabetes attributable to family history and clinical obesity; glucose monitoring and diet modification are required.

Assessment

These assignments can be performed in written format, which can be assessed for content and communication qualities. An alternative, more challenging approach is to use this activity as an oral presentation in front of the class or a small group so that verbal and nonverbal communication styles can be assessed. Peer evaluation and self-evaluations of oral presentation rubrics are useful and provide valuable feedback regarding communication and sensitivity.

LEARNING ACTIVITY 4: DOUBLE-ENTRY JOURNAL

Objectives

1. To promote critical thinking about class materials, including in-class or reading assignments
2. To encourage self-reflection regarding professional behaviors
3. To stimulate alternative perspectives

Description

After a reading assignment or in-class activity, record ideas and arguments you find most meaningful and/or controversial as well as an explanation of the personal significance of the idea and/or argument.[1] This two-part journal entry will enable you to articulate your perceptions on each topic in a confidential manner.

Tip: Numerous scenarios can be used with this learning activity. Be creative; use this frequently throughout each course or clinical assignment to engage in reflection and application. This activity will help you sort out your feelings and/or perceptions about a wide range of topics related to the athletic training profession. Your instructor may even have you bring in selected topics for the class to consider in their journal entries.

Assessment

A journal rubric is most effective for this activity. The goal is to express feelings and perceptions on the basis of class or clinical content. The evaluation should be based on expression, rather than on content, because no "right" answer to this activity is possible. A unique approach is to also go back through the entries for a given period and identify any themes that emerge. This will alert you to potential biases or trigger points that will guide you in future professional decisions.

LEARNING ACTIVITY 5: PROFILES OF ADMIRABLE INDIVIDUALS

Objectives

1. To identify qualities and traits in individuals who serve as role models
2. To understand how a person's qualities shape their professional behavior
3. To facilitate an understanding of professional and personal values

Description

Write a brief, focused profile of someone in the field whose values, skills, or actions you greatly admire.[1] Be specific and express why you feel those values, skills, or actions are admirable.

Assessment

As a writing assignment, this activity can be assessed on writing skills and completion of the task rather than content. Feedback on the connections between the selected values, skills, and actions and the professional practice of athletic training will be provided and serves as a valuable evaluative activity.

Tip: Alternative ways of using this activity include providing a list of people to consider and decide who are admirable, rank a variety of profiles by importance, write profiles for people who are not admirable, and create a composite list of qualities from a collection of profiles that reflect desired professional behaviors for the athletic training professional. Lastly, compare your profile with the profile you created for this activity. How similar are they? What do you need to do to become like this person?

LEARNING ACTIVITY 6: MISCONCEPTION/PRECONCEPTION

Objectives

1. To acknowledge bias in perceptions in professional practice

2. To facilitate dialogue among peers relative to how bias affects professional behaviors
3. To encourage reflection on personal values and behaviors

Description

Review the following case scenarios, and respond to the corresponding questions or statements.[1]

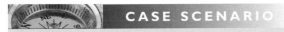

CASE SCENARIO

An Asian-American athletic trainer applies for an assistant athletic training position at an institution that is greatly lacking diversity. She is awarded the position over many other equally qualified individuals.

- Did the athletic trainer receive the appointment because of her minority status?
- Are institutions required to hire minority candidates when all other qualifications are equal?

CASE SCENARIO

An athletic training student reports that he was in a drug rehabilitation program during his high school years and still attends Narcotics Anonymous meetings on a regular basis. This student has a sincere interest in pharmacologic research and asks if the ATEP director can help him get an internship at a pharmacy or research laboratory.

- Is having this ATS in a setting where pharmacologic agents are readily available a risk?
- Should this student not have access to the physician's office in the athletic training room because locked medications are stored there?

CASE SCENARIO

A certified athletic trainer is openly gay and has the assignment of men's basketball. An athletic training student is also assigned men's basketball and has the opportunity to travel with the men's team with the certified athletic trainer for the upcoming away tournament. He will have to room with the certified athletic trainer because the team will not pay for an additional room for him to travel.

- Should the student be apprehensive about traveling with the team?
- Should the student be permitted by the ATEP director to travel knowing that he will have to share a room with the certified athletic trainer?

CASE SCENARIO

The age difference between faculty/clinical supervisors and students is sometimes relatively slight. A collegiate professor, graduate assistant, or clinical supervisor could be 25 years old and the college athletic training student could be 22 years old.[10]

- Should a faculty member (outside the ATTR curriculum) date an athletic training student?
- Should an affiliate instructor who will never supervise the athletic training student again in a clinical setting date an athletic training student who has completed her rotation at that venue?

Assessment

As a personal activity, a simple evaluation reflecting the ability to identify personal bias is appropriate. Identification of strategies to avoid bias is also a viable assessment approach.

Tip: An interesting approach if you are tentative about your own bias is to identify misconceptions or preconceptions that you think others may have and support these ideas with the appropriate justification.

Another fun activity is to complete the activity as a preclass assignment, have group discussion, and then complete it again as a postclass assignment to see if your thinking has changed. Often group discussion helps you acknowledge the subtle biases that you did not realize you possess.

LEARNiNG ACTIVITY 7: DECISION TREE

Objectives

1. To visualize the processes by which you make decisions
2. To understand the impact of the decisions you make along each path
3. To encourage critical reflection on the reasons why you chose the paths for each decision

Description

Use the decision tree shown in Figure 10-1 while moving through a decision-making process.[1] Analyze the following case, and create a pathway to select your responses.

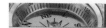

CASE SCENARIO

Does Being Ethical Pay?

Regular assignments are required in class that sometimes are due at inconvenient times. They are graded A through F. The instructor is quite strict about missing assignments. You wonder whether the instructor might not know the difference if you copy the answers from a friend.

The decision tree shown in Figure 10-1 will help you look at the various options encountered along this decision-making course. Should you do your own work, copy the answers, or not do the assignment at all? Fill in the lines provided as you think about the different paths along the way.

After careful consideration of all alternatives and completion of each of the lines, which solution did you choose? Why did you choose this alternative? How does it relate to your values systems? Are grades or ethical behaviors more important? How can you balance these?

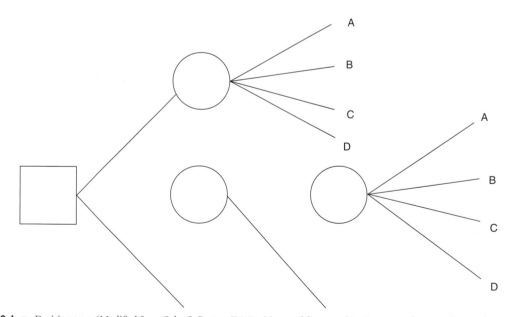

Figure 10-1 ■ Decision tree. *(Modified from Cahn S, Pastore JM: Decision modeling: an objective approach to moral reasoning,* Teaching Bus Ethics *7:329-340, 2003.)*

Assessment

Consideration of viable alternatives and processing the reward versus the risk of each path on the tree is the objective of this activity. Assessing how you complete the chart with consideration for the ability to delve into deeper implications for selected actions is critical. Assigning a point value for the ability to generate viable options with consideration of the cost-benefit ratio is a good approach. Peer evaluation is also helpful because it will help you see what others were thinking and alternatives that you may not have considered.

LEARNING ACTIVITY 8: THINK ABOUT . . .

Objectives

1. To identify the importance of beliefs, values, and norms in professional behaviors
2. To emphasize the role of your value system in the professional socialization process
3. To identify ways of addressing cognitive dissonance

Description

Analyze the following questions and scenarios and be able to express them to your peers. Make connections to foundational behaviors for professional practice as you progress through these activities.[2]

- Can you identify key values for the athletic training profession?
- Values can be personal, social, political, economic, religious, or social. Identify an example of each of these value categories, and discuss how these values affect your life and career choice.
- Identify whether you agree with the following statements, and explain why or why not:
  - My attitude affects my behaviors.
  - My behavior affects my attitude.
  - Your attitude affects my behaviors.
  - Your behavior affects my attitude.
- Dissonance is created in the presence of internal tension. Dissonance usually is resolved by avoidance, denial, or change. Identify a situation in your professional preparation that has caused you dissonance, and identify which strategy you used to resolve that dissonance.

- Think of an example for each of the strategies listed above as they relate to your clinical experiences. How do your personal values shape your response?

Assessment

Because the assignment involves critically reflecting on situations that have occurred in the past, this activity often is assessed by a reflection rubric. Examination of the level of critical thinking and reflection is more important than the content of the responses.

LEARNING ACTIVITY 9: COMMUNICATION ACTIVITY (ROLE PLAYING)

Objectives

1. To demonstrate effective communication styles in conflict situations
2. To stimulate prompt, effective communication (thinking on your feet)
3. To illustrate multiple perspectives on each scenario

Description

Each of the following scenarios describes the roles, situation, and facts of the case. You will be assigned a role by your instructor and will have only 3 minutes to prepare for your role. Each role-playing scenario is slated for a 5-minute interaction.[5]

After the role playing, your instructor may assign you a written reflection or have a group activity to identify issues relative to communicating in a sensitive, ethical manner.

CASE SCENARIO

Budget Cuts
The characters: The head athletic trainer, who believes denying payment for athletic-related medications for nonscholarship athletes is unethical; and the athletic director, whose budget has been cut and decides that financial support will not be provided to any nonscholarship athletes.

The athletic director sends the head athletic trainer a memo stating that your institution will no longer be providing financial coverage for any medication (general medical or athletic injury–related) for any nonscholarship athlete.

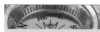

CASE SCENARIO

Negligence and Loss of Eligibility
The characters: The assistant athletic trainer, parent, and athletic director.

A parent contacts the institution regarding what she perceives to be unacceptable medical coverage. She claims that the assistant athletic trainers' unwillingness to provide appropriate and timely care to her son after his anterior cruciate ligament surgery has caused him to develop joint adhesions. As a result, he will miss the remainder of his senior season and will lose his last year of eligibility. She demands that you get him a medical "red shirt" (an additional year of eligibility because of extenuating medical conditions) and that the school pay for damages.

Background Information

The athlete is a 22-year-old male gymnast who injured himself at the beginning of the season. He received an aggressive surgical repair of his injury in an attempt to give him an opportunity to participate in conference and nationals after the season, but he was noncompliant with rehabilitation

The assistant athletic trainer is responsible for the sport and oversees all aspects of the sport. The assistant athletic trainer made numerous attempts to get the athlete to be compliant with his rehabilitation and documented noncompliant behavior.

The parent is ill informed of the conferences policies and procedures regarding medical red shirts. She is easily excitable and irrational regarding her son's responsibility in the success of his rehabilitation.

The athletic director supports the athletic training staff but is trying to placate the parent because she is a donor. The athletic director is trying to see if any "strings can be pulled" to make this situation go away.

CASE SCENARIO

Inappropriate Conduct
The characters: An athletic training student, the head coach, and a graduate assistant coach

An athletic training student is addressing inappropriate sexual conduct from a coach. The student claims that the graduate assistant coach has made inappropriate comments and contact with her on an away road trip. The graduate assistant and athletic training student were assigned to share a room.

Background Information

The student is a senior athletic training student who has a reputation of hanging out with the coaching staff and having a beer or two with them. The graduate assistant coach has been known to be a sexually forward person. She feels that the student (who is the same age as she is) seemed to be receptive to her and sees nothing wrong with what she has done. The head coach's philosophy is "if I don't see it, then it didn't happen." The head coach does not like having to spend money on taking an athletic training student to serve with the health care team and would be just as happy to see the athletic training student stay at home.

Assessment

Assessment for this task can be approached from multiple perspectives. A group discussion (looking at participation by using one of the rubrics in the appendixes or a self-created rubric) is a viable option because it will stimulate discussion relative to the case, body language, and professional behaviors that emerge. An additional option is to critique each person's role individually in regard to professional communication and behaviors displayed. A journal assignment also can help you reflect on how you felt in the role and/or how you perceived others' behaviors.

Tip: You can also create scenarios that can be role played in class, or if in-class time is limited, these may be assigned as essay activities. Lastly, this activity can be videotaped to perform self- or peer assessment.

SUMMARY

The activities listed in the chapter were designed to help you recognize how who you *are*—your personal identity—shapes how you *act* as a professional in the field of athletic training. Working through activities that force you to look deeply at what you stand for will assist you along your professional discovery journey. The goal of these activities is not to generate correct responses because many of the activities have a wide range of responses. Instead, the goal is to process the information and respond to acknowledge and identify factors that guide you as you make decisions and interact in the profession. What you do and how you do it affect those around you. By processing this information in a practice setting, you will be better prepared to face these challenges as you encounter them in real-life scenarios.

REFERENCES

1. Angelo TA, Cross KP: *Classroom assessment techniques: a handbook for college teachers,* San Francisco, 1993, Jossey-Bass.
2. Arnold LE, Sullivan D: *Department of the Army: consideration of others (CO2) handbook: lesson number 17: values, attitudes, behaviors and self-awareness.* Leadership Division, Human Resources Directorate Office of the Deputy Chief of Staff for Personnel (website): http://chppm-www.apgea.army.mil/co2/CO2_book/Lp17.htm. Assessed July 17, 2007.
3. Cahn S, Pastore JM: Decision modeling: an objective approach to moral reasoning, *Teaching Bus Ethics* 7:329-340, 2003.
4. Gardiner A: You signed the waiver: NATABOC-exam confidentiality, *Athl Ther Today* 10:54-55, 2005.
5. Hale CC, Peer KS: *Classroom activity for communication skills.* Unpublished classroom activity for "Professional Development in Athletic Training" course, Kent State University, Fall 2004, Kent, Ohio.
6. Jenson GM, Richert AE: Reflection on the teaching of ethics in physical therapy education: integrating cases, theory, and learning, *J Phys Ther Educ* 19:78-85, 2005.
7. Mensch JM, Mitchell M: Enforcing professional standards or violating personal rights? *Athl Ther Today* 9(3):28-29, 2004.
8. Miller MA: A clinical quandary, *Athl Ther Today* 8(3):40-41, 2003.
9. Mitchell M: From humor to harassment: how context changes everything, *Athl Ther Today* 10(4):38-39, 2005.
10. Ruggiero VR: *Thinking critically about ethical issues,* Mountain View, Calif., 1997, Mayfield Publishing.

CHAPTER **11**

Professional Awareness and the Cultivation of Professional Identity

ETHICAL CONCEPTS

Affective taxonomy

Ethical standards

Foundational behaviors of professional practice

Professional attributes

Professional identity

Professional values

Technical standards

Value analysis

Values conflict

LEARNING OBJECTIVES

After reading this chapter, the student should be able to do the following:

1. Describe professional identity in athletic training.

2. Identify personal characteristics of expert athletic trainers.

3. Appraise and compare your work ethic with those of expert athletic trainers.

4. Evaluate your typical personal relationship with a patient-athlete and how it compares with the relationship expressed by expert athletic trainers.

5. Discuss why professional passion appears important in athletic training.

6. Explain why professional values are important.

7. Describe how professional values are passed down to the next generation.

8. Identify important values of athletic trainers working in the Great Lakes Athletic Trainers' Association, also known as District 4.

9. Identify values in the National Athletic Trainers' Association Code of Ethics.

10. Compare the professional values of nursing, physical therapy, and medicine.

11. Explain values-based behaviors.

12. Explain how professional values shape foundational behaviors of professional practice.

PRINCIPLE 3: Members shall maintain and promote high standards in their provision of services. 3.1 Members shall not misrepresent, either directly or indirectly, their skills, training, professional credentials, identity, or services.

—NATA Code of Ethics[13]

A profession is a unique culture.[6] Broadly speaking, the profession of athletic training and the resulting cultural expression encompass two significant standards: (1) technical standards (cognitive competencies and clinical proficiencies) and (2) ethical standards (values and interpersonal skills). The combination of these two standards creates the professional identity, or the image of athletic training (Figure 11-1). The identity crystallizes through reiteration of positive, competent, and consistent interactions with the patient-athlete and other professionals and is reflected in the foundational behaviors of professional practice.[14]

TECHNICAL STANDARDS

Being a competent professional is more than applying the right knowledge and skills, it also means a commitment to set core values.[15]

For many years, the technical standards (cognitive competencies and clinical proficiencies) have been the primary focus of athletic training education. Although the focus of this text is on professional ethics, a brief outline of the technical standards is of value given their importance in the professional identity of athletic training. Box 11-1 identifies the content areas in which technical standards in entry-level athletic training originate.[14]

ETHICAL STANDARDS

Athletic training isn't just what we do, it is who we are, a way of life.[24]

Much has been written in athletic training about the technical standards describing essential *knowing* and *doing* elements, but little attention has been given to *being* a certified athletic trainer. Ethical standards embrace two interrelated concepts: values and interpersonal skills. Both concepts inform foundational behaviors of professional practice.

Professional attributes of athletic trainers provide a backdrop to a more focused discussion on the ethical standards. The attributes of the certified athletic trainer

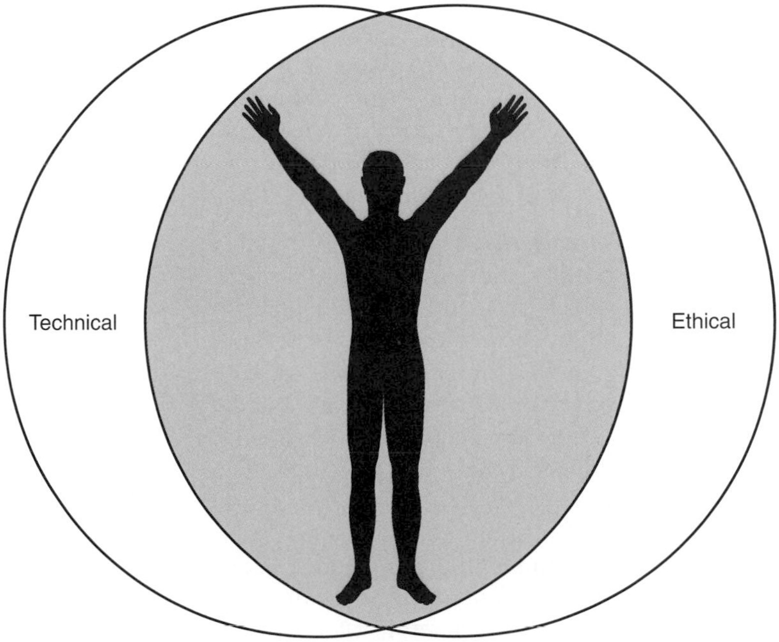

Figure 11-1 ■ Technical and ethical standards form professional identity.

Technical

Ethical

AREAS IN WHICH TECHNICAL STANDARDS ORIGINATE

Risk management and injury prevention
Pathology of injuries and illnesses
Orthopedic clinical examination and diagnosis
Medical conditions and disabilities
Acute care of injuries and illnesses
Therapeutic modalities
Conditioning and rehabilitative exercise
Pharmacology
Psychosocial intervention and referral
Nutritional aspects of injuries and illnesses
Health care administration
Professional development and responsibility

Data from National Athletic Trainers' Association: *Athletic trainer educational competencies,* ed 4, Dallas, 2006, National Athletic Trainers' Association.

define specific qualities of this unique professional; typically they are best understood by observing the professional in action. Little has been written about professional attributes. However, perhaps, the most powerful and recorded authentic portrayal of the professional attributes comes from the voices of male athletic trainers who have been identified as experts with prolonged engagement (20 years) at National Collegiate Athletic Association Division I universities.[11] Relative to professional attributes, three themes were expressed: (1) personal characteristics, (2) personal philosophies, and (3) personal relationships.

Personal Characteristics. Characteristics such as loyalty, generosity, and a strong work ethic helped these individuals succeed in a field where they must put others above themselves. According to ATC 1, "One of the things that I pride myself on is being loyal. If someone works for me and does a good job, I'll do anything I can to help them for the rest of my life. I make that promise to them. If they're loyal, then I return that to them as many times as I can." In addition, ATC 7 said, "I've had a unique opportunity to give something back to the school. At the same time, the institution has come back and done some things for me. So, it became a two-way street. I guess my final goal at

[the university] would be to make sure that I left this place in a better condition than when I came."

Personal Philosophies. The work ethic and philosophies of the participants have resulted in the development of a great passion for their work. As ATC 2 said, "For the last 15 years, I haven't worn a watch. The job has never been about how much time I spend at work. I go to work, do my job, and go home when everything is done. If you start looking at the clock and worrying about the fact that you're putting in 14 to 15 hours a day, you won't last very long." Another athletic trainer (ATC 7) said, "Years ago the philosophy was that the job wasn't done until the job was done and practice wasn't over until everyone went home. Now because of clinical environments and educational controls, the 'good old boys' have a hard time recognizing there is a 40-hour week. I'm probably one of those."

The athletic trainers truly cared about the athletes. As ATC 1 said, "To me, and I mean this with all my heart, an athletic trainer is a person who cares more about the athlete than he does himself. The athlete comes first over you. That doesn't mean he's first over your religion or your family; it means he's first over you. Athletes know if you really care. I take my time and pay attention to them."

The athletic trainers made their availability to the athletes a priority. Their professional philosophies were based on a service-oriented concept. As ATC 1 explains, "I've been an athletic trainer a long time now, almost 30 years, and I haven't missed a day of work, not one. My responsibility is to be there for those athletes, and that's my job. They expect me to be there with them all the time." According to ATC 2, "I went in and opened the training room at 7 in the morning and closed at 7 or 8 at night. The coaches thought the sun rose and set with me. It wasn't because I knew everything but it was because I was willing to put in the time. I think that that's true with most successful athletic trainers. I think you can make up for what you don't know by working hard and being interested. Spending time with kids and being available to them is very important."

The personal characteristics of the participants have made their careers more successful and fulfilling. However, the ATCs could not have accomplished everything alone. They received support and direction from the personal relationships they have created inside and outside the sporting environment.

Personal Relationships. The development of a bond between the ATC and the athlete is inevitable while working in an athletic training environment. There is a mutual respect for one another. Relationships that are created can last a lifetime. The following are statements made by ATC 1 and 2, respectively: "As a student, I noticed how much the athletes respected our head athletic trainer, and I noticed how much he cared for them in return. I thought the way they treated him, and the fact that athletes would come back years later to see him, was something special. There was a special bond that he had with the athletes. He taught me to respect the athletes and care for them. The very special bond that we have with athletes as athletic trainers is hard to find anywhere else. I'm not sure everybody has that bond, but I think some of us do."

"Being involved with the athletes on a day-to-day basis is what keeps me going. That has made it really easy to stay interested and motivated. It's certainly not money, glamour, or prestige. When a kid comes back on campus and the first place that he comes into is the athletic training room, it says a lot. That's what I will miss the most. Having that relationship with the athletes where they depend upon you and respect you. It's always been a family to me. They become my children."

In a profession where a great deal of time is spent with others, the demanding work environment can limit the time that is spent at home. As ATC 7 states, "Growing up in a small community, my children respected what I did and at the same time resented what I did. I was there at the big events, but the day-to-day battles and struggles in their lives were basically handled by their mother. We always went on the basis that what I brought was quality and not quantity. I would have liked to spend some more time with them so they could understand better where I was coming from. They had the opportunity to get an education. I think they had a good support structure, and they both turned out to be good kids."

Some of the ATCs made special compromises to accommodate both family and work, as illustrated by the following statement by ATC 2: "I have three boys, and they are very much a part of what I do. They can come in and spend time with dad. They love to do that. Sometimes they come out to the field for practice. So even though I'm working 90 hours a week, they are not spent exclusively away from the family. My family is very much involved in a lot of what I do." One athletic trainer (ATC 4) has changed his views on the amount of time spent at work versus time spent at home. "I don't feel that putting in over 70 hours a week is the way to function anymore. There is more to life than work. It was fine when it was just me or my wife and I, but when you start a family you have a commitment to them as well. In order to be able to give of yourself to them, something has to be sacrificed. I have lessened my availability in the athletic training room to be available to my family. When you look at things in proper perspective, the first thing is your faith, then your family, and then your job. If you keep life in that perspective, something has to give, so I started altering that in my life. I do my job to the best of my ability. I try to be honest and fair with my athletes and my coaches. I think it is important to keep your life in balance."

Meaningful experiences and personal attributes can be influential in the development of an athletic trainer. Without direction, however, these experiences and qualities can go undeveloped. All of the participants had the benefit of a number of mentoring role models to guide, encourage, and teach them.[11]

Although a limitation of the study is that the subjects are all male and working in the intercollegiate athletic training practice setting, it provides a glimpse into some important and authentic professional attributes in athletic training. Box 11-2, which details the values and beliefs of Ray Ramirez, head athletic

COMBINING FAMILY AND CULTURE IN ATHLETIC TRAINING

Education, a strong work ethic, and compassion describe a successful athletic trainer. Add to that list a commitment to heritage, devotion to family, and high standards for leadership, and you are describing the New York Mets head athletic trainer, Ray Ramirez. Raised in Puerto Rico, Ramirez learned the fundamentals of building a successful career from his parents, who have continued to be his unending inspiration.

As a past member of the Professional Baseball Athletic Trainers' Society (PBATS) executive committee, Ramirez continues to lead by example for the younger membership. Combining his strong passion for athletic training and his Latin background, Ramirez has been an active member of the Rookie Career Development Program. As part of the program, he is able to leverage his background to build relationships with Latin players. His fluent Spanish helps comfort young Latin athletes who enter the league, and their similar backgrounds create bonds stronger than baseball and medicine.

Ramirez is also able to educate Latin intern athletic trainers on the intricacies of medicine in major league baseball. He leads by example as he mentors young athletic trainers through the Foreign Athletic Trainer Program. "Students in Puerto Rico tell me that they are an athletic trainer because of me," said Ramirez. "That is overwhelming. So it is important to me to help those individuals work toward meeting their career goals."

During the off-season, Ramirez focuses on spending time with his kids and returning to Puerto Rico to visit his parents. He relaxes by listening to salsa and learning to play the guitar. Despite his success in major league baseball and his current role with the Mets, Ramirez has not forgotten the importance of his family, his Latin roots, or his colleagues, like Kent Biggerstaff and Jeff Cooper, who helped him along the way. Those values have been a driving force behind his success as an athletic trainer in major league baseball.

From Professional Baseball Athletic Trainers Society: Ray Ramirez, New York Mets head athletic trainer: combining family and culture in athletic training, *The Annual Publication of the Professional Baseball Athletic Trainers Society* 19(1), 2006.

trainer for the New York Mets, further supports the beliefs and observations of expert intercollegiate athletic trainers.[16]

These voices from competent athletic training professionals articulate the significance of the resolute work ethic coupled with a professional passion and tireless commitment to service in caring for the patient-athlete. Clark[5] addresses the importance of the professional voice in that it provides the framework for professional socialization and thus professional identity formation.[5] Given that each profession has its own distinctive voice or identity providing a unique world view, each profession embraces different values that are implicitly embedded in ethical standards and expressed in foundational behaviors of professional practice.

The available literature in athletic training captures the importance of the tireless work ethic and the passion for the profession. The attributes and essence of the athletic training professional provide a distinguished backdrop as ethical standards are explored through the lenses of values and interpersonal skills. Moreover, the knowledge of values and interpersonal skills informs foundational behaviors of professional practice.

ETHICAL APPROACHES: PROFESSIONAL VALUES

Values, as one quality of a professional group, impart exclusiveness. In general, values give shape, meaning, and direction to life as well as influence professional behavior, attitudes, and beliefs. Furthermore, professional values are at the heart of every professional decision and action. They support a framework to facilitate excellence in clinical judgments, a spontaneity in practice, and a sense of professional commitment.[22,25] The acquisition and internalization of professional values that are congruent with those espoused by the professional body shape the professional identity.[27]

The extent to which a professional has adopted and internalized professional values is analogous to wading in water (described earlier by John Schrader in Chapter 1).[21] Clark provides meaning for three different levels parallel to values immersion[4]:

1. Wading ankle high. Compliance—the professional acts in a particular way to gain positive feedback.

Table 11-1	PROFESSIONAL CORE VALUES IN NURSING, PHYSICAL THERAPY, AND MEDICINE
Profession	**Professional Core Values**
Nursing	Altruism, esthetics, equality, freedom, human dignity, truth, justice
Physical therapy	Accountability, altruism, compassion/caring, excellence, integrity, professional duty, social responsibility
Medicine	Trustworthiness, integrity, discernment, compassion, conscientiousness

Data from American Association of Colleges of Nursing: *Essentials of college and university education for professional nursing*, Washington, DC, 1986, American Association of Colleges of Nursing; American Physical Therapy Association: *The APTA vision sentence for physical therapy 2020 and APTA vision statement for physical therapy 2020*, www.apta.org/AM/Template.cfm?Section=Advance_Search&section=Policies&template=/CM/ContentDisplay. cfm&ContentFileID=3252. Accessed August 1, 2005; and Beauchamp TL, Childress JF: Principles of Biomedical Ethics, New York, 2001, Oxford University Press.

2. Wading waist high. Identification—the professional chooses certain behaviors but not values.
3. Full immersion. Internalization—the professional accepts the norms and values of the professional role because he or she believes in them.

Professional Values in Health Care

The formation and internalization of a professional identity through acquisition of values that are congruent with those espoused by the profession facilitates professional development.[27]

In health care, the mark of excellence within a collective body is the degree to which the members share congruent values.[26] Similar professional values in each health care group inform a predictable and consistent action (behavior) and decision. Table 11-1 reveals that conventional health care professions (e.g., nursing, physical therapy, and medicine) have articulated their own unique set of core values that impart a sense of professional distinctiveness.[1-3]

Given that professional identity goes well beyond role and well beyond technical skill and competence, perhaps the tie that binds the professional to the profession is something much more inherent, such as professional values. According to Wilson,[27] the acquisition and internalization of professional values that are congruent with those espoused by the professional body shape the professional identity. Unlike other health care professions, athletic training has yet to explore and discover professional values.

Chapter 9 discussed several major value systems; within major systems are values that can be bundled into exclusive subsets. Similar to the personal value system, the professional value system is a major system with exclusive subsets of values bundled together to give rise to a unique occupational group, such as law, business, medicine, and health care. The unique professional value subset contributes to the distinctiveness of a professional group.

Health care professionals make many value-laden decisions leading to right action. Values relating to health care are moral in nature. Moral values focus on human rights, integrity, and welfare—in other words, how others ought to be treated.[17] Furthermore, these moral professional values fortify ethical standards—including professional code of ethics and the prima facie health care principles of autonomy, beneficence, nonmaleficence, and justice—and guide the foundational behaviors of professional practice.

Professional Values in Athletic Training

The ideal and real in the sense of professional practice are rooted in a strong and lasting value system.[10]

In general, the athletic training membership has grown considerably since its inception in 1950. Today, there are more than 30,000 members of the NATA. In the early years after the association's foundation, membership numbers were significantly lower and the professional legacy was easily passed from one generation to another by word of mouth. Given the rapid influx of athletic trainers into the association over the last 20 years, the informal ways of passing the traditions of athletic training to the next generation may need to be reevaluated. To ensure that the membership is on the

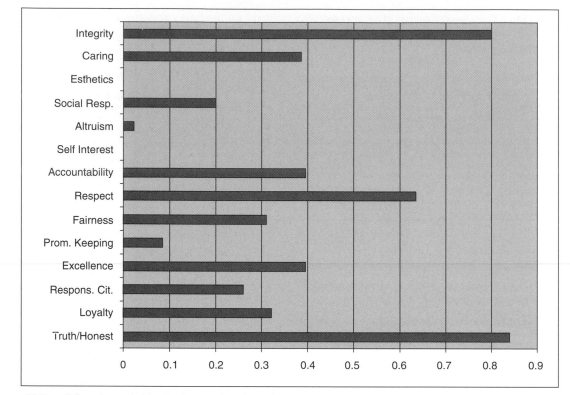

Figure 11-2 ■ Values chosen (%) by GLATA members (n = 95) in summer 2005.

same page, professional distinctiveness hinges on identifying and explicitly articulating one singular set of professional core values so that consistent and predictable patterns of professional practice and behaviors become linked to professional athletic training identity.[5]

No published research relative to professional values exists in the profession of athletic training. Therefore preliminary research was conducted by the authors (Schlabach and Peer) in the summer of 2005 after the Great Lakes Athletic Trainers' Association's (GLATA) business meeting.[20] GLATA is also known as District 4 (D4). A survey instrument was developed according to the values clarification criteria of Raths et al[18] (Table 9-2). It required the subject to choose values freely from alternatives. The list of values presented to subjects originated from values implicit in the NATA Code of Ethics as well as values explicit in health care principles and professions.[1-3] In the event that the list of values was not all inclusive, the subject

had an opportunity to add a value. A convenience sample was used. Surveys were distributed to volunteers (n = 95), and the response rate was approximately 63%. The subject pool consisted of 45 men and 50 women, with an average of 19 years of professional experience. The average age of the subject pool was 42 years old, and a comparable number of respondents represented each setting (e.g., university, clinical/industrial, high school). Participants represented all states of GLATA. Completed surveys remained anonymous and confidential.

The frequency in which GLATA members (n = 95) chose from the list of 15 values was expressed in percent (number of times one particular value was selected out of 95). Based on percent, the results (Figure 11-2) indicated that the top five values were (1) truth/honesty (85%), (2) integrity (81%), (3) respect (64%), (4) accountability and excellence (40%), and (5) caring (39%). District 4 membership clearly found the discovery of professional values to be

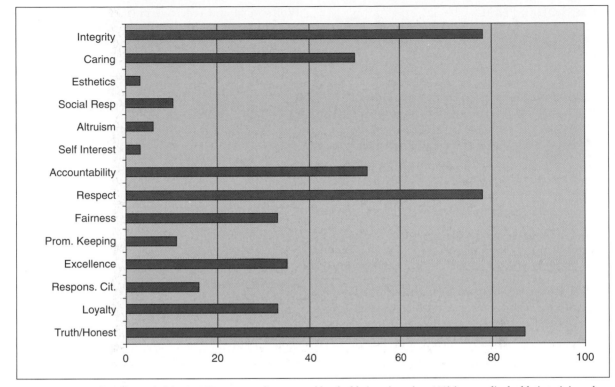

Figure 11-3 ■ Values chosen (%) by GLATA program directors and head athletic trainers (n = 109) in accredited athletic training education programs in fall 2006.

important and that the professional body should explicitly articulate professional core values. Because professional values guide behaviors and motivate professional attitudes and beliefs, the discovery of athletic training's common *core* professional values may plausibly unify professionals across role, setting, and population served and one singular professional identity in athletic training will emerge.

Furthermore, Schlabach and Peer discovered important professional values among program directors and head athletic trainers in GLATA.[19] A similar professional values instrument developed according to the criteria established in Raths et al[17] was mailed to all program directors and head athletic trainers (n = 150) employed in Commission on Accreditation of Allied Health Education Programs accredited programs in District 4. The response rate was 73%. Results (Figure 11-3) indicate that truth/honesty (87%), integrity (78%), respect (78%), accountability (53%), and

caring (50%) are important values to program directors and head athletic trainers employed by accredited athletic training education programs.[19]

From the combined samples of District 4 athletic trainers, the evidence suggests that truth/honesty, integrity, respect, caring, accountability, and excellence are central values. This preliminary research provides insight into relative professional values. Well over 95% of the surveyed membership responded that professional values are extremely important, and 68% believe it is extremely important for the professional body, NATA, to explicitly articulate professional values. According to the literature in other health care fields, identity and explicit articulation of common core values serve to cultivate moral character and high-quality service. Furthermore, articulation will advance professional standing as a unified health care profession with a singular mission and the attempt to gain the public's trust as a health care provider.

PROFESSIONAL PEARL

Leadership begins with one's values. Leaders of character stay where they are valued, where they grow, and where they are respected. It is my goal to create such an environment by being a good listener, understanding my people, being creative in positive problem solving, and making sure that everyone in the organization feels a significant part in the process. Leaders of character get what they want when they help others get what they need.

—Julie Max, the first female president of NATA (2000-2004), 2006 Hall of Fame Inductee, and co-head athletic trainer at California State University, Fullerton, Calif.

FOUNDATIONAL BEHAVIORS OF PROFESSIONAL PRACTICE AND PROFESSIONAL VALUES

Until one believes what s/he does is best or right, behavior will be marked by inconsistencies and tensions that accompanies the need to decide the right thing to do with insufficient information.[7]

The fourth edition of the *Athletic Training Educational Competencies* underscores the importance of foundational behaviors of professional practice.[14] Given that knowledge informs behavior, the cognitive competence in professional role and responsibility, as outlined in Table 11-2, channels the professional in training to act in an appropriate manner. Foundational behaviors of professional practice are further refined, distinguished, and guided by professional values stemming from the NATA Code of Ethics (Figure 11-4).

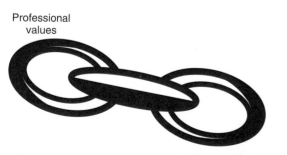

Professional values

Foundational behaviors of professional practice

Figure 11-4 ■ Professional values are linked to foundational behaviors of professional practice.

Professional and reflective practice experiences continue to distill foundational behaviors. Over time, the distinct identity of the athletic training professional is conveyed through consistent patterns of foundational behaviors of professional practice.

Table 11-2 outlines seven significant foundational behaviors relative to professional practice. The foundational behaviors are further delineated into specific cognitive and psychomotor learning objectives. Thus knowledge informs behavior. Professionals in training are expected to further refine the foundational behaviors during professional practice as certified athletic trainers. Perhaps the most important aspect of the foundational behaviors of professional practice is their capacity to foster trust.[7] Box 11-3 defines and underscores the importance of trust.

The intersection of professional values and behaviors is the NATA Code of Ethics, which embodies professional values-based behaviors.[7] Like many professional codes, the NATA Code of Ethics is a mixture of what may be called rules of etiquette and professional courtesy as well as rules about matters of deep ethical concern. In essence, the code reflects implicit values through explicit principles, as revealed in Box 11-4. Furthermore, the Code of Ethics unifies the professional conduct of a culturally diverse membership with differing moral philosophies.[23] A code of ethics is considered one of the hallmarks of a profession.

Although professional values are implicit, professional values–based behaviors are transparent,

---

Box 11-3

TRUST AND TRUSTWORTHINESS

Trustworthiness is not an inner character trait or self-involved interest in being a good person; trust and trustworthiness are not generic virtues that can be developed without context and then applied to practice. To be trustworthy means to meet others with a relational focus with attentiveness and responsiveness that can lead to many different actions, of which truth telling and promise keeping are only two possibilities.

From Day LJ, Stannard D: Developing trust and connection with patients and their families, *Crit Care Nurse* 19:66-71, 1999.

Table 11-2 FOUNDATIONAL BEHAVIORS OF PROFESSIONAL PRACTICE	
Foundational Behaviors	**Cognitive and Psychomotor Learning Objectives**
Primacy of the patient	• Recognize sources of conflict of interest that can affect the patient's health • Know and apply commonly accepted standards for patient confidentiality • Provide the best health care available for the patient • Advocate for the needs of the patient
Teamed approach to practice	• Recognize unique skills and abilities of other health care professionals • Understand the scope of practice of other health care professionals • Understand and execute duties within the identified scope of practice for athletic trainers • Include the patient (and family, where appropriate) in the decision-making process • Demonstrate the ability to work with others in creating positive patient outcomes
Legal practice	• Practice athletic training in a legally competent manner • Recognize the need to document compliance with laws that govern athletic training • Understand the consequences of violating the laws that govern athletic training
Ethical practice	• Understand and comply with the NATA *Code of Ethics* and the Board of Certification's *Standards of Practice* • Understand the consequences of violating the NATA *Code of Ethics* and the BOC's *Standards of Practice* • Understand and comply with other codes of ethics, as applicable
Advancing knowledge	• Critically examine the body of knowledge in athletic training and related fields • Use evidence-based practice as a foundation for delivery of care • Understand the connection between continuing education and the improvement of athletic training practice • Promote the value of research and scholarship in athletic training • Disseminate new knowledge in athletic training to fellow athletic trainers, patients, other health care professionals, and others as necessary
Cultural competence	• Understand the cultural differences of patients' attitudes and behaviors toward health care • Demonstrate knowledge, attitudes, behaviors, and skills necessary to achieve optimal health outcomes for diverse populations • Demonstrate knowledge, attitudes, behaviors, and skills necessary to work respectfully and effectively with diverse populations and in a diverse work environment
Professionalism	• Advocate for the profession • Demonstrate honesty and integrity • Exhibit compassion and empathy • Demonstrate effective interpersonal communication

predictable over time, and ageless.[26] Thus values-based behavior develops consistency in the foundational behaviors of professional practice and cultivates public trust because it conveys predictability in the professional therapeutic relationship.

PROFESSIONAL VALUES CONFLICT AND TRANSFORMATION

. . . practice requires complex cognitive and interpersonal skills, an extensive knowledge base, and the capacity for improvisational performance, where complex factors including disease state, unique patient and environmental needs, and ethical considerations, are integrated.[23]

Conflict and dilemma are part of the certified athletic trainer's professional life. A certified athletic trainer can use many approaches to resolve conflict. Relative to values conflict, a dilemma exists when two or more competing and contradictory values exist in the deliberation of the right course of action. Such conflict indicates a readiness to start learning beyond the receiving and responding phases of Krathwohl's affective taxonomy. This taxonomy (Table 11-3) is ordered according to the principle of internalization.[7] The goal of all athletic training educational programs is to develop a curriculum that progresses the profes-sional in training toward the last phase of affective development, characterization.

The development of affective competence is important in clinical practice because it facilitates (1) mature interpersonal relationships characterized by sensitive and appropriate communication skills, (2) adherence to the highest standards of the profession, and (3) confidence in knowledge and skills. When values are internalized, characterization becomes apparent and predictable and consistent clinical judg-ments emerge.[5]

Working through a moral dilemma by using a professional values approach determines how patients, athletes, and others *ought* to be treated.[17] A moral con-flict requires the certified athletic trainer to use moral sensitivity and reasoning. Metcalf[12] provides a system-atic way to evaluate a values conflict by using value analysis (Box 11-5).

Processing dilemmas by using a professional values approach facilitates predictability and compe-tence in clinical judgments and decision making. Irving and Snider[10] affirmed that

> Finally, the study and adoption of professional values should include an additional lesson. Stu-dents should be taught appropriate and honor-able ways to resolve the tensions and issues that can be expected to arise between work values and professional values. This is more than a survival technique. It is a cogent method through which reason can be brought to bear in those situations

---

Box 11-4

VALUES IMPLICIT IN THE NATA CODE OF ETHICS

PRINCIPLE 1: Values: respect, caring

Members shall respect the rights, welfare, and dignity of all.

PRINCIPLE 2: Values: social responsibility, accountability

Members shall comply with the laws and regulations governing the practice of athletic training.

PRINCIPLE 3: Values: caring, accountability, excellence

Members shall maintain and promote high standards in their provision of services.

PRINCIPLE 4: Value: integrity

Members shall not engage in conduct that could be construed as a conflict of interest or that reflects negatively on the profession.

Modified from the National Athletic Trainers' Association: *Code of ethics*, Dallas, 2005, National Athletic Trainers' Association, http://www.nata.org/codeofethics/code_of_ethics.pdf. Accessed July 5, 2007.

Table 11-3   KRATHWOHL'S AFFECTIVE TAXONOMY

Stage	Affective Learning Objectives
Receiving	Shows awareness, willingness to hear
Responding	Attends to and reacts to a particular phenomenon
Valuing	Attaches to a particular object, phenomenon, or behavior and ranges from simple acceptance to the more complex state of commitment
Organization	Organizes values into priorities by comparing different values, resolving conflicts between them, and creating a unique value system, ultimately evolving toward a personal and consistent philosophy
Characterization	Has a value system that controls their behavior, which is pervasive, consistent, predictable, and most important, characteristic of the learner

Data from Krathwohl DR, Bloom BS, Masia BB: *Taxonomy of educational objectives: the affective domain, handbook II,* New York, 1964, McKay.

Box 11-5

VALUE ANALYSIS TEACHING METHOD

1. Identify and clarify the value question
2. Assemble purported facts
3. Assess the truth of purported facts
4. Clarify the relevance of the facts
5. Arrive at a tentative value decision
6. Test the value decision

Modified from Metcalf L: *Values education: rationale, strategies and procedure,* Washington, DC, 1971, National Council for the Social Studies.

in which values are threatened. This may well serve the purpose of reducing the perceived polarity between ideal and real professional practice.

SUMMARY

Professional identity is foundational because it conveys unique professional values and identity trust.[5,12,26] Therefore professional awareness of the technical standards, as well as the values and interpersonal skills embedded in the ethical standards relative to professional practice, yield athletic training's distinctive professional identity. Technical standards of professional practice have been articulated in professional programs for many years. The fourth edition of the NATA *Athletic Training Educational Competencies* advances ethical standards by outlining the foundational behaviors of professional practice.[14] What may not be as

transparent are professional values that underpin these foundational behaviors. At best, a glimpse of the professional values is revealed in the NATA Code of Ethics. However, the implicit nature of the values woven into the code may lead to multiple interpretations. Over time, confusion and misunderstandings relative to professional values may emerge.

Today, the inherent characteristics embedded into the ethical standards of the profession are being passed down from one generation of professionals to another generation by word of mouth through the socialization process. Because of the significant increase in the number of certified athletic trainers over the last 2 decades, consideration should be given to an explicit and formalized approach in the communication of the profession's distinctive attributes so that one singular professional identity is conveyed to the next generation and, in turn, to the public.

Preliminary research relative to professional values suggests that truth/honesty, integrity, respect, accountability, caring, and excellence are important values to a certified athletic trainer. Given that values drive behavior, professional values are firmly linked to the foundational behaviors of professional practice.

In the next section, attention turns to the second component that fortifies ethical standards, namely, interpersonal skills in the professional therapeutic relationship. Important considerations of this type of relationship include cultural sensitivity and boundary issues. Public trust hinges on the combined elements of technical and ethical standards.

REFERENCES

1. American Association of Colleges of Nursing: *Essentials of college and university education for professional nursing,* Washington, DC, 1986, American Association of Colleges of Nursing.
2. American Physical Therapy Association: *The APTA vision sentence for physical therapy 2020 and APTA vision statement for physical therapy 2020* (website): www.apta.org/AM/Template.cfm?Section=Policies_and_Bylaws&TEMPLATE=/CM/ContentDisplay.cfm&CONTENTID=36073. Accessed July 9, 2007.
3. Beauchamp TL, Childress JF: *Principles of biomedical ethics,* New York, 2001, Oxford University Press.
4. Clark C: The professional socialization of graduating students in generic and two-plus-two baccalaureate completion in nursing programs, *J Nurs Educ* 43:346-352, 2004.
5. Clark PG: Values in health care professional socialization: implications for geriatric education in interdisciplinary teamwork, *Gerontologist* 37:441-452, 1997.
6. Cromie JE, Robertson VJ, Best MO: Work-related musculoskeletal disorders and the culture of physical therapy, *Phys Ther* 82:459-473, 2002.
7. Davis CM: Affective education for the health care professions, *Phys Ther* 61:1587-1593, 1981.
8. Day LJ, Stannard D: Developing trust and connection with patients and their families, *Crit Care Nurse* 19:66-71, 1999.
9. Garret TM: *Health care ethics principles and problems,* Englewood Cliffs, NJ, 1993, Prentice-Hall.
10. Irving JA, Snider J: Legal and ethical issues: preserving professional values, *J Prof Nurs* 18:5, 2002.

11. Malasarm R, Bloom GA, Crumpton R: The development of expert male National Collegiate Athletic Association Division I certified athletic trainers, *J Athl Train* 37:55-63, 2002.

12. Metcalf L: *Values education: rationale, strategies and procedure,* Washington, DC, 1971, National Council for the Social Studies.

13. National Athletic Trainers' Association: *Code of ethics,* Dallas, 2005, National Athletic Trainers' Association (website): www. nata.org/codeofethics/code_of_ethics.pdf. Accessed July 5, 2007.

14. National Athletic Trainers' Association: *Athletic trainer educational competencies,* ed 4, Dallas, 2006, National Athletic Trainers' Association.

15. Olthius G: Professional competence and palliative care: an ethical perspective, *J Palliative Care* 19:192-198, 2003.

16. Professional Baseball Athletic Trainers Society: Ray Ramirez, New York Mets head athletic trainer: combining family and culture in athletic training, *The Annual Publication of the Professional Baseball Athletic Trainers Society* 19(1), 2006.

17. Purtilo R: *Ethical dimensions in the health care setting,* ed 4, Philadelphia, 2005, Saunders.

18. Raths LE, Harmin M, Simon S: *Values and teaching,* Columbus, Ohio, 1978, Charles E. Merrill.

19. Schlabach GA, Peer KS: *Professional values: the comparison between program directors and head athletic trainers in CAATE accredited athletic training education program in the Great Lakes Athletic Trainers' Association.* Presented at the Athletic Trainers' Education Conference, Jan. 12-14, 2007, Dallas, TX.

20. Schlabach GA, Peer KS: *The value of professional ethics,* presented at the GLATA Annual Meeting and Symposium, March 8-10, St Charles, Ill., 2007.

21. Schrader J: Professionalism, one member's perspective, *NATA News* 9:1, 1997.

22. Sieglar MA: Professional values in modern clinical practice, *Hastings Ctr Rep* 30:S19-S23, 2000.

23. Sisola S: Moral reasoning as a predictor of clinical practice: the development of physical therapy students across the professional curriculum, *J Phys Ther Educ* 14:26-35, 2000.

24. Thompson C: Editorial: Once certified, always competent, *J Athl Train* 35:17-18, 2000.

25. Weis D, Schank MJ: An instrument to measure professional nursing values, *J Nurs Scholarship* 32:201-205, 2000.

26. Weis D, Schank MJ: Professional values: key to professional development, *J Prof Nurs* 18:271-275, 2002.

27. Wilson SC: *The perception of values and the process of professional socialization through classroom experiences among baccalaureate nursing students* [dissertation], 1995, Ball State University, Muncie, Ind.

CHAPTER 12

The Professional Therapeutic Relationship

LEARNING OBJECTIVES

After reading this chapter, the student should be
able to do the following:

1. Define trust, and compare it to identity trust.
2. Discuss how professional socialization develops
   professional identity.
3. Describe the role of the socializing agent in the
   development of professional identity.
4. Explain the fiduciary relationship and discuss
   how it is influenced by trust.
5. List important interpersonal skills that have
   been identified in the athletic training literature.
6. Define culture.
7. Discuss the ethnocentric perspective, and
   explain how it may express itself in an athletic
   training room.
8. Briefly describe the history of athletic training
   from a cultural perspective.
9. Identify important considerations when
   communicating with another person.
10. Describe the boundaries in the fiduciary
    relationship.
11. Discuss some questions that can be asked to
    assess exploitation.
12. Compare the athletic trainer/patient-athlete
    relationship in unstructured and structured
    settings.
13. Describe the notion of sexual harassment.
    Explain Title VII, and compare it to the NATA
    Position Statement on sexual harassment.

Rehabilitation outcomes are greatly enhanced by high satisfaction among patients. Also, third-party reimbursement depends on quality care, which is in keeping with outcomes-based rehabilitation. Equal treatment of athletes is a professional responsibility to which all athletic training professionals should aspire and is identified in the National Athletic Trainers' Association (NATA) Code of Ethics. Treating all athletes with dignity and respect, providing emotional support, and considering each athlete's individual perspective, no matter the sport, are just a few of the strategies to increase satisfaction without increasing staff, supplies, or equipment. (p. 55)[29]

Chapter 11 described the identity of the athletic training professional as evolving from the combination of technical and ethical standards. Professional values and interpersonal skills underpin ethical standards. To build on professional values, the first ethical component, this chapter examines interpersonal skills, the second ethical component communicated in the professional therapeutic relationship.

In the profession of athletic training, trust is at the heart of the professional therapeutic relationship in the provision of services to the patient-athlete. Trust is to have faith in the honesty, integrity, and competence of another person.[5] The essence of values and trust is best expressed by 2004 NATA Hall of Fame inductee Clint Thompson.

PROFESSIONAL PEARL

My tenet has always been to be as effective as possible, as an individual and athletic trainer, to the many different populations of people with whom I dealt. If one is effective, by definition one produces, or is capable of producing, an intended result of having a striking effect.

While we are all less than perfect, a true awareness of one's value system will put us in a position to evaluate our decisions when dealing with others. One's values are the bedrock of consistency in dealing with those whom we come in contact. If those values do not include an overwhelming number of moral values (e.g., truth, honesty, loyalty, responsible citizenship, excellence, promise keeping, fairness, respect, accountability, altruism, social responsibility,

aesthetics, caring, integrity), one's effectiveness is less than maximum.

In my mind, consistency leads to trust, a vitally important characteristic that opens the door to maximizing effectiveness. In an intercollegiate athletic training setting, with the multiplicity of populations with which to deal, the demands of being effective require a myriad of ways to communicate with an athlete, a coach, an administrator, a head or assistant athletic trainer, an athletic training student, a physician, a parent, etc. My overt belief in truth, honesty, fairness, respect, integrity, and accountability not only allows me to enjoy a very comfortable daily existence but allowed me to experience a very long and successful career as an athletic trainer.

—Clint Thompson, 2004 NATA Hall of Fame inductee, served as the head athletic trainer for Michigan State University, East Lansing, Michigan, and Colorado State University, Fort Collins, Colorado, and as the program director at Truman State University, Kirksville, Missouri, as well as adjunct clinical professor at the Kirksville College of Osteopathic Medicine, Kirksville, Missouri. He is a previous editor of the *Journal of Athletic Training* and served the profession in countless ways.

The bond between the athletic trainer and the patient-athlete is the professional therapeutic relationship. The primary goal for members of this professional body is to promote healing. The professional therapeutic relationship embodies the belief that no one will be exploited or used for the benefit of another. Trust is fragile; once earned it must continue to be nurtured through consistent patterns of acceptable foundational behaviors of professional practice.[5]

Identity trust is a type of trust that underpins professional identity. Professional identity emerges from being a member of the athletic training profession from whom a patient-athlete expects a certain level of care through predictable and acceptable foundational behaviors of professional practice. The patient-athlete learns identity trust. In other words, healthy relationship experiences with one certified athletic trainer project and establish trust with another certified athletic trainer because trust is based on the athletic training identity—that is, professional identity. Thus identity trust is extremely important because it is a reflection of the culture of the athletic training profession and all that it stands for in its delivery of health care services.

Socialization is the developmental process in which students gain insight into the identity and internalize the distinctive qualities of the certified athletic trainer. The area of professional socialization in the health care disciplines was initiated in the 1960s when social psychologists studied adult socialization and focused specifically on medical education.[12] Health care continued to explore other equally important aspects of professional socialization (e.g., attitudes, values, and beliefs). Socialization develops and advances professional identity through the interaction of the certified athletic trainer with the patient-athlete in the practice setting.[27] Socialization stage theory suggests three developmental stages: (1) the anticipatory, exploratory phase; (2) the professional, formal education phase; and (3) the organizational, practice-setting phase.[15,21]

Socializing agents influence professional identity formation. For example, socializing agents impart a sense of professional distinctiveness by modeling technical and ethical standards that are exclusive to members of the profession.[2,28] Because each health care profession socializes new members differently, the agent, who socializes the promising athletic training student into the profession, should be able to convey the technical and ethical standards of a certified athletic trainer accurately. Intuitively, the agent should be an experienced certified athletic trainer to impart an authentic professional understanding to the promising student as he or she transitions to the professional role.

Socialization is a dynamic and interactive developmental process and encourages identify formation. As tensions, uncertainty, and dilemmas surface, reflection ensues, experience manifests, practice changes, learning takes place, awareness dawns, and new opportunities to rework one's professional identity are presented. Like a clay sculpture, professional identity is a piece of work that gets remolded and reshaped and reworked over the lifespan of a professional's career by refining adequacy and practice. The process of reworking identity and norms of practice is both reflective and dynamic.[27] It becomes more efficient with each new iteration.[14] The attainment of new experiences in a variety of work-related environments allows the professional to learn, mature, and develop increased levels of adequacy. Furthermore, the degree to which a new experience reshapes the professional depends on the length of professional engagement and the amount of time devoted to critical reflection. The reflective prac-

titioner enjoys grappling with moral dilemmas and those gray areas that create the uncertainty, ambiguity, insecurity, and tension of professional practice.[2]

PROFESSIONAL PEARL

Give people the gift of your time. Be willing to listen to people and hear what they say. Be attentive when someone is talking to you. Put down what you are doing and give him or her your complete attention. Maintain eye contact and make that person understand he or she matters to you.

—Kathy Schniedwind, 2004 NATA Hall of Fame inductee, worked at Illinois State University in Normal, Illinois, for 30 years. Schniedwind climbed through the ranks to become head athletic trainer halfway through her career. "Schnied," as her friends call her, has diligently served the profession in many ways, including serving on the National Collegiate Athletic Association Competitive Safeguards Committee, the Research and Education Foundation board, and the NATA College/University Athletic Training Student Committee.

INTERPERSONAL SKILLS

The point at which professional values, morals, and ethical principles meet is the nurse-client relationship.[26]

The interpersonal skills involved in the relationship between the certified athletic trainer and the patient-athlete and other colleagues require appropriate verbal and nonverbal behaviors. To reiterate and underscore, trust is the essential factor in the professional therapeutic relationship evolving from a feeling of faith and confidence. In medicine, the trusting relationship is the fiduciary relationship that a doctor establishes with a patient.[20] By extension, the relationship that an athletic trainer develops with the patient-athlete is fiduciary as well and is referred to as the professional therapeutic relationship.

Trust can be described as a relationship among people that consists of truth, honesty, and consistency relative to competent care.[3] The power differential between the athletic trainer and the patient-athlete cannot be overlooked, which puts the patient-athlete in a vulnerable position. In the athletic setting, the athlete's ability to return to play is largely based on the certified athletic trainer's evaluation of the situation. Interpersonal skills are critical in conveying honest, accurate, and reliable information to the patient-athlete to ensure competent care. Box 12-1 highlights

IMPORTANT INTERPERSONAL SKILLS

Maintain an atmosphere that allows expression of opinions.
Encourage people to feel free to ask questions.
Convey an open, approachable demeanor.
Be accessible.
Exhibit a genuine interest.
Demonstrate confidence.
Provide support and encouragement.
Form appropriate and professional relationships.
Appropriately advocate for the patient-athlete.
Demonstrate respect for culturally diverse patient-athletes.

Modified from Weidner TG, Henning JM: Development of standards and criteria for the selection, training, and evaluation of athletic training approved clinical instructors, *J Athl Train* 39:335-44, 2004, and Lauber CA, Toth PE, Leary PA, et al: Program directors' and clinical instructors' perceptions of important clinical-instructor behavior categories in the delivery of athletic training clinical instruction, *J Athl Train* 38:336-341, 2003.

important interpersonal skills that have been cited in the athletic training literature.[13,32]

The certified athletic trainer must always be committed to the patient-athlete's well-being and promote his or her interests regardless of financial arrangements, the health care setting, and other potentially discriminating factors. In short, the certified athletic trainer is in a position of trust and must not compromise the professional therapeutic relationship.

CONSIDERATIONS OF THE PATIENT-ATHLETE/CERTIFIED ATHLETIC TRAINER RELATIONSHIP

Culture

In the 1990s the United States became the most culturally diverse nation in the world. The shift toward a more ethnically diverse population has driven the need to develop culturally competent health care professionals. Educational programs of study in medicine and health care often instruct by using Western, Eurocentric ideologies. This unicultural understanding leads to narrow-mindedness and an ethnocentric approach—a belief in the superiority of one's own cultural group.[9,23]

Culture refers to the shared values, beliefs, traditions, customs, and practices of a particular group. Different cultures have different value systems. Awareness of cultural values helps attain positive health outcomes as well as instill public trust.[9,11,23]

GOOD TO KNOW

Ethnocentrism

Because of the amount of cultural diversity surrounding and within human societies, the belief of individuals that their culture is the best is not uncommon. However, attempting to understand why cultural diversity exists would be more beneficial, as would be attempting to understand what the differences are in any group (cultural diversity). However, simply because someone is from a particular cultural group does not necessarily mean that he or she has the same cultural beliefs as the group.

In the United States, sick people may see a doctor, but in other countries or other groups in the United States, sick people may see an herbalist, shaman, or homeopath. For some, using two health care systems at the same time can be beneficial. For example: a returning athlete tells you he injured his shoulder over the summer and one of his parents, who is from Mexico, wanted him to see the *curandera* (a healer). The athlete participated in specific treatment given by the healer. The other parent took him in to have radiographs taken (typical Western medicine). You can tell the athlete feels caught between two worlds, especially when he states his shoulder is still sore. How do you handle this?[25]

Even though an individual is part of a certain culture (e.g., Italian, Irish, African-American), he or she also may become part of a subcultural group (college student), where the norms of the subculture may be quite different from the main culture. For example, a college student leaves her home in the southern part of the United States and goes to school in the north. She calls all individuals older than her Miss or Sir, because it is a sign of respect in the south, but she no longer eats the same type of food she ate at home.

Historically, athletic trainers were predominantly white, male professionals employed by a university who treated predominantly white, male student athletes. Two significant federal mandates caused cultural changes in the athletic training: (1) desegregation and civil rights in the 1960s and (2) Title IX, Education Amendments of 1972. Thus, as with society as a whole, the profession had to come to terms with multifaceted humanistic, political, and sociocultural issues. Paul Geisler, ATC, writes:

Athletic trainers working in the clinical and industrial settings have perhaps the most challenging and diverse patient population with which to work. Typically, the patient population at these settings is very diverse—socioeconomically, culturally, educationally, ethnically, and religiously and, as such, different from the young and athletic population seen by many ATCs and athletic training students in the college and university settings. In these contemporary settings, the potential is high for uninitiated athletic training professionals to encounter a sizable proportion of patients who do not speak English as the first language, are immigrants of different status with regard to citizenship, or represent various levels of cultural and linguistic illiteracy. Because of the difficult life experiences that many marginalized people and so-called blue-collar workers have encountered, many patients encountered in these settings may be disillusioned and disheartened about their social status and promise for social advancement. This feeling of resignation can often be accompanied by a strong, inherent distrust of those people in positions of authority, knowledge, and power-college-educated professionals in particular. Establishing a trusting relationship with these patients, especially for white, male ATCs, can oftentimes be difficult, painful, and nonproductive. Being aware of, and exposed to, the culture of whiteness and the perspectives of the marginalized others who exist in society and having the confidence to confront these issues are critical components of the daily working lives for ATCs in the clinical and industrial settings. Medical schools and physical therapy education programs have certainly realized the importance of this complex pedagogic and social phenomenon, and with the recent evolutionary trends in our profession, so too must athletic training education programs.[8]

Certified athletic trainers need to become effective in managing the issues surrounding race, class, ethnic, sex, sexual orientation, and religious diversity. As a profession, athletic trainers must demonstrate cultural competence to ensure public trust.

GOOD TO KNOW

A lack of communication can lead to misunderstanding and a lack of respect for persons whose cultural values are different from one's own.

The following are some keys to communication:

1. Determine if the patient-athlete is fluent in English or if an interpreter is needed.
2. Ask how the patient-athlete would prefer to be addressed.
3. Speak directly to the patient-athlete, but be aware that certain cultures are patriarchal and the male makes the final decision.
4. Avoid slang or technical terms, which may be misunderstood or not understood.
5. Use open-ended questions to give the patient the opportunity to give you as much information as possible.
6. Be aware that in certain cultures making eye contact is not appropriate.
7. Determine the reading ability of your patient-athlete before you send him or her home with written information about treatment.
8. Be aware of the language you use and the jokes you make, which could be offensive in different cultures or to the opposite sex.

Boundaries

In particular, legal and ethical behavior . . . [is] considered the most important, applicable, and crucial. . . . [U]nsatisfactory legal and ethical behavior would justify eliminating the ACI from the clinical education program.[33]

Boundaries are the limits of fiduciary, therapeutic relationships. In all types of structured athletic training settings, power differentials exist between the certified athletic trainer and the patient-athlete. Obviously the injured patient-athlete is vulnerable and the certified athletic trainer assumes a position of power in his or her role as the health care provider and must maintain the professional therapeutic relationship. Intimate relationships have the potential to be exploitive relationships.[24] The health care provider must avoid an intimate relationship with the patient. The certified athletic trainer must maintain the professional therapeutic relationship and not cross boundaries. Questions in Box 12-2 are useful in evaluating the professional therapeutic relationship.[20,21]

Debate exists regarding whether a health care provider can or ought to have an intimate relationship with a patient-athlete after care has been given and the professional therapeutic relationship no longer exists. Two polar thoughts on this subject exist in health care: that such an act is ethical and unethical.[24] Obviously, this issue presents two extreme views. Any emotional issue always has a middle ground, and some suggest a waiting period of 6 months at termination of therapy. Some professionals have argued that waiting minimizes the potential for exploitation.

Without a doubt, intimate relationships are complex. The ethics become even murkier when the relationship is between a certified athletic trainer and patient-athlete and when disparity exists in power, status, and emotional defenselessness. To determine the ethics or nonethics of an intimate relationship with a former patient/athlete, the certified athletic trainer should consider the questions outlined in Box 12-2. Moreover, this issue becomes further clouded when the relationship involves the promising athletic training *college* student and *college* patient-athlete. The best advise is to always follow the rules and regulations of the athletic training facility. And when in doubt, seek counseling from an immediate supervisor and/or human resources representative.[24]

Fiduciary Relationships in Practice Settings

Certified athletic trainers work in structured and not-so-structured environments, usually determined by the practice setting. For example, hospitals and clinics

---

Box 12-2

ASSESSING EXPLOITATION: QUESTIONS TO CONSIDER IN THE PROFESSIONAL THERAPEUTIC RELATIONSHIP

Does the patient-athlete seem vulnerable?

Is the age difference between the athletic trainer and the former patient-athlete substantial?

Is the patient-athlete considerably poorer or less educated than the athletic trainer?

Does the patient-athlete have significant psychiatric or psychological problems?

Does the patient-athlete have problems with substance abuse?

Has the patient-athlete been the victim of abuse, especially sexual abuse?

Is the patient-athlete particularly lonely or extremely shy?

Is the patient-athlete suffering from a recent separation or divorce, death of a loved one, or economic difficulty?

Is the patient-athlete undergoing psychological adjustment to a significant illness or injury?

Is the certified athletic trainer's behavior consistent with the NATA Standards of Practice and the NATA Code of Ethics?

Is the certified athletic trainer considering the patient-athlete's needs as the top priority, or could a conflict exist between the certified athletic trainer's needs and the client's needs?

Would the certified athletic trainer want other people to know about this behavior or interaction with the patient-athlete?

Would the certified athletic trainer support another certified athletic trainer having the same relationship with the patient-athlete?

Could the certified athletic trainer be using the patient-athlete to meet personal needs for social support or financial gain?

Is the certified athletic trainer preoccupied with the patient-athlete?

Is the certified athletic trainer perceived to be giving preferential care to the patient-athlete?

Modified from Sisola SW: Patient vulnerability: ethical considerations for physical therapists, *Phys Ther* 11:46-51, 2003, and RNABC: RNABC policy statement: nurse-client relationships: establishing professional relationships and maintaining appropriate boundaries, *Nurs BC* 33(11):13, 2001.

typically are considered structured settings, with little social engagement and many rules and regulations, whereas athletic training rooms at the high school, college, and professional levels are less-structured settings and could be described as social, with fewer rules and regulations. The structure of the environment is an important aspect when examining the notion of relationship with the patient-athlete.

Given that the less-structured athletic training settings reflect a more relaxed environment and may appear to be social in nature, mixed messages may be conveyed to the athlete. Furthermore, the environment's social nature may be further compounded because certified athletic trainers intentionally strive to develop a social support system so that athletes feel secure while the athletic trainer works to prevent, treat, and rehabilitate athletic injuries.[29] Kidding and joking around are commonly part of the social antics in these settings; however, no one (athlete, athletic training student, and the certified athletic trainer) has the license to be offensive. Balancing the social and professional aspects that facilitate and maintain the fiduciary relationship can be challenging to both the professional in training and the certified athletic trainer in a less-structured setting.[18,24,26]

Furthermore, not-so-structured settings may suggest gray professional boundaries. Certified athletic trainers and athletic training students must be ever vigilant when working with high school– and college-age athletes, who may not display professional matu-

rity. A general rule of thumb to follow is that if one's actions, behaviors, and/or words are offensive to one person in the setting, then they are offensive to one too many (Table 12-1).[16]

Sexual Harassment

Sexual harassment is not uncommon in the health care setting. Violation of sexual boundaries has a devastating result on the professional therapeutic relationship as well as the professional collegial relationship.[19] Trust, that fragile element in all relationships, shatters.[4]

Under Title VII of the Civil Rights Act of 1964, sexual harassment includes unwelcome sexual advances, requests for sexual favors, and other verbal or physical conduct of a sexual nature constitute sexual harassment when (1) submission to such conduct is made either explicitly or implicitly a term or condition of an individual's employment, (2) submission to or rejection of such conduct by an individual is used as the basis for employment decisions affecting such individual, or (3) such conduct has the purpose or effect of unreasonably interfering with an individual's work performance or creating an intimidating, hostile, or offensive working environment that is perceived by the victim to be abusive or hostile.

This encompasses two separate forms of harassment: (1) quid pro quo and (2) hostile environment. Quid pro quo occurs when a power differential exists and a form of harassment involves a situation in which the submission to sexual advances or request is condi-

Table 12-1   EXAMPLES OF INAPPROPRIATE SEXUAL INNUENDOS

Example	Description
Offensive comments	Sexual innuendo; derogatory jokes or remarks; flattering; suggestive remarks on physical appearance; expressions of sexual interest
Inappropriate staring	Leering
Unwelcome touch	Unwelcome kissing; grabbing; fondling; touching breasts or genitals
Unwelcome gifts	Expensive wine; flowers (e.g., red roses on Valentine's Day)
Offensive requests and displays	Requests for inappropriate touch or home or dormitory room visits (disguised as part of therapy)
Unwanted persistent invitations	Repeated requests for dates; unwanted telephone calls at home

Modified from O'Sullivan V, Weerakoon P: Inappropriate sexual behaviours of patients towards practising physiotherapists: a study using qualitative methods, *Physiother Res Int* 4:28-43, 1999.

tional to keeping a job or job benefits. The hostile environment harassment is apparent when the workplace environment is made offensive through sexual innuendo even though no economic loss occurs.[7,30]

GOOD TO KNOW

The Center for Women Policy Studies states that one of every two women will experience sexual harassment at some point in her life.

Sexual harassment can occur even if the behavior is not directed specifically at someone because the behavior creates a hostile work environment.

Simply because the offender says that he or she has been making these comments for years and no one has said anything does not mean the behavior is not sexual harassment. Remember that sexual harassment is something people do not want to admit to or are afraid to talk about.

Can men be sexually harassed? Although 90% of sexual harassment is directed toward women, men have the same protection as women by law.

Sexually explicit material that is visible at work can create a hostile work environment.

The computer has given people an opportunity to send improper jokes and watch pornographic materials at work. Most employers do not allow this.

Sexual harassment can be physical (touching), verbal (unwanted sexual comments), or nonverbal (obscene gestures).

If you are being sexually harassed, tell a supervisor. It is not your fault; the harasser is at fault. Others probably feel just as you do. Practice how to tell someone that what he or she is saying is offensive. Keep a record of the date, time, and exactly what happened. Do not suffer alone.

You can learn more at the Web site for the Human Rights Commission, www.hrc.org.

Violations of Title VII are not just reported by women. In fiscal year 2005, the Equal Employment Opportunity Commission reported that 12% of the 12,679 charges of sexual harassment were made by men.[7] All employees and employers should recognize the steps in preventing sexual harassment (Box 12-3).

Given the social nature of some athletic training settings, boundaries can be blurred. In 1994, the NATA Women in Athletic Training Committee developed a survey to study issues related to certified female athletic trainers; this was followed up 1 year later with a survey designed to examine issues related to certified male athletic trainers. One thousand randomly selected female certified athletic trainers were selected from the NATA database. Thirty-seven percent of the women reported that they had been a victim of sexual harassment in the work setting. In support of this observation, 41% of 1000 randomly selected certified male athletic trainers believed that women were victims of sexual harassment. Since the 1990s, much has been done by the profession to raise awareness of this offense. In fact, Women in Athletic Training developed a sexual harassment brochure to alert the membership about the seriousness of this misdemeanor. The NATA position statement relative to sexual harassment is shown in Box 12-4.[17]

Athletic trainers are social professionals, and they work in a setting that requires patient-athletes to disrobe partially or fully. Because of this, the professional must take measures to ensure that their professional behaviors communicate nothing more than competence and trust. Humor, comments, and/or incidental physical contact can be misconstrued. Sexual harassment is not about *intent,* but rather *perception.* So even if the certified athletic trainer had no intention of being offensive, that does not matter in a court of law. As athletic trainers know, prevention is the first step in addressing this serious offense.[31]

SUMMARY

Professional values and interpersonal skills unite to create the ethical standards in athletic training and are evidenced in the NATA Code of Ethics and conveyed in foundational behaviors of professional practice. Moreover, as professional awareness becomes transparent, engagement in the professional therapeutic relationship reveals the importance of the establishment

Box 12-3

STEPS EMPLOYERS CAN TAKE TO AVOID SEXUAL HARASSMENT LAWSUITS

1. If your company does not have a sexual harassment or discrimination policy, get one fast! The policy should communicate that the company takes a "zero tolerance" approach toward sexual harassment. Have an attorney review it, and ensure it gets distributed to all your employees either through the employee handbook or in memo form. Have the employees sign a form to acknowledge that they received and read the policy. The policy should be verbally communicated to all new employees and can even be posted in the workplace. If you have employees whose primary language is not English, have the sexual harassment policy translated or communicate to them in their primary language.

2. Provide different routes that employees can take to file complaints, such as calling a hotline, contacting the human resource department, or contacting their supervisor. Also, the employee should have the option of talking with a male or female company representative.

3. Conduct sexual harassment training, even if it is only composed of reading material or watching a videotape; something is better then no training at all.

4. Conduct yearly meetings with your supervisors to review the sexual harassment policy and make sure that they understand that an employee does not need to suffer negative consequences to make a claim of sexual harassment. Inform the supervisors that even mild to moderate sexual jokes or statements can create an atmosphere of hostility that will make some employees uncomfortable and lead to the creation of an environment where sexual discrimination could develop. The supervisor should also be directed to always inform upper management of any sexual harassment complaints he or she receives from employees. Supervisors should never promise confidentiality with an employee when the information relates to sexual harassment.

5. Conduct a yearly sexual harassment survey among your employees. The survey can be done anonymously and should be distributed with a copy of the company's sexual harassment policy. The survey can simply ask the employees (male and female) if they have experienced any form of sexual harassment during the past year. Why do a survey? The results of the survey tell a court that your company is actively engaged in preventing and correcting sexual harassment. Remember, the Supreme Court has recently determined that employers can be held liable for incidents of sexual harassment that they are unaware of. So, one method of defense, if necessary, can be to demonstrate to the court or a jury that your company conducts yearly meetings with supervisors and also conducts a yearly sexual harassment survey to attempt to uncover sexual harassment violations before they cause problems for your employees.

6. Conduct investigations promptly and thoroughly. After the dispute is resolved, a follow-up should be done with the employee to ensure that no one has suffered retaliation. Make sure your sexual harassment policy spells out clearly that retaliation against an employee filing a sexual harassment complaint is illegal and will not be tolerated.

7. Treat same-sex harassment, and men reporting harassment, the same as you would for a woman reporting her male supervisor being sexually inappropriate.

8. Always document the results of any sexual harassment complaint or investigation. Also document any corrective action that you asked the employee or supervisor to take. Follow up on any corrective action so you can document if the employee fails to take advantage of your company's polices and procedures or any corrective action that your company takes to prevent the sexual harassment from occurring again in the future.

9. Inform all employees that they are obligated to report sexual harassment that they experience or witness.

From Employer-Employee.com: *Sexual harassment and discrimination,* (website): www.employer-employee.com/sexhar1.htm. Accessed April 19, 2006.

Box 12-4

NATA POSITION STATEMENT ON SEXUAL HARASSMENT

Workplace Discrimination and Harassment

Equal opportunity in the workplace means that the workplace is free of both discrimination and harassment. Workplace discrimination occurs when an employment decision is made on the basis of race, color, gender, creed, religion, national origin, age, gender (including pregnancy), disability, veteran/military status or any other status protected by law. Workplace harassment occurs when there is unwelcome conduct based on the protected categories noted above; the harassment may create a hostile work environment (which means that a reasonable person finds the environment hostile) or may be a quid pro quo situation (where a benefit or detriment is conditioned on submission to the offensive conduct). Equal opportunity also means that the workplace is free from retaliation for reporting or participating in investigations of discrimination and harassment

Additional information about this subject is available at the Web site maintained by the Equal Employment Opportunity Commission that can be found at www.eeoc.gov.

NATA encourages its members to create and maintain workplaces free of discrimination and harassment and to report any unlawful behavior to the appropriate parties at their workplace.

From the National Athletic Trainers' Association, www.nata.org/index.htm.

of trust between the patient-athlete and certified athletic trainer. Trust matters with every patient-athlete, with every colleague, and with every student. It is fragile; once trust is earned, it needs to be nourished through continuous attention and consistent patterns of verbal and nonverbal behaviors that reflect competent skills of professional practice. Boundaries of the professional therapeutic relationship can at times be gray. Crossing the boundary in a professional therapeutic relationship is forbidden. Awareness of boundaries helps the promising student realize potential practice dangers and opportunities to prevent such an occurrence. Furthermore, attentiveness to the foundational behaviors of professional practice facilitates proficiency within the ethical framework of professional practice.

Athletic training students should regularly take time to immerse themselves fully into challenging learning experiences, whether related to the classroom or athletic training setting. This involves devoted reflection and examination of athletic training issues through a number of perspectives. Regular reflective activity cultivates important professional skills such as independence, leadership, critical thinking, commitment, communication, personal management, collaboration, and professional distinctiveness.[1,6,12] In short, being a competent professional is a lifelong process, eventually morphing into a well-defined distinctiveness and a resolute commitment to the profession.[10]

REFERENCES

1. Bruhn JB: Being good and doing good: the culture of professionalism in the health professions, *Health Care Manag* 19:47-59, 2001.
2. Clark P: Values in health care professional socialization: implications for geriatric education in interdisciplinary teamwork, *Gerontologist* 37:441-452, 1997.
3. Cruess RL, Cruess SR, Johnston SE: Professionalism and medicine's social contract, *J Bone Joint Surg* 82:1189-1195, 2000.
4. Davidhizar R, Erdel S, Dowd S: Sexual harassment: where to draw the line, *Nurs Manag* 29:40-44, 1998.
5. Day L: Stannard D: Developing trust and connection with patients and their families, *Crit Care Nurse* 19:66-71, 1999.
6. du Toit DD: A sociological analysis of the extent and influence of professional socialization on the development of a nursing

identity among nursing students at two universities in Brisbane, Australia, *J Adv Nurs* 21:164-171, 1995.
7. Employer-Employee.com: *Sexual harassment and discrimination* (website): www.employer-employee.com/sexhar1.htm. Accessed April 19, 2006.
8. Geisler P: Multiculturalism and athletic training education: implications for educational and professional progress, *J Athl Train* 38:141-155, 2003.
9. Gray DP, Thomas D: Chapter 15: critical analysis of "culture" in nursing literature: implications for nursing education in the United States, *Ann Rev Nurs Educ* 3:249-273, 2005.
10. Hewson K, Friel K: A unique preclinical experience: concurrent mock and pro bono clinics to enhance student readiness, *J Phys Ther Educ* 18:80-87, 2004.

11. Jones MJ, Bond ML, Cason CL: Where does culture fit in outcome management? *J Nurs Care Quality* 13:41-51, 1998.

12. Koenig K, Johnson C, Morano CK, et al: Development and validation of professional behavior assessment, *J Allied Health* 32:86-94, 2003.

13. Lauber CA, Toth PE, Leary PA, et al: Program directors' and clinical instructors' perceptions of important clinical-instructor behavior categories in the delivery of athletic training clinical instruction, *J Athl Train* 38:336-341, 2003.

14. MacIntosh JA: *Reworking professional identity: processes and perceptions of experienced nurses* [dissertation], 2002, The University of New Brunswick, New Brunswick, NS, Canada.

15. Mensch J, Crews C, Mitchell M: Competing perspectives during organizational socialization on the role of certified athletic trainers in high school settings, *J Athl Train* 40:333-341, 2005.

16. Murray M: From humor to harassment: how context changes everything, *Athl Ther Today* 10:38-39, 2005.

17. National Athletic Trainers' Association: *Women in athletic training survey* (website): www.nata.org/members1/committees/watc/watc_membersurvey/watc_membersurvey/surveywomen.htm. Accessed April 17, 2006.

18. O'Sullivan V, Weerakoon P: Inappropriate sexual behaviours of patients towards practising physiotherapists: a study using qualitative methods, *Physiother Res Int* 4:28-43, 1999.

19. Pehrson KL: Boundary issues in clinical practice as reported by Army social workers, *Mil Med* 167:14-23, 2002.

20. Pellegrino E, Thomasma D: *The virtues in medical practice,* New York, 1993, Oxford University Press.

21. Pitney WA: The professional socialization of certified athletic trainers in high school settings: a grounded theory investigation, *J Athl Train* 37:286-293, 2002.

22. RNABC: RNABC policy statement: nurse-client relationships: establishing professional relationships and maintaining appropriate boundaries, *Nurs BC* 33:11-13, 2001.

23. Shaw-Taylor Y, Benesch B: Workforce diversity and cultural competence in healthcare, *J Cultural Diversity* 5:138-147, 1998.

24. Sisola SW: Patient vulnerability: ethical considerations for physical therapists, *Phys Ther* 11:46-51, 2003.

25. Spector RE: *Cultural diversity in health and illness,* ed 6, Upper Saddle River, NJ, 2004, Prentice Hall.

26. Steckler J: Examination of ethical practice in nursing continuing education using the Husted model, *Adv Pract Nurs Q* 4:59-65, 1998.

27. Stiller C: Exploring the ethos of the physical therapy profession in the United States: social, cultural, and historical influences and relationship to education, *J Phys Ther Educ* 14:7-17, 2000.

28. Teschendorf B, Nemshick M: Faculty roles in professional socialization, *J Phys Ther Educ* 15:4-11, 2001.

29. Unruh S, Unruh N, Moorman M, et al: Collegiate student-athletes' satisfaction with athletic trainers, *J Athl Train* 40:52-56, 2005.

30. US Equal Employment Opportunity Commission: *Title VII of the Civil Rights Act of 1964* (website): www.eeoc.gov/policy/vii.html. Accessed April 17, 2006.

31. Velasquez BJ: Sexual harassment: a concern for the athletic trainer, *J Athl Train* 33:171-177, 1998.

32. Weidner TG, Henning JM: Development of standards and criteria for the selection, training, and evaluation of athletic training approved clinical instructors, *J Athl Train* 39:335-344, 2004.

33. Weidner TG, Henning JM: Importance and applicability of approved clinical instructor standards and criteria to certified athletic trainers in different clinical education settings, *J Athl Train* 40:326-333, 2005.

CHAPTER 13

The Development of Moral Behavior: Step 2—Moral Reasoning

LEARNING OBJECTIVES

After reading this chapter, the student should be able to do the following:

1. Define moral reasoning.
2. Describe the three stages of Kohlberg's theory of moral reasoning.
3. Explain some of the concerns that have been raised about Kohlberg's theory.
4. Identify another name for Kohlberg's postconventional, just-orientation approach and explain its focus.
5. Define principles and describe how they are used in athletic training.
6. Describe principle-based ethics.
7. Compare absolute duties to prima facie duties.
8. Describe Beauchamp and Childress's principle-based approach.
9. Discuss and compare the four prima facie principles, substantive rules, authority rules, and procedural rules.
10. Describe Beauchamp and Childress's reflective equilibrium.

In Chapter 9, the first step in Triezenberg and Davis's[27] three-step model of moral behavior, moral sensitivity, was examined. The next step in the development of moral behavior is moral reasoning (Figure 13-1).

Moral reasoning is the ability to make judgments based on standards of right and wrong.[14] This type of reasoning seems to improve with age and education. An understanding of Kohlberg's moral development theory sheds light on the notion of moral reasoning.

MORAL DEVELOPMENT

The fact that man knows right from wrong proves his intellectual superiority to other creatures; but the fact that he can do wrong proves his moral inferiority to any creature that cannot.
—MARK TWAIN

As the child matures, the development of a system of values, ideas, and attitudes advances to help the individual do good and right. Moral development cultivates this awareness.

As part of professional preparation, the athletic training student will be inspired by educators, mentors, and friends.[17] Accordingly, the student's technical and ethical competence, along with foundational behaviors of professional practice, will be influenced and cultivated to reflect acceptable professional insight, skill, and behavior distinctive of a certified athletic trainer. Although the technical standards encompassing the athletic training knowledge and clinical skills may be readily apparent to the promising student, ethical standards consisting of values and interpersonal skills may appear vague.

Well before the student enrolls in an athletic training education program (ATEP), he or she has been ushered into the stages of moral development, which entails a systematic maturation of attitudes, beliefs, and values that determine right from wrong and good from bad. Family and religion largely influence a child's personal morality.[15]

A number of perspectives examine moral development, such as clinical psychology, cognitive-development psychology, social learning theory, and social psychology. The most widely recognized theory on moral development in the health care professions is presented by the cognitive psychologist Lawrence Kohlberg. The stages of Kohlberg's moral development explain moral reasoning. Kohlberg believed that cognitive development is a co-requisite to moral development and draws on Piaget's theory of cognitive development.[6,8]

Piaget's Cognitive Theory

Piaget's cognitive theory relating to moral development suggests a two-stage, age-related maturation. Before the age of 10 or 11 years, children view rules as fixed and absolute, handed down by adults and/or some supreme spiritual being. Younger children tend to make moral judgments based on expected consequences. After age 10 or 11 years, children view rules as relative and used to instill cooperation among adults. The older group understands that rules are not sacred and can change, if everyone agrees. Moral judgment in older children gives significant consideration to intent.[6]

Kohlberg's Theory

Kohlberg's theory of moral development embraced the work of Piaget and extended it to examine adolescence by studying boys at the age of 10, 13, and 16 years from middle and lower-class communities in Chicago.[26] The theory suggests that moral reasoning is age related. Kohlberg identified three levels of moral development, with each level containing two stages.

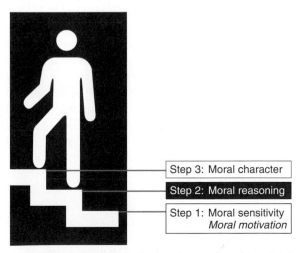

Step 3: Moral character

Step 2: Moral reasoning

Step 1: Moral sensitivity
Moral motivation

Figure 13-1 ■ Moral behavior is a three-step model; step 2 is moral reasoning.

- Level I: preconventional (ages 2 to 7 years)
  - Stage 1, obedience and punishment stage: denotes that rules are to be obeyed or a punishment will occur.
  - Stage 2, individualism and exchange stage: suggests that "if you scratch my back, I will scratch your back." This stage is characterized by a realization that no single right way is handed down by authorities.
- Level II: conventional (ages 7 to 12 years)
  - Stage 3, interpersonal relationships: reflects an interest in good behavior by conforming to expectations to gain approval.
  - Stage 4, the maintenance of social order: focuses on rules, duties, and respect for authority. Many adults do not develop beyond this level, according to Kohlberg.
- Level III: postconventional (ages 12 years and older). During this stage, individuals lead autonomous lives based on personal moral principles.
  - Stage 5, individual rights and social contract: reflects a need to examine what society ought to value.
  - Stage 6, universal principles: centers on universal principles of justice and human rights.

Kohlberg's theory of moral development evolves from self-centered observations of right and wrong (stages 1 and 2) and advances to the acknowledgement of duty and social responsibility (stages 3 and 4). Many do not move beyond stage 4 of moral development. Individuals who progress into stages 5 and 6 are competent to recognize principled moral reasoning and advance decisions based on universal principles. At the conventional level, the individual places emphasis on being a good person and conforming to societal expectations. Thus moral development transitions from an egocentric perspective to an altruistic perspective.[6,8,23,26]

Considerations of Kohlberg's Theory

Kohlberg's theory of moral development is not without its critics. Keeping in mind that Kohlberg's initial research study consisted of white male subjects, whether the theory on moral development is cross-culturally validated is unknown. Moreover, the theory appears to be gender related. Carol Gilligan[23] argues that gender influences moral development and contends that girls and women respond to moral problems differently from boys and men. Although Gilligan agrees that girls and women develop similarly in terms of stage complexity, she argues that women examine moral problems through the lens of care and responsibility, as opposed to rules, rights, and abstract universal principles. Thus the "feminist" approach considers moral problems from the consideration of care to a person or group within the perspective of the unique relationship. Although gender and culture appear to be morally relevant factors when dealing with moral issues, the ability to make moral judgments is an attribute that changes over time and is influenced by experience.[17,23]

PRINCIPLED MORAL REASONING

Only principled moral reasoning can clarify and verify the moral truths.
—SIDNEY CALLAHAN[7]

After a year or so of preprofessional experience in the ATEP, during which professional identity is being cultivated, students should begin to examine ethical issues using Kohlberg's postconventional, justice orientation approach to moral reasoning. This approach also is called principled moral reasoning and encourages contemplation about ethical obligations to guide decision making and behaviors. Principled moral reasoning reflects Kohlberg's postconventional reasoning. At this level of moral reasoning, students learn they have an increasing duty to consider obligations, responsibilities, and rights.[2] They must judge and justify a decision regarding an ethical dilemma by using the principled approach to moral reasoning. The emerging professional should detach himself or herself and weigh and consider the principles of the National Athletic Trainers' Association (NATA) Code of Ethics as well as the prima facie principles and other moral health care principles discussed later in this chapter.

In general, principles are universal and impartial.[2] In relation to rules, a principle may be thought of as a first rule from which all other rules originate. One example is the golden rule, which states "do unto others as you would have them do unto you," and can be thought of as a principle from which other rules originate. Another example includes the principles of the

NATA Code of Ethics, which are, of course, specific to athletic trainers. Additional moral principles (e.g., the prima facie principles) have been established as first rules in biomedical and health care ethics. To understand better the process of moral deliberation with the principled approach, the English philosopher W.D. Ross indicates that the four prima facie principles are binding unless overridden by a competing principle.[24]

The universal nature of moral principles means they are not explicit and cannot alone explain why a particular ethical position is significant. The usefulness of moral principles is that they serve as markers to define important concepts and help shape and encapsulate an ethical position. Moral principles do not narrow the deliberations but rather broaden them—and require professional sensitivity along with an appreciation of the grayness of professional life.

Principles

In matters of principle, stand like a rock; in matters of taste, swim with the current.
—Thomas Jefferson

Chapter 9 discussed the importance of professional, institutional, and program rules, policies, and procedures to guide and manage appropriate conduct of a professional in training. Policies and procedures are secondary and tertiary rules derived from important principles.

Important principles of health care also serve to direct professional action. Principles are universal rules of conduct and are revealed in values. Relative to human relations, principles identify which types of conduct, intentions, and motives are forbidden, obligatory, or allowed.[11,16]

PROFESSIONAL PEARL

One NATA Hall of Fame Inductee conveys the effect of living by one's principles:

"Principle I: always, always, make the health and welfare of the athlete your number one priority. Principle II: never, ever let anyone or anything prevent you from fulfilling principle I. There will never be anyone who can challenge your decisions if you live by these two principles. It cost me the only position I ever wanted in my entire career, but I still feel good that I never let anyone or anything interfere with my number one priority: the health and welfare of my athletes."

—Robert Behnke, NATA Hall of Fame Inductee, 1990, has held numerous teaching and athletic training positions throughout Indiana and Illinois, including the University of Illinois in Champaign, Illinois, and Indiana State University in Terre Haute, Indiana. Dr. Behnke served the profession in many ways. As the chair of the Professional Education Committee, he was instrumental in garnering the American Medical Association recognition of athletic training as a health care profession.

This professional situation emphasizes how principles inform decisions and behaviors (Figure 13-2).

Principles

Foundational behaviors of professional practice

Figure 13-2 ■ Principles are linked to foundational behaviors of professional practice.

ETHICAL APPROACHES: PROFESSIONAL HEALTH CARE PRINCIPLES*

*There are often different **ethical approaches** to implementing projects. Those favoring particular prioritizations of values may regard other approaches not as unethical but as affording different weight to ethical **principles** and values. The role of ethical analysis is to require proponents to articulate the **principles** or values at stake and to justify why they have elevated or subordinated each of them.*[10]

The enormous problems associated with health care delivery, reimbursement, technological advancements, managed care, and changes in practice environments have created ethical and moral challenges to patient care for all health care professionals. The profession of athletic training is not immune to such challenges. Although the ethical issues confronting the athletic training profession may be far removed from some of the more complex issues commonly associated with

*The remainder of this chapter was contributed by Regis Turocy.

health care ethics (e.g. withholding or withdrawing treatment, abortion, cloning),[5] the unique relationships among the certified athletic trainer, the athlete, the physician, the employer, coaches, and parents can carry significant ethical challenges. For example, a simple case of shoulder pain could be riddled with ethical questions concerning informed consent, autonomy, conflicts of interest, nonmaleficence, and justice. These topics are discussed later in this chapter.

In a broader context, several unique issues that could confront the athletic trainer include the following: (1) limits of confidentiality, (2) use of medical means for enhancing athletic performance, (3) impediments to obtaining informed consent, (4) the application of medical arts to enable dangerous behavior, (5) preference for enhanced short-term performance over long-term well-being, (6) medical advertising, (7) fair resource allocation, (8) special concerns for the pediatric athlete, and (9) loyalty to the athlete versus the organization.[5] Although the magnitude of decision making for these ethical issues differs, the constant that should be present in all ethical decision making is the ability of the athletic trainer to apply some method to his or her ethical decision-making process. These decisions may affect a single athlete or an entire community. As an example, the following case scenario is provided.

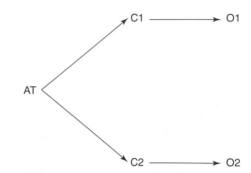

Figure 13-3 ■ A schematic of an ethical dilemma.

This case illustrates a typical ethical dilemma. The athletic trainer (AT, or agent) is confronted with two actions: maintain confidentiality and autonomy (choice 1 [C1]), which may cause serious injury (outcome 1 [O1]), or adhere to your duty to protect from further harm (choice 2 [C2]), which could save his life (outcome 2 [O2]). Figure 13-3 schematically diagrams this ethical dilemma.

Purposeful action, in response to this dilemma, requires some guidelines to help the AT select the appropriate course of action for this particular situation. This chapter provides the AT with a principle-based approach to ethical decision making.

Principle-Based Ethics

Simply stated, ethics is the critical and reflective analysis of what is good and bad about a person's actions as a moral agent when confronted with ethical problems. Sometimes the differentiation between good and bad decisions is fairly straightforward; competently taking care of athletes is a good action, whereas providing incompetent care is a bad action. However, other ethical situations may be more complex and involve both good and bad consequences. In the case scenario above, the AT can honor the athlete's confidentiality, which is a good thing; however, as a result, the athlete may experience significant physical damage while participating, which would be a bad thing.

The history of health care ethics has seen the development of numerous theories that can be used to assist the AT in choosing the appropriate moral action. Many of these theories place an emphasis on moral obligations or duty (e.g., deontology, absolute rules; utilitarianism, the greatest good for the greatest number; and

CASE SCENARIO

A major university recruited one of country's top running backs to play football and offered him a full scholarship. Without this scholarship, the athlete could not afford to attend the school. Before his senior year, he had three concussions that required hospitalization. During his senior year he did not sustain a concussion but complained of concussion-like symptoms on occasion. During his on-campus evaluation, he falsified medical information and did not reveal his history of concussions. He was given a "clean" medical examination by the team physician. On his return to school, he confides to you, the athletic trainer, about what transpired and demands your confidentiality.[4] How do you arrive at your decision?

rights, liberal individualism).[9] These principles and rules that guide moral duties are considered *moralities of law,* which are focused on principles, rules, and rights as "action guides that we have a duty to observe and respect."[9] Examples include not killing, fulfilling promises, telling the truth, paying debts, and not stealing. Another theory that has dominated contemporary health care ethics professes a common set of principles that everyone is obligated to follow to determine what the AT is morally obligated to do. These principles are not absolute but are prima facie binding, meaning an obligation to follow unless overridden by a competing principle. If the principles conflict with one another, then the good and bad outcomes of the action must be balanced against one another to decide which course of action the AT is morally obliged to follow.

Principle-based ethics had its beginnings in the early twentieth century as described in a textbook by W.D. Ross, *The Right and the Good.*[24] In this book, Ross attempts to investigate the morality of the good; in other words, what ought to be done or not done. He suggests that moral choices do not consist of absolute principles (deontology) or producing the most good (utilitarianism), but rather should consist of prima facie duties (obligatory principles).[24] These duties include the duties of (1) fidelity (keep promises), (2) reparation (for wrongful acts), (3) promoting justice (fair distribution), (4) beneficence (promote the good), (5) self-improvement (improve our own condition), and (6) nonmaleficence (not to injure others).[24] Unlike absolute duties that are binding no matter the situation, prima facie duties allow choices between conflicting principles.[23] For example, in health care, the prima facie duty of fidelity (confidentiality) is binding if no other duty conflicts. However, if by following the principle of fidelity harm is caused to another, then the principle of nonmaleficence would outweigh fidelity and be the correct moral action for the AT to follow.

In an attempt to make normative ethics more acceptable to adherents of different philosophical, ethical, religious, political, cultural, or social stances, Thomas Beauchamp and James Childress reformulated Ross's notion of prima facie obligations and developed a "principle-based, common morality–based" theory that was pluralistic and universal.[3] This approach to ethical analysis has been more commonly referred to as the "Georgetown Mantra" or "principlism."[3] The underpinnings of this theory begin with a common morality shared by members of a society "that is unphilosophical common sense and tradition."[3] This common morality provides the framework for the development of principles and rules, and the framework serves as a guideline to help determine the "correct" moral action that should be followed. The principles are as follows[3,23,25]:

- *Autonomy:* This principle respects the individual's rights to self-determination and self-governance. In health care, the principle of autonomy emphasizes that when fully informed and capable, an individual has the right to decide which treatment options are best for his or her individual circumstances. Autonomy also involves the right to refuse treatment. Although in theory the principles have no set priority, the principle of autonomy is provided a priority status within U.S. culture because of the country's emphasis on individualism. Autonomy's prioritization should be nurtured because self-rule is what makes morality possible.[13]

  For the athlete autonomy involves respecting his or her decision-making capabilities regarding treatment and the AT's respect for the decision about what treatment is in the best interest of the athlete. These autonomous decisions must be voluntary and independent of any other influences. Today, a major concern with autonomy in the sports medicine arena is the notion of informed consent. When an athlete is being treated, the principle of autonomous decision making requires that he or she is given true informed consent; however, because of the treatment environment, informed consent often is considered implied, presumed, or persuaded. The AT must recognize the manipulative potential of a sports medicine environment and be prepared to serve as the athlete's advocate and act only in his or her best interest.

- *Beneficence:* This principle refers directly to the covenant that all health care providers are obligated to use their skills in the best interests of the patient (athlete). It has an ancient Judeo-Christian foundation in the parable of the good Samaritan. At all cost, the AT's obligation is to prevent harm or remove harm when identified. A brief example would be when an AT does not adhere to proper antimicrobial cleansing techniques within the athletic training room, creating the development and spread of methicillin-resistant *Staphylococcus aureus*.

- *Nonmaleficence:* This is the core principle of every health care provider: to do no harm (*primum non nocere*). Although pain may be caused by treatment, it must not be intentional. This principle also covers acts of omission (failure to act). For example, if the AT does not attend to the responsibility of ensuring proper fluid replacement during extreme hot weather conditions and an athlete is eventually harmed, the AT has breached the principle of nonmaleficence. Athletic training can never allow room for harm.

- *Justice:* This principle cultivates the fair treatment of the individual or group. It involves the fair distribution of benefits, burdens, and economic costs of treatment at a societal level (distributive justice) or individual level (comparative justice). As an example, consider the following contradiction in sports medicine: How does the AT justify the immediate access of expensive diagnostic tests (e.g., computed tomography, magnetic resonance imaging) given that a professional athlete is injured when 45 million Americans do not have health insurance or access to health care? Where is the justice associated with these decisions?

Several rules have evolved from these core principles to assist and guide moral actions[3]:

1. Substantive rules:
   - Veracity: Truth telling; compels the individual to act in a certain way
   - Confidentiality and privacy: Ensures that the release of private information about the athlete is authorized

- Fidelity: Faithfulness; involves competency, respect, adherence to the NATA Code of Ethics and honors the covenant between the AT and athlete
- Informed consent: Involves providing the athlete with all the factual information necessary to make appropriate medical decisions for his or her benefit
2. Authority rules (authority for decisions):
   - Surrogate authority: Establishes authority for substitute decision maker
   - Professional authority: Who can make decisions to override the patient's decision?
   - Distributional authority: Who determines the fair distribution of resources?
3. Procedural rules: Procedures to follow when actions cannot be decided by substantive or authority rules

These principles and rules, taken together, provide action guidelines that bring a framework of objectivity, not abstract theory, to moral reasoning. They are devoid of identity preferences and have as their primary concerns the patient-athlete's values and well-being in mind.

Conflict and Transformation

Many of the problems encountered in health care ethics take the form of a dilemma in which two of the principles conflict. Another significant aspect of principlism is the strategy they propose when two of the principles conflict. Because the principles and rules are considered prima facie and have no intrinsic priority, some guidance for choice must be possible. Beauchamp and Childress state that judgment in these cases requires a "weighing and balancing" of the norms through "reflective equilibrium"[3]—the good and bad effects of the particular circumstance are carefully examined and analyzed. They also provide prima facie conditions that must be met to justify giving priority to one principle over another. These justificatory conditions are as follows[3]:

- Substantial reasons to act on the overriding norm rather than the infringed norm.
- The moral objective justifying the infringement is realistic.

- No morally preferred alternative action is possible.
- Choice minimizes the infringement commensurate with the goal.
- The agent seeks to minimize the negative effect of the infringement.

This balancing strategy of conflict resolution provides a theoretical framework of ethical flexibility designed to consider compromise, mediation, or negotiation.[3] The following case scenario illustrates this balancing strategy.

CASE SCENARIO

You are the AT of a small division II school that has a starting tailback with unbelievable potential (scouted heavily by the National Football League). Toward the end of his senior year, he confides in you that he has tested positive for HIV because of a summer liaison with an old girlfriend. He does not want his coach, team physician, teammates, present girlfriend, or family to know. He does not plan to seek medical attention. How would you balance your conflicts?

In today's health care environment, a great deal of emphasis is placed on respecting patient autonomy and confidentiality. In the case study above, the athlete has the right to choose what he believes to be the best option for him. He also is the sole decider regarding to whom this medical information is transmitted.[1] Also, because of the AT's fiduciary responsibility to those he cares for, the athlete is correct to assume that his confidence will be upheld. On the other hand, the AT knows that withholding this information could cause harm to the athlete, his present girlfriend or others he may have had sexual relations with, the team physician, and/or his teammates. As the AT weighs the good and bad effects of this situation and reflects on the justificatory conditions that allow one principle to override another, the principle of nonmaleficence appears to trump the athlete's autonomy and confidentiality. The AT therefore is morally obligated to speak to the team physician about the athlete's HIV status.

When confronted with ethical problems or dilemmas, the AT has available numerous normative ethical approaches to help in deciding which moral action to pursue that produces the most good. Knowing how to apply these theories to health care practice is often difficult for the AT. In an attempt to provide a solid starting point for moral judgment, the principle-based, common morality–based ethics that use four widely accepted general principles and specific rules allow the AT to analyze ethical dilemmas and arrive at consensus. However, in the complex world of health care moral reasoning, a mixture of multiple theoretical approaches, principles, rule, rights, virtues, passions, and experience is used to convert an ethical dilemma into appropriate moral action (Figure 13-4).[22]

Other Important Supplemental Documents

ATs have two other "principled" documents that can provide guidance when confronting an ethical problem and help substantiate moral judgment in a particular case. One such document is the NATA Code of Ethics. A professional code of ethics defines the morality of a profession and represents the articulated consensus of the professional community about its identity. The standards established are compatible with the common morality of society and therefore are closely linked to principle-based ethics. For example, the principles of autonomy, beneficence, nonmaleficence, and confidentiality are the foundation of principle 1 in the NATA Code of Ethics: "Members shall respect the rights, welfare, and dignity of all." Veracity and honesty are the foundation in principle 2, justice in principle 3, and fidelity in principle 4.[20] Although not frequently used, the principles woven into the Code of Ethics can help defend moral positions when applicable.

The other documents that the AT may find useful when gathering supportive information for his or her moral decisions are the "Foundational Behaviors of Professional Practice," found in the NATA's *Athletic Training Educational Competencies,*[19] and the Board of Certification Standards of Practice.[21] One of the behavioral standards that comprises the common values or morality of the profession is ethical practice. This behavior is a fiduciary responsibility and compels the AT to a role morality agreed on by the members of his or her profession and the society in which they serve.

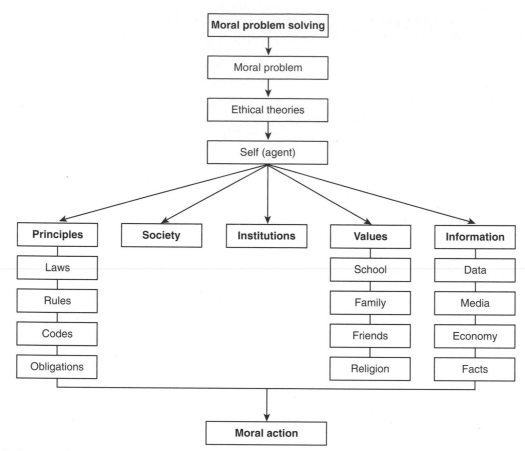

Figure 13-4 ■ Moral problem-solving process.

SUMMARY

Almost all theories converge to the conclusion that the most important ingredient in a person's moral life is a developed character that provides the inner motivation and strength to do what is right and good (p. 323).[12]

The adherence to principles to guide an active consciousness in the complex ethical world of health care is important to moral life. In the health care professions, these principles are instrumental in preventing the loss of public trust, which is a huge concern in today's practice environment. As a moral compass, principles have a universality that appeals to any religion, culture, or belief system—not as absolute rules but as a framework for appropriate moral actions. However, in a complex ethical society, principles alone do not encompass every situation. To use principles alone would cause moral decision making

to "choke" and not meet the true needs of those with whom ATs work. To maintain an "open airway," moral decision making also involves a virtuous character, common sense, and emotional responsiveness.[3] Professional virtues such as compassion, integrity, truthfulness, trustworthiness, competence, and justice are critical attributes.[3] The moral being of the AT is a product of these virtuous attributes and is developed from the characteristics nurtured in the profession's Code of Ethics, educational guidelines, rich tradition, competent practice, and position as advocate for the athlete. All of this, in combination, provides the AT with the inner voice necessary to make sound moral judgments when confronted by any ethical challenge.

Read through the following case studies and use the principles discussed in this chapter while reflecting on the questions.

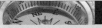

CASE SCENARIO

A baseball player was hit in the eye with a pellet from a pellet gun when he was a child. He has only peripheral vision in that eye. You (the AT) recommend that he play with protective eyewear. He states that he cannot play with something on his face. The coach thinks that playing with sport goggles would bother him and, because he never played with them in high school, he sees it as "no big deal." His parents are comfortable with him not playing with goggles.

How do you resolve this situation?

CASE SCENARIO

A 19-year-old female long-distance runner has been losing more weight than you would like to see. Your concerns are confirmed by a conversation with a teammate and roommate, who are also concerned about her weight loss. You confront the athlete and she agrees to go to the nutritionist for counseling. After several meetings with the nutritionist, this individual is diagnosed with a serious eating disorder. When confronted by you and the nutritionist regarding your concerns and that the recommendation for her to see the team physician, the athlete refuses. She states emphatically that you (the AT) and the nutritionist are not to discuss her case with anyone—the team physician, the coach, or her parents. She promises to continue to see the nutritionist. You and the nutritionist thought this was better than nothing, and she continued counseling. However, the athlete's condition worsened. She continued to lose weight. She began to miss classes and failed to keep her appointments with the nutritionist.

Are you legally bound to confidentiality in this situation?

CASE SCENARIO

During Friday's football game, a 16-year-old defensive back experiences a head injury in which he is confused but has no loss of consciousness or cognitive function. The confusion clears within 15 minutes, but he continues to report a headache. He is removed for the remainder of the game. He is seen in the training room on Monday by the team physician. Results of a neurological examination are normal, but he continues to report a mild headache, loss of appetite, mild sleep disturbance, and difficulty concentrating in class. Because these symptoms continue, the team physician disqualifies him from the upcoming Friday night championship game. The parents are livid with the decision and take their son to his personal physician, who clears him for the game.

As the AT, what do you do?

REFERENCES

1. American Medical Society for Sports Medicine: *HIV and other blood-borne pathogens in sports* (website): www.newamssm.org/hiv.html. Accessed February 1, 2006.

2. Andrews DR: Fostering ethical competency: an ongoing staff development process that encourage professional grow and staff satisfaction, *J Continuing Educ Nurs* 35:27-36, 2004.

3. Beauchamp T, Childress JF: *Principles of biomedical ethics,* New York, 1994, Oxford University Press.

4. Berstein J, Perlis C, Bartolozzi AR: Ethics in sports medicine, *Clin Orthop Relat Res* 378:50-60, 2000.

5. Berstein J, Perlis C, Bartolozzi AR: Normative ethics in sports medicine, *Clin Orthop Relat Res* 420:309-318, 2004.

6. Burkhardt MA, Nathaniel AK: *Ethics and issues in contemporary nursing,* Clifton Park, NY, 2002, Delmar.

7. Callahan, S: The bonds of family, *Hastings Ctr Rep* 29(3):44, 1999.

8. Davis CM: Affective education for the health care professions, *Phys Ther* 61:1587-1593, 1981.

9. Devettere R: *Practical decision making in health care ethics: cases and concepts,* Washington DC, 1995, Georgetown University Press.

10. Dickens BM: The challenges and opportunities of ethics, *Am J Public Health* 95(7):1094, 2005.

11. Gillon R: Medical ethics: four principles plus attention to scope, *Br Med J* 309:184-188, 1994.

12. Gillon R: Defending "the four principles" approach to biomedical ethics, *J Med Ethics* 21:323-324, 1995.

13. Gillon R: Ethics needs principles—four can encompass the rest—and respect for autonomy should be "first among equals," *J Med Ethics* 29:307-312, 2003.

14. Ham J: Principled thinking: a comparison of nursing students and experienced nurses, *J Continuing Educ Nurs* 35:66-73, 2004.

15. Kanner S, Langerman S, Grey M: Ethical considerations for a child's participation in research, *J Specialists Pediatr Nurs* 9:15-24, 2004.

16. Limentani AE: The role of ethical principles in health care and the implications for ethical codes, *J Med Ethics* 25:394-399, 1999.

17. Maldonado N, Efinger J, Lacey CH: Shared perceptions of personal moral development: an inquiry in social research, *Int J Hum Caring* 7:8-19, 2003.

18. Mathes M: Ethical decision making and nursing, *Medsurgical Nurs* 12:429-432, 2004.

19. National Athletic Trainers' Association: *Athletic training educational competencies,* ed 4, Dallas, 2006, National Athletic Trainers' Association.

20. National Athletic Trainers' Association: *Code of ethics* (website): www.nata.org/codeofethics/code_of_ethics.pdf. Accessed July 17, 2007.

21. National Athletic Trainers Association Board of Certification: *Standards of practice* (website): www.bocatc.org/atc/STD. Accessed March 14, 2006.

22. National Health Museum: *Moral problem solving* (website): www.accessexcellence.org/LC/SER/BE/beethicsmap.html. Accessed March 12, 2006.

23. Purtilo R: *Ethical dimensions in the health professions,* ed 4, Philadelphia, 2005, Saunders.

24. Ross W: *The right and the good,* London, 1930, Oxford University Press.

25. Scott R: *Professional ethics: a guide for rehabilitation professionals,* St Louis, 1998, Mosby.

26. Sisola SW: Moral reasoning as a predictor of clinical practice: the development of physical therapy students across the professional curriculum, *J Phys Ther Educ* 14:26-35, 2000.

27. Triezenberg HL, Davis CM: Beyond the code of ethics: educating physical therapists for their role as moral agents, *J Phys Ther Educ* 14:48-59, 2000.

CHAPTER 14

Learning Activities: Linking Content to Practice

In addition to superior clinical skills, outstanding clinicians possess highly developed professional behaviors (p. 27).[3]

The activities in this section are designed to help the student apply knowledge of ethical theory and principles to real-life situations. An understanding of the theoretical framework and the terminology commonly associated with ethics helps incorporate it into professional practice. Furthermore, and equally important, these activities help the student connect personal identity and emerging professional identity. These concepts are integrally related, and acknowledgment of their reciprocity shapes the student's journey through the career of athletic trainer.

As before, honest responses to each of the activities in this unit prompts reflection on the self as a professional. While participating in these activities, recognize that movement from personal to professional identity includes the role of others in one's moral development. Many activities involve interaction with peers and are not as scripted as the earlier activities; as such, they may create some dissonance. That is all part of the journey into the profession.

ACTIVITIES FOR APPLICATION: LINKING CONTENT TO PRACTICE

LEARNING ACTIVITY I: ANALYTIC MEMO

Objectives

1. To articulate a professional message concisely
2. To examine how what you say can be interpreted
3. To demonstrate how perceptions affect professional behaviors

Description

Write a 1- to 2-page analysis of a problem in memorandum format.[1] Your instructor will identify from whom and to whom the memo will be written from the following case scenarios. This memo should be succinct and written with appropriate professional language.

CASE SCENARIO

Analytic Memo I

You are the head athletic trainer at a high school, and you are writing your memo to the athletic director.

The topic is recent budget cuts in the school district that will mandate no overtime hours (in excess of a 40-hour work week) for any employee. You currently receive hourly wages for any time exceeding 40 hours in any given week at a rate equal to normal pay. You are quite concerned that you must now choose which sport to cover or not cover and/or whether to work overtime for no additional pay.

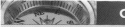

CASE SCENARIO

Analytic Memo 2

You are an athletic trainer employed by a private physical therapy clinic, and you are writing your memo to the owner/head therapist.

The topic is a recent mandate by the head therapist to have athletic trainers' notes co-signed by physical therapy aides in the absence of a licensed physical therapist. You are disturbed by this trend because aides have only a 2-year degree and you have completed a master's degree. Furthermore, the clinic refuses to use athletic training billing codes for which you could sign your own notes.

CASE SCENARIO

Analytic Memo 3

You are an athletic trainer employed at General Autoworks and you will be writing your memo to the case manager, who is a registered nurse.

The topic is the issue of return-to-work releases. As an athletic trainer, you work diligently to return the employee back to work as safely and effectively as possible. However, the case manager encourages you to be a bit more conservative in approach to rehabilitation and treatment because an employee does not have to return to work in 3 weeks when he or she has technically been released for 6 weeks from work. The case manager reports that employees are expressing dissatisfaction with having to return sooner than they anticipated. The employees are successfully completing functional capacity examinations and functional tests that indicate they can safely return to work.

Assessment

The goal of this exercise is to assess your ability to integrate concepts relative to the dilemmas presented in the case argument. Although grammar and language are critical in written communication, those items are not the primary focus. One way to address the content (argument) is to have a peer evaluate the memo. With a peer evaluation rubric, you and your peers can provide each other substantive feedback. Additionally, working in pairs allows one person to write the original memo and the other to respond in memo format, which further develops the critical issues and communication style necessary when encountering these ethical dilemmas.

This activity can be addressed by the group by distributing the memo to the class and having the class ask questions for clarification. However, this activity is best suited for a written format.

LEARNING ACTIVITY 2: APPLICATION CARDS

Objectives

1. To create scenarios that apply to basic ethical theories and principles
2. To examine the multiple applications of various theories and principles
3. To appreciate the real-life nature of the cognitive content present in ethics education

Description

After the introduction of an ethical theory or principle, create an index card and provide a real-life application of that theory or principle.[1] You will be asked to make the connection between the theory and/or principle and what you have encountered in your personal and professional life.

List of Theories and Principles for Cards

Piaget's cognitive theory	Benefit
Kohlberg's theory of moral development	Social benefit
	Paternalism
Autonomy	Honesty
Beneficence	Lawfulness
Nonmaleficence	Veracity
Justice	Role fidelity

Assessment

Assessment relative to the use and explanation of the application is at the core of evaluating this activity. A conceptual understanding of the actual terms and the direct application of these terms is critical in developing professional behaviors. Peer assessment is helpful in reinforcing each other's understanding of the term.

Tip: Although this activity can be performed individually, forming pairs or small groups may help you feel more comfortable with the applications. Furthermore, this activity can serve as a preclass assignment as a preparatory tool or used to begin discussions for in-class activities. In addition, after class discussion, this activity can be used as a journal activity.

LEARNING ACTIVITY 3: CATEGORIZING GRID

Objectives

1. To review key terms and concepts relative to ethical theories and/or principles
2. To demonstrate cognitive understanding of the relations among selected theories and/or principles
3. To connect related concepts to terms commonly used in ethics education

Description

Use the following grid to categorize the scrambled list of corresponding information.[1] Sort the list in a 3-minute time period.

Values	Principles

List of Items to Match

Beneficence	Loyalty
Fidelity	Nonmaleficence
Honesty	Promise keeping
Justice	Respect for others
Autonomy	Veracity
Fairness	

Assessment

Because this activity includes correct and incorrect responses, a simple assessment for accuracy is vital. Peer assessment may also be used to provide constructive feedback to help understand the information.

Tip: An alternate option for using this grid as a study tool is to look at the categories but not the items for the scrambled list to encourage recall of critical elements.

LEARNING ACTIVITY 4: EVERYDAY ETHICAL DILEMMAS

Objectives

1. To acknowledge that dilemmas occur in everyday activities in the athletic training profession
2. To question what is seen in practice to encourage critical reflection about professional behaviors
3. To demonstrate an understanding of basic ethical decision-making processes

Description

Consider one of the following everyday ethical dilemmas or one posed by your instructor or one of your peers.[1] Resolve this case in an anonymous fashion.

CASE SCENARIO

Everyday Ethical Dilemma 1

As an athletic training student, you are asked to volunteer for a weekend softball tournament. The certified athletic trainer in charge of softball asks if you will help her with the tournament; many teams will be playing, and it will be a great learning experience for you. The tournament will last all day and not conclude until approximately 8 PM. You have plans to go to the lake with your friends for the entire day. You do not want to disappoint the athletic trainer by not volunteering because you respect her as a professional, but you really want to go to the lake with your friends. What do you do?

CASE SCENARIO

Everyday Ethical Dilemma 2

You are assigned to report to the athletic training room for your basketball rotation immediately after your 1 PM class. However, you always go to the student hub to grab lunch before reporting for your clinical assignment because you have class continuously from 8:00 AM to 1 PM without a break. You have done this all semester without fail. One day, the graduate assistant athletic trainer happens to see you at the hub and indicates that you are to be at the athletic training room immediately after class. She indicates she is going to tell your supervisor that you are not reporting as assigned. What do you do?

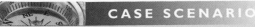

CASE SCENARIO

Everyday Ethical Dilemma 3

You are an athletic training student who is assigned to a local high school as one of your rotations. You are currently a junior in college. During your time at the high school, you establish a friendship with a high school student who is a senior. When you are done with your rotation, you and this student begin dating. This is disclosed to the supervisor at the university by the high school clinical instructor. What do you do?

Assessment

Being able to identify the ethical dilemma and address the means by which you would address the situation professionally are central to this activity. Assessment could be directed toward classifying the response to a corresponding principle. You may also be assessed by creating a dilemma and addressing the response of your peers. Additionally, approaching the dilemma from another person's perspective helps distinguish multiple perspectives.

LEARNING ACTIVITY 5: FOCUSED AUTOBIOGRAPHICAL SKETCHES

Objectives

1. To encourage self-reflection and analysis of personal traits
2. To promote critical thinking about socialization in the profession
3. To examine the relation between personal and professional identities

Description

Choose one of the following topics and write a focused autobiographical sketch relative to the topic, including a statement of how this sketch affects you personally and professionally.[1] This sketch need not be lengthy but should be concise and represent key qualities about you relative to any or all of the following topics.

Selected Topics

Leadership	Patient advocate
Mentoring	Responsible citizen
Integrity	Team player
Empathy	Health care provider
Public speaking	Teacher
Role model	Student

Assessment

Because this activity is deeply reflective, careful assessment regarding your ability to express your perceptions and tie them to professional development is essential. However, be sure to acknowledge the disclosure required to complete this task. Connections between the personal and professional self may be reflected in many forms in this type of activity.

Tip: You may also approach this activity from a different person's perspective by writing what others might say about you. This activity can also be completed by writing about someone else in the class as if you were that person.

LEARNING ACTIVITY 6: INVENTED DIALOGUE

Objectives

1. To demonstrate the critical link between communication and the development of a professional identity
2. To encourage interaction to reflect the importance of tone, inflection, and nonverbal cues in the communication process
3. To engage in a dialogue that simulates real-life settings and dissonance

Description

Choose one of the following topics, and write one quote on an index card to be given to the student who is "in character."[1] You may create your own quotes in a sequential dialogue in combination with quotes from others. Many quotes will be woven together to create the dialogue. This person will use direct quotes provided on the cards as well as personally created quotes in the interaction with the other character. Although some elaboration is permitted, you must stay close to the quotes as you enter into the "scripted dialogue" with the other character. The other character can respond in any way; the cards are created for your character only.

Selected Topics

1. You are an African-American athletic trainer who recently overheard the head coach of your assigned sport make a racial slur.
2. You are a female athletic trainer at a local high school, and the athletic director refuses to provide an athletic training space for football that is not in the football locker room.
3. You are an athletic trainer of the Jewish faith, and your employer fails to recognize your religious holidays as holiday release time (and holiday pay). You must take these holidays as vacation or personal time.
4. You are an athletic trainer who is in the last 4 weeks of a high-risk pregnancy. You have an overseas trip approaching within 2 weeks, and you are fearful of taking the trip with the team because of the possibility of early labor.

After each person in the class writes one quote for you to use, you will be given a few minutes to pull together the quotes to create your dialogue. The teacher will assign someone else to play the other character.

After approximately 5 to 7 minutes per case, discussion will occur regarding the reaction of the group to the quotes used in the dialogue.

Assessment

Group participation rubrics identify the contributions of each group member. Identification of key components relative to the concepts being presented is at the core of this activity. Being able to discuss the rationale for why the quotes were ethically responsible or not is a good gauge for this activity.

LEARNING ACTIVITY 7: WHAT IS THE PRINCIPLE?

Objectives

1. To reinforce the understanding of selected ethical principles
2. To relate specific principles to selected examples
3. To draw connections between ethical theory and practice

Description

Choose one of the following cases, and identify which principles are being applied to each case.[1] Provide supporting facts specific to the case in your response.

CASE SCENARIO

Case 1

You are working closely with the field hockey team, and one of the athletes discloses to you that she has been treated with medication for depression. During the season, however, she chooses not to take her medication because her symptoms are less intense and she enjoys the game and thrill of the competition. She does not express any threat to herself or others; she simply notifies you that she does not take her medication during season. Which principle is applied here? Why?

CASE SCENARIO

Case 2

You are the athletic trainer in an outpatient physical therapy clinic. You know that several people on your staff are dissatisfied with how the work schedule has been arranged. As it stands now, the person with the most seniority gets to choose which shift to work (7 AM to 4 PM, 8 AM to 5 PM, or 9 AM to 6 PM). This person always wants to come in early on the 7 AM shift so that he can leave earlier. The evening shift usually runs overtime because patients who have 5:30 PM schedules are seldom done by 6 PM. As the athletic trainer in charge of scheduling the staff, you mandate that the shifts will be on a rotating basis, with each staff athletic trainer working one early day and at least one late day. This would mean the athletic trainer with the most seniority now has two 7 AM shifts, one 8 AM shift, and two 9 AM shifts. Each of the other staff has a similar schedule. Which principle is applied here? Why?

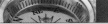

Case 3

You are the athletic trainer assigned to cover a wrestling tournament. A high school athlete has recurrent subluxations of his left shoulder. After two matches and immediately before the final match, the athlete's shoulder subluxates and he cannot get it back in place in the fashion he typically uses. He asks you to reduce the shoulder for him so that he can participate in the finals. You refuse. Which principle is applied here? Why?

CASE SCENARIO

Case 4

You are the athletic trainer at a collegiate baseball game. You are the home team and are hosting the conference championship game. A player from the other team—the star pitcher—comes to you before the game to ask for a massage on his throwing arm. They did not bring a certified athletic trainer to the game. The player from the other team discloses that without the massage, his pitches are typically slower and less accurate. You choose to perform therapeutic massage on this athlete as if he were one of your own athletes. Which principle is applied here? Why?

Assessment

Evaluation of this activity is based on the nature of the task. If the task is an individual task, then assessing the accuracy and rationale for each response is appropriate. If completed as a group activity, a group activity assessment rubric can help provide valuable input.

Tip: An interesting twist to this activity is to provide the principles and then provide examples from your clinical experiences or personal experience. This typically will yield interesting stories, which are powerful learning tools.

LEARNING ACTIVITY 8: STATEMENT OF ASSUMPTIONS

Objectives

1. To illustrate the assumptions that each person holds relative to any situation
2. To increase awareness of the impact of assumptions in professional settings
3. To encourage careful reflection on personal bias and assumptions in the profession

Description

Identify your assumptions about the following case. Because the case provides limited information, rely on your own personal assumptions. This activity has no right or wrong answers, so write freely about what you assume.

CASE SCENARIO

A Latino steelworker reports to your clinic with a worker's compensation claim against his company for a back injury sustained during work. His physical examination is inconsistent with this history and mechanism of injury. He discloses his dissatisfaction with his employer and makes reference to using this time off to catch up on the vacation time he did not receive earlier this year due to understaffing. He also frequently talks about his friend, an attorney, who is going to "go after the employer like a bulldog."

List your initial assumptions about this case. Try to generate at least six assumptions based on the information provided for you.

After creating the list, identify the reasons why you assumed what you did based on the information provided in the case. Lastly, identify how these assumptions can affect your professional identity.

Assumption	Rationale	Affect on Professional Identity

Assessment

This activity may be used as an individual activity, particularly because it presents personal bias that may affect professional behaviors, which may be embarrassing. This activity should be evaluated on the basis of the ability to connect how bias can affect professional behavior. This connection must be present. Feedback in the form of comments from peers or your instructor will be helpful with a follow-up journal activity (using a journal rubric for guidance) to help reflect after acknowledging that these assumptions exist.

LEARNING ACTIVITY 9: INTERVIEW

Objectives

1. To identify key personal and professional values
2. To facilitate professional communication with superiors
3. To integrate conceptual knowledge into daily professional activities

Description

Perform an interview of one of your clinical supervisors to establish his or her input on professional behaviors and the professional identity.[2] This interview should have two parts and be scheduled with the supervisor for times that will be uninterrupted so that you have the undivided attention of the supervisor during the interview.

The first interview should be open ended. Ask your supervisor to discuss a concrete incident that involved an ethical dilemma. No questions are needed to follow up this portion of the interview. It is designed to capture the supervisor's story.

At the conclusion of part one, summarize the scenario and identify any theories or principles described in the interview. Obviously, they will probably not be identified by the exact terms, but the essence is what you should detect. Also identify specific values that you perceive your supervisor held while resolving this dilemma. Any other factors, such as patient-clinician interaction and/or organizational structure, that may have had an effect on the resolution of this case should be highlighted in the documentation as well.

The second part of the interview, performed on a different day, should be more structured. It should involve sequential, specific, and structured questions regarding the following hypothetical case. This will help you identify the decision-making frameworks used by your clinical supervisor.

CASE SCENARIO

Mr. Jones is seen by the physician for progressive neurological deficits after several months of symptoms. This patient had a fatal neurological disease that would quickly progress and completely disable this patient. Additionally, the patient was recently diagnosed with Hodgkin's disease. The patient and the family wish to receive treatment for the Hodgkin's disease, although it will probably not have an effect until well after the neurological disease fully deteriorates the nervous system and leaves the patient in a permanent disabled state. You are the athletic trainer charged with discussing the plan for maintaining balance and gait during the treatment protocol for the Hodgkin's disease. What do you do?

Ask and record responses to the following questions:

- What is the ethical dilemma here?
- Where do you seek information regarding resolution of this case?
- What are the alternatives for this case?
- What are the consequences of your actions?
- What theory or major ethical principle did you use to resolve this case?
- What values are important to you as you consider resolution of this case?
- What makes this case and how you solved it different from the one we discussed last week?

After recording the responses of the supervisor, write a reflection or summary of your perceptions. Discuss each element listed in the questions relative to your perceptions of how the responses reflect professional behaviors and professional identity.

Assessment

This activity is designed to allow interaction with your supervisor to see how complex ethical issues can become in the athletic training profession. Use this as a writing activity to reflect on the information you gained during the interview. Group discussion can follow to reflect further on the broad range of dilemmas facing athletic trainers and the diverse ways in which professionals respond to the same case. A group participation rubric is beneficial in assessing this activity.

LEARNING ACTIVITY 10: STRENGTHS I SEE, STRENGTHS OTHERS SEE

Objectives

1. To identify personal and professional strengths
2. To recognize personal and professional strengths in others

3. To exemplify how others' perceptions of you affect you professionally

Description

On a full sheet of paper, create a form like the one below to identify your personal and professional strengths. Write as many strengths as you can in 10 minutes, then fold the paper and circulate it to fellow classmates. They will then record strengths (personal and professional) that they see in you. They should not flip the paper over to read your own strengths, and their comments should be anonymous (they should not write their name or initials by the comments).

Sample: SIS-SOS Activity

Name _____

Personal Strengths I See	Professional Strengths I See

Name _____

Personal Strengths Others See	Professional Strengths Others See

Once the paper circulates through the entire class, it should come back to you. As a follow-up activity, write a journal reflection that summarizes how you felt about this activity and what you and others had to say about your personal and professional strengths. This activity should be highly reflective and link directly to how your professional identity is affected by what you read and wrote during this activity.

Assessment

A journal rubric is most appropriate for this activity. Perceptions relative to how the statements affect the professional identity are central to this reflection. Being able to make the connection between what others say about you and how you react to their comments is a critical component of professional socialization.

SUMMARY

Establishing your professional identity can be complex and may create some uneasy feelings. Being able to relate to your personal identity—your values, beliefs,

and morals—provides a compass to your professional identity. Because professionals in athletic training do not work in isolation, others have an effect on your behaviors. Professional behaviors reflect the professional identity you have created for yourself. Professional identity may change depending on the job setting; however, personal identity remains constant and guides you in any setting. As you grow into the profession, you will see the importance of having strong personal and professional identities to steer you through the challenges you will certainly face. Do not shy away from these challenges; approach them with confidence and clarity, knowing that you have thought about and know who you are and what you stand for.

The next phase of your journey involves the discovery of how your personal and professional identities tie into organizational identity. The process for understanding and connecting with the organizational identities in athletic training again requires self-reflection. After an introduction to key concepts related to organizational identity, you will once again be challenged to complete learning activities that will provide continuity and clarity from your previous work.

REFERENCES

1. Angelo TA, Cross KP: *Classroom assessment techniques: a handbook for college teachers,* San Francisco, 1993, Jossey-Bass.
2. Grundstein-Amado R: Ethical decision-making processes used by health care providers, *J Adv Nurs* 18:1701-1709, 1993.
3. MacDonald CA, Cox PD, Bartlett DJ, et al: Consensus on methods to foster physical therapy professional behaviors, *J Phys Ther* 16:27-36, 2002.

CHAPTER **15**

Moral Theory: Deontology, Teleology, and Virtue Ethics

LEARNING OBJECTIVES

After reading this chapter, the student should be able to do the following:

1. Define normative ethical theories.

2. Compare deontology and teleology, and discuss how these action-based theories are incorporated into the athletic training education program.

3. Discuss virtue ethics and compare it with action-based moral theories.

4. Explain moral reflections, and describe the perspectives of deontology, teleology, and virtue ethics in athletic training.

5. Explain how moral philosophy guides foundational behaviors of professional practice.

6. Describe Potter's ethical triangle, and compare it with Beauchamp and Childress's reflective equilibrium.

Normative ethical theories are approaches derived from the disciplines of theology and philosophy. They serve as a framework to reflect on ethical issues. These philosophical approaches attempt to provide action guides. In other words, they attempt to provide direction to the practical question, "what ought I do?"[4,20] In general, three normative ethical theories have developed. Two of the three theories concentrate solely on the actions a person performs and are referred to as *action-based theories*. The third theory is different in that it centers on the character of the person and is referred to as *virtue ethics*.[6-8,11,19]

Consider the following case scenarios.

CASE SCENARIO

Bobby is a talented wide receiver at East Coastal University. He likely will be drafted into the National Football League. He and his team worked very hard to become the first-place team in the Atlantic Ocean Athletic Conference and will be playing against the *USA Today* No. 1 football team on New Year's Day. The university has never seen this kind of attention and excitement. On the field, Bobby is a no-nonsense, focused, hard-working athlete, and he has been working intensely as he prepares for the New Year's Day game. Off the field, Bobby enjoys socializing with other college students. A week before the team was to leave for the New Year's Day game, Bobby was drinking beer with other college students at the local tavern. Ron, the team's athletic training student, stops by the tavern to pick up some grilled burgers to take home to his fraternity brothers when he observes Bobby hoisting a beer to his lips. The East Coastal University Athletic Department has a no-tolerance policy for athletes drinking alcoholic beverages.

How should Ron respond?

CASE SCENARIO

Susie is a high school shot putter. She dreams of becoming a veterinarian. Susie's parents have told her that the only way that she could go to college is if she gets an athletic scholarship. Susie has worked extremely hard all season—up at 5 AM lifting weights, going to classes, attending a 3-hour afternoon practice, and studying hard. A friend of hers on the wrestling team suggested that she take some "supplements" to improve her performance. He indicated that they were safe and that he takes them all the time. Nonchalantly, she takes the bottle and starts to take the pills regularly. Two months later, Kelly, the team's certified athletic trainer, pats her on the back and says, "Susie your performance has really improved." Susie responds, "Thanks, I think the pills are helping." Kelly was curious and asked to see the bottle. Kelly identified the pills to be legal but a banned substance in the state's interscholastic athletic society.

How should Kelly respond?

ACTION-BASED THEORY

Normative ethics involves two duty-based theories: deontology and teleology. *Deontology* is the Greek word for duty and is a school of thought that considers that the *means* justifies the *end*. In contrast, the Greek word *teleos* means end or purpose. Thus the moral theory of teleology deems that the *end* justifies the *means*.

Deontology

Duty-oriented ethicists feel that the basic rightness or wrongness of an act depends upon its intrinsic nature rather than upon the situation or the consequences. This position is often described as a deontological theory, taken from the Greek word for duty (p. 25).[6]

Deontology underscores the importance of a person's duties and obligations, or what a person ought to do. This theory suggests that decisions should be determined by a person's duty to act and the rights of others. Deontology is in direct opposition to teleology.

Immanuel Kant (1724-1804) is the most influential Western philosopher and advanced the theory of deontology by suggesting that *reason* is the highest principle that ultimately concludes in *goodwill*. Universal principles that are binding for all people under all conditions are the basis of Kant's moral philosophy. Central to Kant's philosophy is the categorical imperative. The term *categorical* implies absolute and without exception, and the term *imperative* means command to act. An action is thought to be right when it satisfies the categorical imperative. Finally, Kant declared that persons should be treated with respect. He viewed people with absolute value because of their capacity to make rational choices. Kant emphatically noted that people should not be used or taken advantage of as a means to an end.

Principles, Principles, Principles

Sections I and II of this text have identified several types of principles. Principles honor the notion of reasoning and justify right action, depending on the approach. Principles are found in the following:

1. National Athletic Trainers' Association (NATA) Code of Ethics, which lists principles arbitrarily. Honoring the conduct required of all principles is right. Thus principles in a code serve as guides to develop rules of conduct. Box 15-1 provides Principle 1 and some (but not all) of the rules of conduct related to that principle. The NATA Code of Ethics clearly identifies in the prelude that the principles

---

Box 15-1

NATA PRINCIPLE I AND RULES OF CONDUCT

Members shall respect the rights, welfare, and dignity of all.
1.1 Members shall not discriminate against any legally protected class.
1.2 Members shall be committed to providing competent care.
1.3 Members shall preserve the confidentiality of privileged information and shall not release such information to a third party not involved in the patient's care without a release unless required by law.

---

are written generally; the circumstances of a situation determine the interpretation and application of a given principle and the code as a whole.

2. The principle approach to moral reasoning, which was reviewed in Chapter 13, weighs and considers all principles. Honoring the prima facie principles is right unless they conflict with an equal or stronger obligation.

3. Deontology, which makes principles absolute and binding. Honoring an absolute principle is right because it is universal and binding under any condition—for example, do not hurt the young.

The Right

In deontological theory, the word *right* is in reference to action. Simply put, *right* suggests good manners in relation to a person's duty, obligation, imperative, principle, or rule.[6,7]

Teleology

In contrast to deontology, teleology is a consequence-oriented theory in which right actions are based on the predicted outcome(s). The ends justify the means. In health care, the most widely used and understood teleologic theory is utilitarianism, which was advanced by Jeremy Bentham (1748-1832) and John Stuart Mill (1806-1876). This moral theory distills all principles into one: Do the greatest good for the greatest number of people. In utilitarian theory the good is identified by utility, which is equivalent to happiness.

The Good: Deontology versus Utilitarianism

Interestingly, in deontology the good is the focus of moral reasoning and is independent from the right (action). In contrast, in teleology an action is only right if it maximizes the good. Furthermore, deontology considers the morality of an action by its rationale, whereas teleology judges the morality of an action based on its consequences.[6,7,10,11,19]

The Utilitarian Framework and Athletic Training

Many athletic trainers use the utilitarian framework of moral reasoning on a regular basis but do not realize it. By mapping out potential outcomes of a particular action, the athletic trainer can weigh and consider the consequences by using a benefit/burden ratio. Table 15-1 illustrates such a concept relative to an athlete's

Table 15-1   UTILITARIAN FRAMEWORK: ANALYSIS OF THE BENEFIT/BURDEN RATIO*

Perceived Benefits (the Good)	Perceived Burdens (the Bad)
Educates athlete's parents about the condition	Space limitations in the athletic training room
Helps the family care for the athlete	Confidentiality and athlete's privacy may be violated
Allows athlete's family to support athlete and athletic training staff	Insufficient staff to meet the needs of the athlete's family because the focus is on the athlete
Removes doubt for the athlete's family about what is happening to their son and reinforces the fact that the staff is doing everything possible	Increased stress on the staff
Reduces fear and anxiety of athlete's parents	Athlete's parents may lose emotional control and interfere with care
Reminds staff of athlete's personhood	Increased performance anxiety of athletic training staff
Sustains connectedness and bonding of the athlete-parent relationship	Event may be too traumatic for athlete's parents
Encourages professional behavior of staff	Increased risk of litigation

*Relative to an athlete's family being present in an intercollegiate athletic training room after their son sustains a serious head injury in a football game.

Modified from Halm MA: Family presence during resuscitation: a critical review of the literature, *Am J Crit Care* 14:494-513, 2005.

family being present in the athletic training room after their son sustained a serious head injury in a football game.

Summary

Deontology and teleology are competing normative, action-based moral theories, and the contrast between the two theories is striking (Table 15-2). As with all theories, their purpose is to provide divergent frameworks to reflect on ethical issues that are part of professional practice.[6-8,10,11,19]

CHARACTER-BASED THEORY: VIRTUE ETHICS

Character is like a tree and reputation like its shadow. The shadow is what we think of it; the tree is the real thing.
—ABRAHAM LINCOLN

Virtue ethics is the third widely used normative theory in professional ethics. Since the 1970s, it has achieved much attention as a viable moral philosophy in health care. Unlike the duty-oriented and consequence-oriented normative, action-based theories that require reasoning for right action, the center of virtue ethics is the character traits of the *moral agent* and associated behaviors (*habits*) consistent in nature. Furthermore, virtue theorists hold that persons should avoid bad character traits and vices, such as vanity and cowardice.[1,6,7,9,12,16]

Historically, virtues were emphasized by Plato, who recognized four cardinal virtues: justice, temperance, wisdom, and courage. Aristotle also supported the theoretical notions and added the concept that virtues are good habits that one obtains. Furthermore, Aristotle believed that a virtue is a mean between two distinct character traits. For example, the virtue of courage falls between cowardice on one end and foolhardiness on the other. Another example is the virtue of loyalty. At one end of the spectrum is blind loyalty, and at the other end disloyalty. Later the Christian virtues of faith, hope, and charity complemented the Greek virtues.[1,6,7,9,12,16] More recently, Alasdair MacIntyre[12] reaffirmed the Greek virtues and added honesty and integrity as important virtues of contemporary society.

The term *virtue* might suggest to some a sense of moral arrogance. However, the Greek word for virtue is *arête,* meaning excellence in relation to a skill or character. *Arete* and function are connected; for example, good athletic tape tears and supports well, or a good team physician is responsible and dependable. Given that virtue ethics also identifies excellent character traits, the attractiveness of this moral theory is that all a person needs to know is that inner qualities of virtues lead to right decisions and actions.[1] Virtue ethics uses no rules or principles to guide conduct. Aristotle referred to this quality as *phronesis*, or practi-

Table 15-2	COMPARISON OF ACTION-BASED, NORMATIVE ETHICAL THEORIES: DEONTOLOGY AND TELEOLOGY	
	Deontology	**Teleology**
Theorist	Kant	Bentham, Mill (utilitarians)
Focus and judgment	*Right* principle. Judges the morality of an action on reason.	*Good* consequences. Judges the morality of an action by consequences.
Premise	Means justify the ends.	Ends justify the means.
Norm	Act always as if actions will become universal law. Treat people with respect.	Act to maximize the good for the greatest number of people.
Moral distinction	Doing something and letting it happen.	Intending something and foreseeing something.
Concerns	A person is ethical if he or she carries out the *right* duties, even if the outcomes are negative. Which principles should be absolute?	A person may be used to achieve an end; may be unfair to minorities. Can outcomes be predicted?

Modified from Purtilo R: *Ethical dimensions in the health professions,* ed 4, Philadelphia, 2005, Saunders.

cal wisdom. Phronesis is more than a sense to act in a particular way; rather, it is a natural tendency to act consistently in a morally directed manner. Thus Aristotle would describe a man of good character as one who is firm, consistent, and steadfast; chooses virtuous acts for their own sake; and tends to choose a virtuous mean.[3,13]

The challenge with virtue ethics is that it does not provide an action guide. Furthermore, reason is not used to facilitate decisions or determine duty. Finally, this theory does not yield results that capitalize on happiness. Nevertheless, virtue ethics encourages the certified athletic trainer to draw upon personal excellence and reminds the practitioner of the importance of a good character in decision making and service to the patient-athlete.

THE MORAL MIX

Consider the two case studies in the beginning of the chapter according to the three moral theories: deontology, teleology, and virtue ethics. How would you respond to Ron's situation and Kelly's situation?

The three moral philosophical approaches discussed above are used to weigh and balance various particulars of an ethical issue. Deontology and teleol-ogy provide concrete direction through the use of rules, principles, duties, and consequences. In contrast, the inherent character traits of the moral agent serve to provide direction in virtue ethics.

All ethical issues require considerable moral reflection to advance good decisions and right action in professional ethics. Given that no one moral criterion exists, the moral agent needs to consider a number of viable decisions and actions as he or she processes an ethical issue. Professional ethics suggests that the moral agent should give credence to all three moral philosophical theories in deliberation.

A certified athletic trainer gives credence to the moral theory of deontology by giving weight to the NATA Code of Ethics (see Box 1-4). The code provides principles and rules for all members to uphold. In essence, the NATA Code of Ethics is an informal social contract that describes what society can expect when a certified athletic trainer interacts with other certified athletic trainers, patient-athletes, and the public. The code is the heart and soul of NATA and cannot be overlooked. Furthermore, the Board of Certification (BOC) provides a code of conduct, called first rules, for members certified by this agency (Box 15-2). The duties of a BOC-credentialed athletic trainer are

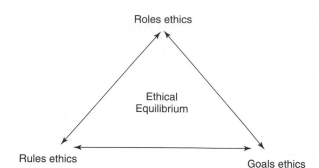

Figure 15-1 ■ Potter's ethical triangle, a multidimensional ethical decision-making framework. *(From Peterson M, Potter RL: A proposal for a code of ethics for nurse practitioners,* J Am Acad Nurse Practitioners *16:116-125, 2004.)*

Box 15-2

BOC CODE OF PROFESSIONAL RESPONSIBILITY

Code 1: Patient Responsibility
Code 2: Competency
Code 3: Professional Responsibility
Code 4: Research
Code 5: Social Responsibility
Code 6: Business Practices

embedded in the Code of Professional Responsibility of the Standards of Practice.[2]

Second, a certified athletic trainer gives credence to the moral theory of teleology by considering the goals of NATA. *Teleos* is the Greek word for goals. Professional bodies develop goals to impart identity, purpose, and direction to members. In athletic training, the NATA Strategic Plan[15] is the cornerstone of the professional body and identifies the mission as well as short- and long-term goals (Table 15-3).[21] Members have a shared, unified commitment when they advocate shared goals.

Finally, a certified athletic trainer gives credence to the moral theory of virtue ethics by becoming aware of his or her professional virtues (values) that result in excellent clinical practice and predictable professional behaviors. In other words, the public will come to

expect that a certified athletic trainer conveys consistent patterns of behaviors, regardless of the context, because these good character traits have been professionally internalized. Furthermore, virtue is more than reflexive or intuitive; it is knowing.

Thus in professional ethics, the deliberation of an ethical issue requires a moral mix of philosophical approaches. Ethical decisions and action in athletic training are considered by the professional in light of the NATA Code of Ethics and BOC Standards of Professional Practice. Potter's ethical triangle (Figure 15-1) suggests a simultaneous flow in moral reflection and the moral repositioning through the use of rule ethics (deontology), goal ethics (teleology), and role ethics (virtue ethics).[21]

FOUNDATIONAL BEHAVIORS OF PROFESSIONAL PRACTICE: PHILOSOPHICAL APPROACHES INFORM BEHAVIOR

The moral philosophical approaches that the certified athletic trainer uses to problem solve and make ethical judgments inform professional behavior. In fact, ethics or moral philosophy is a reflection about morality, and morality pertains to principles of right and wrong behavior.[17] Simply stated, behavior is an expression of moral philosophy. Relative to being a professional member of NATA, the professional body codifies good behaviors in the Code of Ethics.[5] Furthermore, relative to being a promising student in an athletic training education program, the NATA Education Council has

Table 15-3 NATA STRATEGIC PLAN

Strategic Direction	Action Areas
Increasing members' personal satisfaction and professional stature	Fostering emerging leadership Communicating with members Refining education Providing strategies for life balance
Empowering members to use their skills, expertise, and full scope of practice	Maximizing legislative influence Demonstrating the value of the athletic trainer Marketing the profession Guaranteeing financial responsibility

From National Athletic Trainers' Association: *Strategic plan* (website): www.nata.org/consumer/docs/strategicplanupdate_shortoverview.pdf. Accessed February 22, 2007.

Philosophical approaches

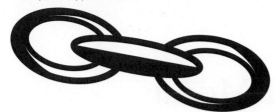

Foundational
behaviors of
professional practice

Figure 15-2 ■ Philosophical approaches are linked to foundational behaviors of professional practice.

outlined good behavior in the foundational behaviors of professional practice.[14] Thus the philosophical approaches (deontology, teleology, virtue ethics) are linked to foundational behaviors (Figure 15-2).

SUMMARY

Much like reflective equilibrium described by Beauchamp and Childress in Chapter 13, Potter's ethical triangle prompts students to consider dilemmas by repositioning themselves through the use of the rules and principles of deontology, goals of teleology, and the role of virtue ethics. Moral reflection encourages awareness of the many moral theoretical frameworks in which moral action and consequences are weighed and considered in ethical deliberation.

REFERENCES

1. Begley AM: Practising virtue: a challenge to the view that a virtue centered approach to ethics lack practical content, *Nurs Ethics* 12:622-637, 2005.
2. Board of Certification: *Code of professional responsibility* (website): www.bocatc.org/atc/Docs/SI-MR-TAB4-355.htm. Accessed June 21, 2006.
3. Clancy RC: Courage and today's nurse leader, *Nurs Admin Q* 27:128-133, 2003.
4. Curtain L: DNR in the OR, *Nurs Manag* 25:29-32, 1994.
5. Easley C, Marks SP, Russel EM: The challenge and place of internal human rights in public health, *Am J Public Health* 19:1922-1926, 2001.
6. Edge RS, Groves JR: *Ethics of health care,* Albany, NY, 1999, Delmar.
7. Gabbard DL, Martin MW: *Physical therapy ethics,* Philadelphia, 2003, FA Davis.
8. Guy ME: *Ethical decision making in everyday work situations,* Westport, Conn., 1990, Quorum Books.
9. Halm MA: Family presence during resuscitation: a critical review of the literature, *Am J Crit Care* 14:494-513, 2005.
10. Lefkowitz J: *Ethics and values in industrial-organizational psychology,* Mahwah, NJ, 2003, Lawrence Erlbaum Associates.
11. Lumpkin A, Stoll SK, Beller JM: *Sport ethics: application for fair play,* St Louis, 1994, Mosby.
12. MacIntyre A: *After virtue,* Notre Dame, Ind., 1984, University of Notre Dame.
13. Martone M: Building character for a new era, *Health Progress* 80:20-32, 1999.
14. National Athletic Trainers' Association: *Athletic training educational competencies,* ed 4, Dallas, 2006, National Athletic Trainers' Association.
15. National Athletic Trainers' Association: *Strategic plan* (website): www.nata.org/consumer/docs/strategicplanupdate_shortoverview.pdf. Accessed February 22, 2007.
16. Olthuis G, Dekkers W: Professional competence and palliative care: an ethical perspective, *J Palliative Care* 19:2-197, 2003.
17. Parkin C: Metaphysics and medical ethics, *J Med Ethics* 21:106-112, 1995.
18. Peterson M, Potter RL: A proposal for a code of ethics for nurse practitioners, *J Am Acad Nurse Practitioners* 16:116-125, 2004.
19. Purtilo R: *Ethical dimensions in the health professions,* ed 4, Philadelphia, 2005, Saunders.
20. Slosar JP: Ethical decisions in health care, *Health Progress* 85:38-43, 2004.
21. Williams D: *Strategic plans are cornerstones* (website): www.nata.org/committees/cic/pdf/strategic_planning.pdf. Accessed June 22, 2006.

Development of Moral Behavior: Step 3—Moral Character

ETHICAL CONCEPTS

Moral behavior
Moral character
Moral courage
Integrity

LEARNING OBJECTIVES

After reading this chapter, the student should be able to do the following:

1. Discuss the importance of moral character.
2. List the characters of a person who lacks moral character.
3. Compare physical courage and moral courage.
4. Explain integrity.
5. Describe how to get out of an unprincipled rut.
6. Discuss why the NATA Hall of Fame inductees convey moral character.

Unlike compliance, which focuses on specific behavior required by law or regulation, ethical behavior is a commitment to moral correctness and honesty (p. 76).[4]

According to Triezenberg and Davis's three-step framework of moral behavior, moral character is the last step (Figure 16-1).[15] The sum of all three steps' components ultimately results in moral behavior (moral action) (Figure 16-2).

MORAL CHARACTER

There are many rites and rituals that can help us improve our moral characters and cultivate a more harmonious world. But first, we must accept one of the basic rules of tribal life—that the motivation for our behavior is grounded, not in what we want to do, but in what we ought to do (p. 12).[3]

The importance of moral character is emphasized in both virtue ethics and moral behavior. Chapter 9 explained the importance of moral sensitivity in identifying moral issues, embedding the notion of moral motivation in moral sensitivity. In Chapter 13, moral reasoning was discussed within the framework of Kohlberg's theory of moral development. The last step of moral behavior is moral character. Although moral sensitivity and reasoning inform behavior, an action may not necessarily materialize. Thus the importance of moral character is significant because it has the ability to initiate action; it is the resolve and courage to follow through. Rest[13] describes moral character as ego strength, perseverance, toughness, strength of conviction, and courage to do right.[13]

A person who lacks moral character has no perseverance, falters under pressure, betrays principles and responsibilities, finds fault in others, lays blame on others, is full of excuses, and simply gives up. Relative to the notion of moral behavior, moral character allows a person to carry out what he or she knows is *right* and *good;* in other words, it ignites moral action.[6,15] Moral courage and integrity are two important aspects of moral character.

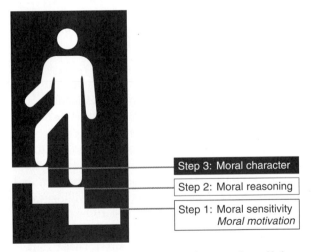

Figure 16-1 ■ The third step in the development of moral behavior is moral character.

PROFESSIONAL PEARL

Who are you really? Your character is who you really are. Your authenticity, your morals, and your ethics are revealed in your character. Your reputation is a matter of public opinion. You have little control over public opinion. But you do have control over your character. I believe that if you take responsibility for your character, your reputation will take care of itself. Reveal who you are by revealing your character.

—Mark J. Smaha, past president of NATA (1988-1992), 1997 NATA Hall of Fame inductee, and former Washington State University—Pullman, head athletic trainer.

Moral Courage

Moral courage is a readiness for voluntary, purposive action in situations that engender realistic fear and anxiety in order to uphold something of great moral

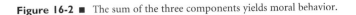

Step 1 (moral sensitivity)	+	Step 2 (moral reasoning)	+	Step 3 (moral character)	=	Moral Behavior (leads to *right* action)

Figure 16-2 ■ The sum of the three components yields moral behavior.

value. Unfortunately, there is no assurance of a successful outcome once one acts on that readiness. A common term to describe courage is "bravery," but when the term "moral" is added to it, the ensuing action must always be with the goal of protecting a moral value that appears threatened (p. 4).[11]

Courage is one of the four cardinal virtues identified by the Greek philosophers. It is often referred to as the most important virtue because it is needed to defend the other three virtues: justice, temperance, and wisdom. Effective leadership requires the courage to hold true to beliefs, principles, and convictions.

Historically, the focus of courage has been on physical courage, meaning the willingness to risk one's life for a higher ideal. In fact, Aristotle suggested that the ability to face danger gladly was the purest form of courage. Such courage is a reactive state in which a person has no time to think. Thus courage is considered a natural disposition. In contrast, moral courage is the willingness to risk disgrace, as well as social ridicule and disapproval, for attending to moral duties. To act with courage requires an individual to be willing to stand in isolation. To expand this concept, great leaders and professionals do not flock together; they have the courage to act alone and stand alone.

Over time, the physical risks associated with physical courage have lessened; today moral courage often is tested. Moral courage is most often witnessed in times of change. The profession of athletic training has experienced much change in the last 20 years, with an assortment of new practice settings, professional preparation, academic program accreditation, research priorities, licensing and regulation, third-party reimbursement, and membership diversity and explosion, to name a few. Many athletic trainers selflessly volunteered to take charge and effect change. The journey was never easy, yet their moral courage was substantiated by their ability to make a significant difference in their profession. These selfless professionals personified ethical fitness because of their well-defined moral values and principles and a deep sense of conviction. When tested, these individuals reacted with valor to take a stand to do what was good and right.[1,11,14]

Integrity

Integrity is an important trait that when combined with moral courage yields moral character. Integrity has many definitions (Box 16-1). A common thread appears to be that integrity is the conviction to hold on to truth and honesty. Furthermore, a person with integrity is ready to carry out his or her duty under adverse circumstances, or when no one is looking, with the purest of motivations simply because it is the right thing to do.

GETTING UNSTUCK

Failure to master integrity results in despair. This is a state of conflict over the way one has lived and continues to live one's professional life. It is the subjective experience of dissatisfaction, disgust, or disappointment, accompanied by the feeling that things could have been done differently if given the chance. There is a feeling of anxiety over the future and a sense of lack of control. The reality of retirement becomes a source of fear and this occupational therapist cannot complete unfinished business or recount the accomplishments of themselves or others (p. 47).[5]

Professionals get caught in an unprincipled rut for a variety of reasons. However, the professional should recognize that the rut is unprofessional and dishonorable. Of equal importance, the professional must understand and realize that it is never too late to get unstuck. To do so takes time, purposeful reflection, and ego courage. The professional must be open and ready for new self-discovery and have a willingness to pull out of the rut and readjust. It starts by putting the ego aside and owning one's irresponsibility, immaturity, and/or unprofessional behavior(s). Then it entails reexamining personal and professional values and principles along with corresponding associated behaviors. Is incongruence present between values and behaviors? Between principles and behaviors? If the answer is yes, then diligent work on aligning values and principles with consistent behaviors will be meaningful. Finally, mulling over challenging professional

Box 16-1

INTEGRITY: WHAT IS IT?

Stephen Covey (1989): "Integrity in an interdependent reality is simply this: you treat everyone by the same set of principles. As you do, people will come to trust you. They may not at first appreciate the honest confrontational experiences such integrity might generate. Confrontation takes considerable courage, and many people would prefer to take the course of least resistance, belittling and criticizing, betraying confidences, or participating in gossip about others behind their backs. But in the long run, people will trust and respect you if you are honest and open and kind with them. You care enough to confront."[2]

Denis Waitley: "Integrity means you do what you do because it is right and not just fashionable or politically correct."[13]

Larry May (1996): "To be a candidate for possession of integrity the person's choices and evaluations must be her own: her identifications with her desires must be neither subject to unconsidered change nor be distorted or confused. Her reasons for action must be genuine."[8]

Marilyn Martone (1999): "Integrity is a 'state of being whole or undiminished.' It is what Aristotle called a 'kind of virtuous activity'—performing noble actions, for example, or working for a society in which people are free to develop to their full potential. Modern philosophers are more likely to define integrity as a person's desire to do his or her best as he or she understands it, even under adverse conditions."[7]

Anonymous: "Integrity is when you do the right thing even though no one is watching."

Jack Kasar (2000): "Integrity is the subjective realization that the choices and decisions made in various professional stages were the best ones possible at those times. It is the evaluation that one is still in control of one's professional life. Just as the student learned trust as successful completion of the first stage, the expert occupational therapist learns that satisfactory retirement is successful completion of the final stage. Integrity bolsters the concept and belief that retirement is the resolution of a successful career; the experience of pleasure in one's own professional achievements; and the expression of pride in the achievements of those that follow them."[5]

---

stretches and learning the hidden lessons is also effective.[15] Thus awareness of the unprincipled rut, along with the willingness and courage to learn and readjust, helps the professional get unstuck.

EXEMPLIFYING MORAL BEHAVIOR: NATA HALL OF FAME

Since 1962, the National Athletic Trainers' Association (NATA) Hall of Fame inductees have epitomized excellence in technical and ethical standards (Figure 16-3). These men and women have been tested and retested, and their moral character is obvious to all. Their ethical disposition of integrity and courage has given them the strength to endure many of the professional challenges and hardships as they paved the way through selfless service. The NATA Hall of Fame inductees are the professionals every student should aspire to become (Box 16-2).[10]

NATA owes its success to the individuals who dedicate themselves to the advancement of the athletic training profession. Each year, the association's Honors and Awards program acknowledges individual achievements in nine award categories. The Hall of Fame is the cornerstone of this program. Induction into the NATA Hall of Fame is the ultimate honor a certified athletic trainer can receive. Selection takes place annually after candidates have completed a rigorous application process. The NATA Board of Directors selects the year's inductees from a pool of nominees evaluated by the Hall of Fame subcommittee. Those individuals receiving the award are selected because they embody the qualities of leadership, service, dedication, scholarly activities, promotion, and professionalism. In so doing, they advance the profession of athletic training.[9] The new class is chosen each spring and is recognized in the summer at the NATA Annual Meeting and Clinical Symposia.

Box 16-2

NATA HALL OF FAME INDUCTEES

1962: Ronald Bevan, Samuel "Doc" Bilik, Wilbur Bohm, David M. Bullock, Mike Chambers, Earl Clark, Chuck Cramer, Frank Cramer, Oliver J. Devictor, Lilburn J. Dimmitt, Carl Erickson, Billy Fallon, Tad Gormley, Jack Heppinstall, Thomas F. Lutz, Frank Mann, Larnard Mann, Michael C. Murphy, George Nelson, Einar Nielsen, Herb Patchin, E. W. Pennock, Michael D. Ryan, Claude Simons Sr., Stanley M. Wallace, Frank Wandle

1964: Elvin C. Drake, Mickey O'Brien, Henry Schmidt

1965: Walter Bakke, Arthur D. Dickinson, A. C. Gwynne, Frank E. Medina, Jules H. Reichel, Lloyd Stein, Eddie J. Wojecki, Edward G. Zanfrini

1966: E. Jay Colville, Charles E. Harper, James E. Hunt, James W. Littlejohn, Allan Sawdy, Steve Witkowski, Alfred J. Wyre

1967: William R. Ferrell, James H. Johnston, William F. Linskey, Werner J. Luchsinger, Naseby Rhinehart, Howard E. Waite

1968: C. A. "Bob" Bauman, Ernest Biggs, Carl Jorgensen, Kenneth B. Rawlinson

1969: Wesley I. Knight, James H. Morris, Richard A. Wargo

1970: Joseph N. Abraham, Delmer Brown, Elmer Brown, Richard K. Cole, Dwayne Dixon, Samuel R. Lankford

1971: Edward A. Byrne, Roland Logan, Charles E. Medlar, Dean B. Nesmith, William B. Robertson

1972: Joseph Blankowitsch, William E. Newell

1974: Edward Block, Anthony F. Dougal, Lincoln Kimura, Ross Moore, Laurence Morgan, Wayne Rideout, Wayne Rudy

1975: Robert H. Gunn, C. Rodney Kimball, Edward A. Sulkowski, Dr. Charles W. Turner

1976: L. F. Diehm, M. Kenneth Howard, Victor D. Recine, Gayle B. Robinson, George F. Sullivan

1977: Warren Ariail, John E. Lacey, Edwin B. Lane, John D. Rockwell, Francis J. Sheridan, Robert C. White

1978: Z. M. Blickenstaff, Martin J. Broussard, Earl J. Porche, Thomas D. Wilson Jr.

1979: Byron Bird, Robert E. Weingart

1980: Bobby Brown, Jim Conboy, Edward A. Coppola, Bruce J. Melin, Sayers J. Miller, Edward J. Pillings

1981: Otho Leroy Davis, Oliver William Dayton, Donald James Fauls, Thomas E. Healion, Fred Hoover, Warren G. Morris, Edward N. Motley, Robert A. Peterson, Buddy Taylor

1982: Francis Boyle, Bobby Lane, Mike Linkovich, Leo Murphy, Joseph Romo, Bruce Vogelsong

1983: Jack B. Aggers, Edgar Harold Biggs, Charles O. Demers, Kerkor Kassabian, Gene Paszkiet, John L. Sciera

1984: Lewis C. Crowl, James E. Dodson, Jim Goostree, Louis K. Grevelle, Walter Grockowski, Fritz Massmann, Joseph Stanitis, Raymond Ulinski, Joe Worden

1985: Larry L. Lohr, Wilford F. Pickard Jr., Jerry Rhea, Paul J. Schneider

1986: Edward R. Abramoski, Henry L. Andel, George C. Anderson, William H. Chambers, Chester A. Grant, Eugene Harvey, Carl E. Nelson, Curtis R. Rylander, William C. Samko, Fred A. Wappel

1987: Joseph R. Altott, Earnest L. Harrington Sr., L. David "Sandy" Sandlin, Frank J. Wiechec

1988: Gary D. Delforge, J. Lindsy Mclean, Leonard D. McNeal, Richard E. Vandervoort

1989: Lawrence J. Gardner, Fred G. Kelley, Charles F. Martin, J. C. Patrick Jr., James A. Wilson, Paul T. Zeek

1990: Robert S. Behnke, Cash Birdwell, Joe Howard Gieck, Roland "Duke" Larue

1991: Phillip B. Donley, Francis John George, Charles Franklin Randall III

1992: Richard F. Malacrea, Alfred F. Ortolani, Troy L. Young

1993: Thomas "Tim" Kerin, Gordon Stoddard

1994: Gary Craner, G. E. "Moose" Detty, Gordon L. Graham, Wesley D. Jordan, Dean L. Kleinschmidt, Dale P. Mildenberger, J. G. "Ken" Murray, Michael E. Nesbitt

1995: Dr. Denis "Izzy" Isrow, Gail Weldon

1996: Robert M. "Bobby" Barton, William Buhler, Paul Grace

1997: Daniel J. Libera, Mark J. Smaha

1998: James Booher, John W. Schrader, James Whitesel

1999: Marjorie J. Albohm, Ronnie P. Barnes, Kent P. Falb, Joseph J. Godek, Dale Googins, Phillip H. Hossler, Donald D. Lowe, James Douglas "Doug" May, Karen R. Toburen

2000: Earlene Durrant, James B. Gallaspy Jr., Richard "Dick" Hoover, Kent Scriber

2001: Donald A. Chu, Andy Clawson, Kenneth L. Knight, Kenneth W. Kopke, Carl Krein, Dennis A. Miller

2002: Peggy Houglum, Kenneth F. Kladnik, Peter Koehneke, Kenneth W. Locker, Sanford "Sandy" Miller, John "Jack" Redgren

Box 16-2

NATA HALL OF FAME INDUCTEES—cont'd

2003: Jack Baynes, Robert Beeten, Ronald Carroll, Robert Moore, David Perrin

2004: Albert Harris Green, William "Bill" Hughes McDonald, William E. Prentice, Theodore "Ted" Quedenfeld, Charles J. Redmond, Kathleen A. Schniedwind, Sue Stanley-Green, Clint Thompson

2005: Gerald W. "Jerry" Bell, Pete Carlon, Kathleen Cerra Laquale, Tony Marek, D. Rod Walters II

2006: Richard Ray

2007: Julie Max, Cynthia "Sam" Booth, Tom Abdenour, Steve Bair

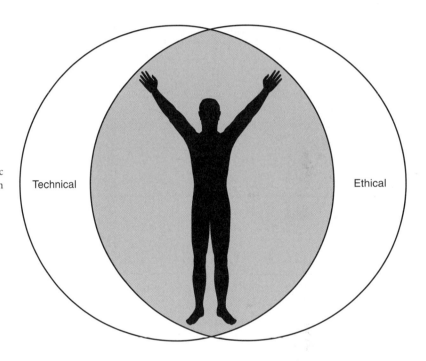

Figure 16-3 ■ In the profession of athletic training, moral behavior is at the intersection of technical standards and ethical standards.

SUMMARY

There is a certain blend of courage, integrity, character, and principle which has no satisfactory dictionary name but has been called different things at different times in different countries. Our American name for it is "guts."
LOUIS ADAMIC[12]

Athletic training is more than simply *knowing and doing* athletic training, as outlined in the athletic training technical standards. *Being* an athletic trainer is also considerably important. The *being* aspect of an athletic trainer is the sum of the ethical competence (values and interpersonal skills) plus technical competence (cognitive competencies and clinical proficiencies). *Being* an athletic trainer is ensured through the development of moral behavior. Moral behavior, the sum total of moral sensitivity, moral reasoning, and moral character, is found at the intersection of technical standards and ethical standards; that is where a person *is* an athletic trainer (see Figure 16-3).[15] Moral behavior is the heart and soul of any profession because that is where the trusting professional therapeutic relationship emerges. And trust does sustain the professional body.

REFERENCES

1. Clancy RC: Courage and today's nurse leader, *Nurs Admin Q* 27:128-133, 2003.
2. Covey S: *The 7 habits of highly effective people,* New York, 1989, Simon and Schuster.
3. Goldstein N: It takes an open tent and a leap of faith, *Newsweek* 144:12, 2004.
4. Gustafson BM: Setting the highest ethical leadership standards ensures a higher standard of results, *Healthcare Financial Manag* 55:76-78, 2001.
5. Kasar J, Muscari ME: A conceptual model for the development of professional behaviours in occupational therapists, *Can J Occup Ther* 67:42-51, 2000.
6. Killen AR: Morality in perioperative nurses, *AORN J* 75:532-541, 2002.
7. Martone M: Building character for a new era, *Health Progress* 80:20-32, 1999.
8. May L: *The socially responsive self: social theory and professional ethics,* Chicago, 1996, University of Chicago.
9. National Athletic Trainers' Association: *NATA award descriptions and criteria* (website): www.nata.org/honors/criteria.htm. Accessed February 15, 2007.
10. National Athletic Trainers' Association: NATA Hall of Fame (website): www.nata.org/honors/hof/index.htm. Accessed April 12, 2006.
11. Purtilo RB: Moral courage in times of change: visions for the future, *J Phys Ther Educ* 14:4-7, 2000.
12. *Quotes by Louis Adamic* (website): www.zaadz.com/quotes/Louis_Adamic. Accessed June 24, 2006.
13. Rest JR: Background: theory and research. In Rest JR, Narvaez D, editors: *Moral development in the professions: psychology and applied ethics,* Hillsdale, NJ, 1994, Lawrence Erlbaum Associates.
14. Rubin SB, Zoloth L: Clinical ethics and the road less taken: mapping the future by tracking the past, *J Law Med Ethics* 32:218-227, 2004.
15. Triezenberg HL, Davis CM: Beyond the code of ethics: educating physical therapists for their role as moral agents, *J Phys Ther Educ* 14:48-59, 2000.

CHAPTER 17

Organizational Awareness and the Preservation of Professional Identity in Context

ETHICAL CONCEPTS

Commitment model
Compliant model
Integrity
Organizational culture
Organizational interpersonal relationship
Organizational moral development
Organizational values

LEARNING OBJECTIVES

After reading this chapter, the student should be able to do the following:

1. Compare the compliant model and the commitment model.
2. Describe organizational culture.
3. Compare the professional therapeutic relationship and the organizational interpersonal relationship.
4. Identify and describe elements of trust in an organization.
5. Describe how values are incorporated into the organization.
6. Discuss the development of organizational integrity by using Kohlberg's stages of moral development.
7. Explain how value incongruence, workplace politics, and workplace bullying can test moral character.
8. Define workplace politics.
9. Describe types of workplace bullying.
10. Compare harassment and bullying.
11. Explain how conflict can help a person grow.
12. Compare a moral problem and an ethical problem.

While this notion of the ethical organization has its merits, it is also one sided. It seems to assume that an organization is or should be led and staffed by "moral heroes" who are strong enough to withstand any dubious influences of peer pressure and organizational climate (p. 26).[12]

In recent years, ethical misconduct in business, government, and health care has necessitated the examination of organizational ethics. The federal government has underscored the need to tackle abuse, fraud, and waste in health care.[9] In health care organizations, tension between care and profit exists. This conflict is real in all types of athletic training settings to varying degrees.

Two distinct models of organizational behavior exist: the compliant model and the commitment model. The compliant model is a system that uses policies, procedures, rules, and regulations to guide behavior. Such a system is akin to the model of rules and regulations in policy and procedure manuals given to professionals in training when beginning the athletic training education program. In contrast, the commitment model reflects deep-seated, shared values, attitudes, and beliefs among members. The National Athletic Trainers' Association (NATA), which is a volunteer organization, is an example of a commitment model. Although the commitment model is more challenging to attain, it sustains itself with little surveillance. A functional organization is suggested to be a blend—that is, an emphasis on the commitment model with compliance (rules and regulations) ambiguously folded in to the system.[19]

Organizations take on lives of their own. An organizational culture affects all aspects of the organizational life with a motto that clearly discloses that "this is the way things are done around here." Organizational culture is a system of shared values and beliefs with control systems to generate behaviors and norms.[4] The organizational culture provides direction, meaning, and a collective energy that moves the entity toward a productive, mediocre, or dysfunctional status.[5] Much like human moral development, organizations develop morally and reflect their culture. In this chapter, organizational ethics is viewed in a familiar framework beginning with (1) organizational values (a similar notion learned in Chapter 9), (2)

moral development of the organization (a similar concept learned in Chapter 13), and (3) moral character of the organization (similar to the discussion in Chapter 16).

ORGANIZATIONAL INTERPERSONAL RELATIONSHIPS

It is in the realm of interpersonal relationships that the culture gap in organizations is most glaring. What is needed is not knowledge but, rather, taking what most people consider to be common sense—treating patients and each other with dignity, respect, and caring—and making it common practice (p. 74-75).[22]

The organizational interpersonal relationship has similar qualities to a professional therapeutic relationship (see Chapter 12). It typically involves the connection with diverse professional groups that share common organizational goals. For some, the tricky part is maintaining a unique professional identity in a multiprofessional organization.

Similar to the professional therapeutic relationship, the organizational interpersonal relationship is built on trust. Furthermore, excellence in leadership requires the development of a trust culture to ensure organizational effectiveness. Table 17-1 identifies elements of a trust relationship in organizations with a diverse group of professionals.[5]

Organizational trust is significant in sustaining the moral posture, effectiveness, and excellence within the entity. The foundation of relationships is trust, which serves to fortify the ties among organizational members. Furthermore, excellence in organizational leadership begins with trust, which conveys all the elements of a trust relationship.[1]

Organizational Values

Organizations with integrity have truly learned that there is no choice but to walk their talk. Their values are true representations of how they want to conduct themselves, and everyone feels deeply accountable to them.[8]

Organizational values are a deep-seated understanding that determines how others should be treated, what actions are acceptable or unacceptable, and whom to

Table 17-1 ELEMENTS OF A TRUST RELATIONSHIP

Element	Examples
Acceptance	Of self and others Of group-made decisions Of group aims Of intrapersonal and interpersonal control Of the need to participate in group action Of differences in others
Assumptions	Issues fall into two opposing camps exemplified by either/or thinking—hard data or soft data, the world is unsafe or safe
Authentic caring	Personal interest Openness to others Willingness to risk close relationships Willingness to serve others
Ethics	Peer relationships Organizational practices Fiscal policy Moral values of the larger society
Leadership	Predictability Consistency Cooperation Service orientation
Individual character	Expect trust Expect honesty in others Expect spontaneous behavior in others Expect openness (not defensiveness)
Predictability	Consistency of action Confidence Actions based on truth

From Fairholm GW: *Leadership and the culture of trust*, Westport, Conn., 1994, Praeger Publishers, p. 106.

trust. Establishing values is an important first step of organizations.

A model developed by Kanji[11] depicts organizational values infusing the vision, mission, strategy, and key issues of the organization (Figure 17-1). The effectiveness of organizational leadership is related to the ability to impart shared values in all components of the organization. Commitment to organizational values is recognized in the structure, awards, rewards, and socialization mechanisms. Shared values are important because they (1) foster strong feelings and personal effectiveness, (2) cultivate organizational loyalty, (3) help develop consensus to meet goals, (4) encourage ethical behaviors, (5) reduce tensions, and (6) encourage pride and teamwork.[11]

Organizational Moral Development

Organizational ethics is fundamentally concerned with fostering the well-being of the organization itself, its associates, those it serves, and the larger community in which it exists, through means that are themselves morally valuable (p. 38).[21]

The development of organizational integrity is not easy. Petrick and Pullins[14] parallel the development of organizational integrity using Kohlberg's framework (Box 17-1). Organizational integrity is realized in the last stage of this developmental theory, but few organizations actually attain it.[14]

Preconventional: Stages 1 and 2

Stages 1 and 2 can be described as the survival of the fittest. The most powerful individuals or alliances

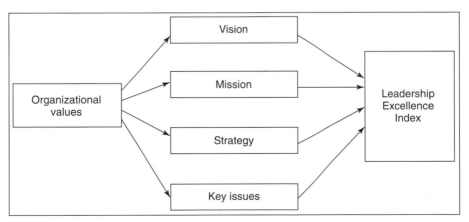

Figure 17-1 ■ The influence of organizational values. (*From Kanji GK:* Measuring business excellence, *London, 2002, Routledge.*)

DEVELOPMENT OF ORGANIZATIONAL INTEGRITY

Stage 1

Social Darwinism: Fear of extinction and the urgency of financial survival dictate moral conduct. The direct use of force is the acceptable norm.

Stage 2

Machiavellianism: Organizational gain guides actions. Successfully attaining goals justifies the use of any effective means, including individual manipulation.

Stage 3

Cultural conformity: A tradition of standard operating procedures and caring groups. Professional peer pressure to adhere to social norms dictates what is right or wrong behavior.

Stage 4

Allegiance to authority: Directions from legal authority determine moral standards. Right and wrong are based on the decisions of those with legitimate hierarchal power.

Stage 5

Democratic participation: Participation in decision making and reliance on majority rule become organizational moral standards. Participative management becomes institutionalized.

Stage 6

Organizational integrity: Justice and individual rights are the moral ideals. Balanced judgment among competing interests shapes organizational character, which in turn determines the rightness or wrongness of behavior.

From Petrick JA, Pullins EB: Organizational ethics development and the expanding role, *Health Care Superv* 11:52-62, 1992.

organization operates with deceit, dishonesty, trickery, and cleverness and resorts to gossip and betrayal to maximize personal gain. Those who are not part of the "in" group are marginalized and learn to distrust others. Good behavior and bad behavior usually are played out in terms of yearly awards, rewards, recognition, and opportunities to advance.[14]

Conventional: Stages 3 and 4

In the next two stages, Petrick and Pullins[14] suggest that organizational behavior is marked by approval seeking and upholding authoritative order. Stage 3 proposes that, to be part of the in group, adherence to the power clique's rules of conduct is required. Thus the mentality of the in group determines what is right. Stage 4 purports that authoritative approval is significantly important. Members of the organization operate by constantly seeking approval from the authority to determine what is right. Organizational socialization is a extremely powerful tool used to indoctrinate new members and maintain the cultural status quo, which limits the ethical development of the organization.

The "in" group mentality in stage 3 can blind the organization to real outside concerns and threats. Furthermore, the subservient behavior to authoritarian rule in stage 4 can perpetuate mediocrity. The negative effects of stages 3 and 4 can impede organizational growth and development. Similar to personal moral development, many business practitioners reason at this level.[14]

Postconventional: Stages 5 and 6

Majority rules (democracy) and principled conviction (justice and individual rights) are the central moral approaches in the determination of right action. Stage 5, majority rules, appears to be forthright and fair except to the minority. At this stage, the excellent contributions of a few can be silenced to the detriment of the organization. Stage 6, the final stage of organizational moral development, honors justice and the minority perspective. At this stage the individual can hold true to his or her professional convictions without fear of punitive measures or reprisals. Consensus is the approach and the right action. At this level all individuals are rewarded justly. Stage 6 occurs when organizational integrity is reached.[14]

determine what is right and wrong. In stage 1, reprimands, as well as cultural isolation, are doled out to those who deviate from the accepted behavior. Power cliques determine what is right and develop the organization's policies and procedures. At stage 2, the

Integrity: The Moral Characteristic of the Organization

Organizations with integrity embrace their organizational values and are outspoken about their characters.[20] These entities "walk the talk" and are ethically fit. Entrenched principles and moral values guide consistent patterns of verbal and nonverbal ethical behaviors. A sense of organizational loyalty and unity emerges. Organizations with integrity promote public trust.

Beyond well-established values and behaviors, characteristics of organizations with integrity include defining a clear purpose, confronting reality, having open agendas, and following through. Defining a clear purpose requires consistency and repetition in communication, transparent motivations, and guiding principles aligned with the organization's values. Such actions eliminate misunderstanding and strengthen trust. The second characteristic of organizational integrity is confronting reality, which encourages knowledge of the organization relative to its services and/or products as well as the employees of the organization. Such revelations—coupled with the willingness to tackle difficult issues—require, at times, brutal honesty. Open agendas, the third characteristic, construct transparent motivations and objectives and sustain a high-trust organizational culture. Finally, follow-through is important because it conveys promise keeping and commitment. Follow-through relative to organizational integrity requires individuals to be open and honest in the event that commitments cannot be made. Life constantly changes, but organizational integrity based on values and the four characteristics provides comforting consistency to diverse groups of professionals.[8,13,16,20]

GOOD TO KNOW

An organization that has a defined set of values and principles demonstrates its desire to serve all members. Behaviors and attitudes acceptable as a professional member of that organization set the standards for treatment of diverse populations.

ORGANIZATIONAL CONFLICT AND TRANSFORMATION: THE TEST OF MORAL CHARACTER

The true test of character is not how much we know how to do, but how we behave when we don't know what to do.
JOHN W. HOLT, JR.[9]

Many organizations uphold high standards of ethical practice. However, some professionals discover that the courage to take the high road of professional practice is daunting in some organizations. Given that professional codes of ethics and standards of practice in athletic training *cannot* be compromised, the foremost question is, how can professionals be resolute in their commitment to uphold their professional values, duties, and responsibilities when they are incongruent with the organization's values and agendas? Insight into potential organizational pitfalls is a good place to start. A professional's moral character is tested by incongruence in workplace and professional values, workplace politics, and workplace bullying.

Incongruence in Workplace and Professional Values

Distress materializes when workplace values are not congruent with professional values, ultimately leading to job stress and/or workplace burnout.[10] Yesterday's theoretical model of burnout simply proposes a mismatch between the person and the workplace. Contemporary conceptualization of workplace burnout is reflected by three components: exhaustion, cynicism, and ineffectiveness.[15]

Certified athletic trainers have a professional responsibility and obligation to abide by the Board of Certification (BOC) Code of Professional Responsibility and Standards of Practice. Professional practice also is further described by the practice acts of each state. Moreover, all members of NATA must abide by the NATA Code of Ethics. Thus relative to athletic training, professional roles and ethical responsibilities are clearly defined by the BOC, NATA, and state licensure regulation, which convey the inherent professional values. The inherent professional values of athletic training always trump organizational values. Accordingly, if value incongruence exists, the certified athletic trainer must find the courage to be unyielding and resolute in upholding the professional values, duties, and responsibilities explicit in the BOC professional credential and NATA membership.

Workplace Politics

Perhaps the least understood and most important area for aspiring leaders to understand is organizational politics is an integral part of any organization's culture.[6]

Insight into workplace politics is important in helping the new professional make good decisions and convey appropriate professional behavior. Workplace politics tests moral character. Awareness of organizational shenanigans helps professionals negotiate some of the potential pitfalls of organizational life.

Workplace politics is complex and has been defined in a number of ways. Sociologists have suggested that workplace politics is a necessary evil, is inevitable, and cannot be avoided. In contrast, the management literature defines it as power or influence that is illegitimate, informal, and dysfunctional. Another definition of workplace politics describes it as a socially influential process that is strategically behavioral for the purpose of serving self-interest at the expense of others' interests.[23] Variables that may initiate workplace politics include scarcity of resources, powerful positions, denial of information, competitive work environments, unclear rewards and advancements, role ambiguity, emotional insecurity, hunger for acceptance, and self-interest.[2] Workplace politics is unhealthy, narrow minded, self-centered, divisive, and, ideally, not sanctioned by the organizational administration. Regardless of the definition, the consequences of workplace politics are personal struggles, inequity, and unfairness.[23]

Getting a sense of the organizational culture is always helpful for the professional. In health care, duties and roles are clearly outlined and defined by the profession and state practice acts. To get a sense of the organization and the potential politics and pitfalls, the professional should detach, observe, listen, read, probe, and reflect. Some important questions to ask in evaluating an organization's politics are listed in Box 17-2. Answers to these questions shed light on how business is done in the organization.[2]

Box 17-2

IMPORTANT QUESTIONS IN EVALUATING ORGANIZATIONAL POLITICS

To whom do key employees report?
Who has the power to veto a decision?
Who asks whose advice?
Who socializes new members?
Who mingles with whom?
Who is marginalized?
Who is the workplace bully?
What is the professional background of middle managers? Executives?
Who is recognized for outstanding work?
What are considered the perks? Who gets them?

Box 17-3

CATEGORIES OF WORKPLACE BULLYING

Threats to professional status (e.g., belittling, humiliation)
Threats to personal standing (e.g., teasing, insults)
Isolation (e.g., withholding information)
Overwork (e.g., impossible deadlines, unnecessary disruptions)
Destabilization (e.g., meaningless tasks, shifting the goal posts)

From Rayner C, Hoel H: A summary review of literature relating to workplace bullying, *J Appl Social Psychol* 7:181-191, 1997.

Workplace Bullying

Most organizations have a serial bully. It never ceases to amaze me how one person's divisive dysfunctional behavior can permeate the entire organization like a cancer.
Tim Field[17]

In the last 6 months of 2005, 2 million people were bullied.[18] Workplace bullying typically involves one member of the workplace targeted by another. Bullying typically involves repeated attacks that grow in intensity. Others in the workplace generally know about the bullying but do not do more than console for fear of retribution. Box 17-3 lists different types of workplace bullying.[18]

The bully may not even realize that he or she is a bully. In fact, he or she often vehemently denies being a bully. Bullies typically are self-centered, immature, and convincing liars but often appear self-righteous. Furthermore, the purpose of bullying is to shield incompetence. Bullies are insecure, and if they can operate without detection, below the radar screen, or have the support of superiors, they prey on strong, competent members of the workplace.

Box 17-4 compares harassment and bullying. In the big picture, the distinction between bullying and harassment may seem insignificant because they both have deleterious psychological and physiological effects.

Stopping workplace bullying may not be easy, But it cannot be condoned in any health care setting. Some organizations have a workplace policy relative to bullying. The best advice for the professional is to confront the bully and document, document, document.

Keep in mind, however, that conflict is part of life. Let conflict teach you about yourself, your profession, and your organization; find the courage, use it, and grow. Curtin[3] writes:

> If the conflict is between what you think you ought to do and what you want to do, you are probably dealing with a moral rather than an ethical problem. If morality consists of the degree of congruence between what one thinks is right and one's actual behavior, then a moral problem by definition is one in which you are inclined to do that which you think is wrong—or, at least, not right. Ethics, on the other hand, is a discipline in which you apply certain principles in order to determine what is the right thing to do in a given situation. Therefore, an ethical problem occurs when you actually don't know what you think is the right thing to do. It is extremely helpful to distinguish between moral and ethical problems because they must be handled differently. An ethical analysis is designed to help you figure out what you think is the right thing to do and why you think it. A moral problem brings you face-to-face with who you are—and just how far you are willing to go to preserve your own integrity (p. 30).[3]

SUMMARY

As with human beings, organizations have many different goals, values, motivations, and beliefs. Furthermore, much like moral development, an organization's moral maturity can be viewed through the lens of Kohlberg's moral development theory and through the behaviors of the professionals working in the organization.

Although most athletic trainers experience the undeniable joy and wonder of professional practice in their workplace, some may not. Awareness of potential organizational pitfalls, such as workplace and professional values incongruence, workplace politics, and bullying, helps the challenged athletic trainer move through a difficult time with courage and integrity. Why the moral character of some professionals is tested to the maximum while others are not is perplexing, but much of the evidence suggests this situation has more to do with the organizational culture rather than the professional himself or herself.

Box 17-4

HARASSMENT VERSUS BULLYING

Harassment can have a physical component or a sexual connotation; this includes sexual intimidation, sexual harassment, or actual assault. Bullying is primarily psychological in nature, at least initially.

Controversy exists regarding whether bullying is related to gender. Some believe that it occurs equally between men and women; however, the actual number of women victims is greater. Women also experience greater rates of sexual harassment.

Harassment, particularly when associated with assault or sexual harassment, can have a criminal element; this tends not to be the case with bullying.

An aspect to both bullying and harassment appears to be gender, with women being victims more often than men. However, women also are perpetrators of these unacceptable behaviors.

"Cyber violence" is currently being reported, with people being harassed and/or bullied by telephone and email.

From Gilmour D, Hamlin L: Bullying and harassment in perioperative settings, *Br J Perioperat Nurs* 13(2):79-85, 2003.

Maintaining professional footing and balance on the high road of professional life can be extremely taxing. Surviving complex workplace culture requires a commitment to moral professional values. The Work, Stress, and Health 1999 Conference even stressed the importance of the organization's support of employee's professional values. Those who are professionally motivated defend, promote, and advocate for their professions during times of adversity in a multiprofessional organization. It may not be easy, but moral character is not cheap. Once the victim of workplace maliciousness appreciates the fact that he or she is not responsible for the immoral behaviors of workplace bullies, the healing process can begin.

Curative approaches to workplace adversity require reality checks. Because colleagues, administra-tors, and/or middle managers may participate in ado-lescent organizational behavior, the human resources department typically is a safe place to seek support. In most organizations this department is equipped to help employees comprehend and cope with the some-times harsh realities of workplace life. Another source for professional guidance can be a certified athletic trainer from another organization. An objective, unbi-ased, and mature outlook may shed much light on a difficult workplace situation.

In brief, being a certified athletic trainer is not always easy. Upholding professional values, duties, responsibilities, obligations, and ethical conduct can be challenging at times. Maintaining footing and balance on the high road of professional life requires a commitment to the profession and moral character.

REFERENCES

1. Bell SE: Ethical climate in managed care organizations, *Nurs Admin Q* 27:133-140, 2003.
2. Chase CR: Corporate politics: the business of health care, *SSM* 8:27-33, 2002.
3. Curtin L: DNR in the OR, *Nurs Manag* 25:29-32, 1994.
4. Dunn MG, Odom RY: Organizational values and value congru-ency and their impact on satisfaction, commitment, and cohe-sion: an empirical examination within the public sector, *Public Personnel Manag* 20:195, 1991.
5. Fairholm GW: *Leadership and the culture of trust*, Westport, Conn., 1994, Praeger Publishers.
6. Frank MS: The essence of leadership, *Public Personnel Manag* 22:381-390, 1993.
7. Healthcare fraud program boasts record returns to the govern-ment, *Healthcare Financial Manag* 57:11, 2003.
8. Johnson JE: Six steps to ethical leadership in health care, *Patient Care Manag* 18:1-6, 2002.
9. *John W. Holt, Jr. quote* (website): en.thinkexist.com/quotation/the_true_test_of_character_is_not_how_much_we/209819.html. Accessed June 22, 2006.
10. Jones-Schenk J: How magnets attract nurses, *Nurs Manag* 32:40-43, 2001.
11. Kanji GK: *Measuring business excellence*, London, 2002, Routledge.
12. McCurdy DB: Creating an ethical organization, *Generations* 22:26-32, 1998.
13. McDermott RJ: American Academy of Health Behavior: a journey and an adventure—incoming presidential address, *Am J Health Behav* 27(suppl 3):S273-S276, 2003.
14. Petrick JA, Pullins EB: Organizational ethics development and the expanding role, *Health Care Superv* 11:52-62, 1992.
15. Poczwardowski A, Grosshans O, Trunnel E: Sustaining enthusi-asm in the classroom: reinvestment strategies that work, *Am J Health Behav* 27:322-344, 2003.
16. Proenca EJ: Ethics orientation as a mediator of organizational integrity in health services organizations, *Health Care Manage Rev* 29:40-51, 2004.
17. *Quotes by Tim Field* (website): www.bullyonline.org/workbully/quotes.htm. Accessed June 22, 2006.
18. Rayner C, Hoel H: A summary review of literature relating to workplace bullying, *J Appl Social Psychol* 7:181-191, 1997.
19. Schleslinger LA: Beyond the carrot and the stick, *Hospital Forum* 28:13-16, 1985.
20. Shaw RB: Organizational integrity, *Executive Excellence* 15:13, 1998.
21. Slosar JP: Ethical decisions in health care, *Health Progress* 85:38, 2004.
22. Sokoloff P: Practicing what we preach, *Health Progress* 87:73-79, 2006.
23. Vigoda E: Internal politics in public administration systems: an empirical examination of its relationship with job congruence, organizational citizenship behavior, and in-role performance, *Public Personnel Manag* 29:185-211, 2000.

Learning Activities: Linking Content to Practice

An attribute of professions . . . is that its members engage in activities with a large element of service to humanity. This raises . . . the problem of the demarcation between personal and professional lives . . . and between a manager's personal ethic[s] and the organization's philosophy and mission. Philosophy and mission are the organization's basic law and guide the development and implementation of policies, procedures, and rules (p. 43).

KURT DARR[3]

During the transition to professional life, students face daily challenges influenced by organizational culture as well as professional standards and behaviors. Organizational culture permeates all aspects of an organization and affects how decisions are made and how dilemmas are resolved. Athletic training professionals should seek an organization that has philosophies and principles that align with their personal and professional identity.

Functioning within an organization requires the development of a strong moral character and moral courage. When faced with challenges, professionals must rely on what is inside and generate the courage to do the right thing to reduce moral conflict. Understanding the impact of organizational features on how to function in a particular setting gives you the ability to resolve conflict and transform yourself into a confident, morally competent professional.

As you complete the following activities and reflect on the assessment options, keep in mind that personal and professional development directly ties in to organizational culture. Many options are provided to encourage reflection on multiple levels regarding how each activity can affect working within a specific organizational culture.

ACTIVITIES FOR APPLICATION: LINKING CONTENT TO PRACTICE

LEARNING ACTIVITY 1: THE NEWSPAPER ARTICLE

Objectives

1. To connect personal and professional identities to organizational culture
2. To examine organizational culture from an informal perspective
3. To identify any potential conflicts between personal and organizational cultures in athletic training

Description

Write a newspaper article or news release (one to two pages) regarding your recent hiring at one of the following athletic training settings:

Setting 1: You are recently hired as the head athletic trainer for the University of Notre Dame.

Setting 2: You are recently hired as the athletic trainer and sports medicine coordinator for NovaCare Corporation.

Setting 3: You are recently hired as the athletic trainer and health educator for Kent Roosevelt High School in Kent, Ohio.

Setting 4: You are recently hired as the athletic trainer for the United Parcel Service company.

Setting 5: You are recently hired as the head athletic trainer and sports medicine coordinator for the X-games.

Setting 6: You are recently hired as the athletic training education program coordinator and director for your current institution.

The document must include personal qualities about you (the new hire) and what you can bring to the organization. You must also include in the article how you (as the new hire) can enhance the organization based on information about the mission and vision of the organization. Be sure to write the document in third person perspective (i.e., do not use "I" statements).

Hint: Information about the organization's culture, mission, and vision can be found by an Internet search.

Assessment

The nature of this activity lends itself well to written feedback. This activity seeks input relative to organizational culture and the ability to articulate how personal qualities and values connect with organizational culture. Peer assessment also is a good option for this activity because it demonstrates cultural perceptions from another person's perspective.

Combining this activity with a journal activity to facilitate further reflection also is useful. A guided entry that addresses issues posed in the following questions also may be used: Did you believe you appropriately addressed your strengths, or did you try to make your strengths match the mission and vision of the organization? Why is having a strong personal and professional identity important before becoming immersed in an organization as a professional? How would the organizational culture in the selected venue affect your professional behaviors? Could you work in this type of setting?

LEARNING ACTIVITY 2: CONCEPT MAPPING

Objectives

1. To recognize concepts related to moral theories and principles[1]

2. To identify key concepts relative to terminology commonly associated with ethics in the workplace

3. To connect conceptual theories to real-life situations in athletic training

Description

Create a graphic depiction of key concepts in relation to other supporting materials. This map should establish connections between related concepts and culminate in addressing professional behaviors.

Choose one of the topics or concepts below to consider. For the first few minutes, record *any* related terms or phrases that come to mind. After listing terms and phrases, create a type of map (linear, circular, or any other form) that illustrates the connections between the selected topic and the terms and phrases you generated.

After plotting these primary associations, take 10 minutes to establish secondary and tertiary connections and associations to build on what you have already mapped. After establishing the secondary and tertiary connections, identify at least one scenario that reflects the connections you just made. As the last step of this activity, address how the foundational behaviors of professional practice—primacy of the patient, teamed approach to practice, legal practice, ethical practice, advancing knowledge, cultural competence, and professionalism—correspond with each terminal connection on your map.

Selected Topics

- Deontology
- Teleology
- Virtue ethics
- Moral character
- Moral courage
- Organizational values
- Sexual harassment
- Position power

Step 1: Think about the key concept.

Step 2: Brainstorm terms and phrases related to the topic, and write them down.

Step 3: Draw a map connecting the terms and phrases.

Step 4: Identify secondary and tertiary connections.

Step 5: Provide concrete, real-life examples linked to the terms.

Step 6: Connect these examples to the foundational behaviors for professional practice.

Step 7: Reflect on the concept map and any organizational features that may have affected your connections.

Assessment

This activity can be assessed by simply analyzing the connections made between the key concepts. Evaluating accuracy in conceptual information is essential. However, the relations established relative to professional behaviors should be much more diverse. Consider the individual application and interpretation of personal and professional identity issues while you perform peer evaluations of your classmates or a self-evaluation.

This activity also can be performed in a small group in which a group participation rubric can guide the assessment. Additionally, a follow-up writing assignment to explain the map can provide valuable insight into the rationale behind the connections that may not be inherently obvious at first glance.

LEARNING ACTIVITY 3: DOCUMENTED PROBLEM SOLVING

Objectives

1. To analyze the steps used in problem solving to gain insight relative to the process[1]
2. To promote critical thinking about how problems are solved
3. To encourage consideration of alternative solutions throughout a problem-solving activity

Description

Create a flow chart to reflect how you solved one of the following problems, documenting how you developed the solution. Provide the rationale for each choice you made as well as which options or choices you did not consider.

CASE SCENARIO

Case 1

You are elected president of the athletic training student organization. You are struggling to get people involved in the activities. Everyone seems to be so busy with clinical assignments and classes that they do not want to be involved in extra activities. How would you promote increased involvement in the student organization?

CASE SCENARIO

Case 2

You are an athletic trainer at a local high school. You have heard through the grapevine that some of the athletes are acquiring steroids from local college athletes and are taking them to enhance performance. You have noticed that some of the athletes are demonstrating signs and symptoms of steroid use, such as increased bulk or size and mood swings. What do you do?

CASE SCENARIO

Case 3

As an athletic trainer employed at a clinic, you are assigned to organize the first-aid provider services mandated by law in your state for all high school coaches. These coaches must document attendance at these seminars to receive their coaching stipends. You are teaching the course, and you notice that many of the coaches are reading the newspaper, text messaging, and planning practices. When you address them, the coaches say all they have to do is attend the seminar; no one said they had to pay attention. What do you do?

Assessment

Part of this activity involves the resolution of the problem. However, more important is the process you use to solve the problem. Group or pair work using a group or peer evaluation rubric (see Appendix B) provides ample opportunity to work through the multiple approaches to problem solving and encourages dialogue among peers. A class presentation describing the problem-solving approach is another viable option. Lastly, after the initial work is completed, comparing the problem-solving approaches used by all the members of the class can be a valuable learning experience when performed as an after-class reflection.

LEARNING ACTIVITY 4: FOCUSED LISTING

Objectives

1. To establish connections between related concepts[1]
2. To promote critical thinking about relations among key terms and concepts
3. To gauge the level of understanding of key concepts and how they fit into larger concepts

Description

After formal presentation of several concepts, choose one of the following key points from the lesson:

Key Concepts

Use the following key concepts for focused listing:

- Moral courage
- Moral intensity
- Professional behaviors
- Values
- Ethical principles
- Code of ethics
- Deontology
- Teleology
- Virtue ethics
- Politics

From this key point, create a list of related terms or ideas that are connected. This technique will be used at various times in a lesson to provide checkpoints for understanding. After listing five to seven connected concepts, define them. Take 3 to 5 minutes to complete this activity in written format.

Assessment

This activity can be performed in class and evaluated by the instructor or peers for accuracy of connections and definitions. It can also be performed as an out-of-class assignment to check after-class understanding. Additionally, if performed in a small group, you can compare others' lists for discussion and ask questions to increase understanding of the key concepts. This activity also serves well in daily use as part of a journal assignment to keep a running log of critical information.

LEARNING ACTIVITY 5: ADVERTISEMENT

Objectives

1. To create a brief portrait of organizational culture
2. To reflect organizational qualities
3. To describe key philosophical elements of a given organization

Description

Write a brief advertisement for one of the following organizations. This advertisement will be published in area newspapers and selected allied health publications. It will be a half-page ad (must fit on half of an 8.5 × 11 inch piece of paper). This advertisement should market the organization and its services. Highlight the role of the athletic trainer in the advertisement. You can create the name and qualities of this organization; be creative.

Organization 1: A newly built, state-of-the-art wellness center adjacent to the local hospital that offers sports medicine services, including aquatic therapy, rehabilitation, sport clinics, gait retraining, and sports massage

Organization 2: A brace manufacturer (e.g., anterior cruciate ligament functional braces)

Organization 3: The National Federation of Rodeo, which is establishing a relationship with Justin Sportsmedicine

Organization 4: Existing sports medicine clinic under new ownership by an athletic trainer that has changed its focus from conservative care with a primarily geriatric population to a sports-focused clientele

Assessment

This activity demonstrates your creative spirit and emphasizes the conceptual understanding of the role of the athletic trainer. Use a rubric (see Appendix B) to evaluate content and creativity to balance this assessment. Peer evaluation of the advertisement also provides a means of reinforcing the multiple roles of the athletic trainer that your classmates may not have considered.

LEARNING ACTIVITY 6: MARKETING BROCHURE

Objectives

1. To promote the athletic trainer as a member of the health care team
2. To demonstrate conceptual understanding of the role of the athletic trainer
3. To promote creativity in communicating the role of the athletic trainer as a professional

Description

Create a trifold marketing brochure for athletic training services that describes one of the following organizations. Select any organization in which an athletic trainer is professionally employed. The role of the athletic trainer as part of the health care team within this organization and the philosophy of this organization must be highlights of this brochure. Be creative.

Select your own organization to market, or choose any of the following:

- An orthopedic physician's office that employs an athletic trainer as a physician extender
- An outpatient physical therapy clinic that employs an athletic trainer in the clinic in the morning and at a local high school in the afternoon
- A private, religious college that employs an athletic trainer as a part-time professor and part-time athletic trainer
- A large hospital corporation that employs an athletic trainer as the director of sports medicine services
- A national pharmaceutical corporation that employs an athletic trainer as a representative for nonsteroidal antiinflammatory medications
- A car manufacturing company that employs an athletic trainer to work with employees receiving workers' compensation

- A large hospital corporation that employs an athletic trainer to work with the local professional basketball team

Assessment

Identification of appropriate services is essential to this activity. Ethical marketing techniques (truth in advertising) also are paramount. Assessment of creativity, impact, and other technical components should provide valuable feedback.

LEARNING ACTIVITY 7: INSTRUCTIONAL MANUAL

Objectives

1. To identify the role ethical principles play in the creation of policies and procedures
2. To appreciate the complexity of establishing policies and procedures that are comprehensive and ethical
3. To think critically about the impact of policymaking on an organizational culture

Description

Create an instructional manual or policy manual for employees at a newly opened sports medicine facility that you, as the athletic trainer, are charged with running. You have an ethnically, religiously, and racially diverse staff consisting of the owner, three physical therapists, three athletic trainers (excluding yourself), two physical therapy aides, two front office staff, and one billing person. The instructional manual must include the following information:

- Organizational mission and vision
- A flow chart depicting the chain of command within the organization
- Personnel policies, including sick, vacation, holiday, break, and personal leave policies
- Dress code and professional behaviors
- Pay structure relative to bonus and merit pay
- Professional development policies
- Communication policies with physicians, parents, clients, and referring allied health care personnel
- Record-keeping policies

As you write each policy, make a connection with one or more of the foundational behaviors of professional practice as part of your rationale.

Assessment

The goal of this activity is to demonstrate the difficulty in writing policies and procedures that are culturally sensitive, fair, and ethical. Consideration of the key elements within each policy is essential; however, the link to the foundational behaviors of professional practice truly reflects a higher level of understanding.

LEARNING ACTIVITY 8: SUMMIT CONFERENCE

Objectives

1. To promote professional communication and interaction
2. To develop critical thinking skills relative to ethical problems
3. To illustrate the complexities associated with ethical dilemmas in the athletic training profession

Description

Divide the class into two teams. Select one of the following ethical dilemmas, and debate it for 15 minutes. The instructor assigns a stance to take on this case. After the debate, negotiate a type of "treaty" to resolve this dilemma. It must be agreeable to both sides.

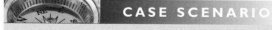
CASE SCENARIO

A student in the athletic training education program is called by the clinical instructor on a Saturday afternoon to report to a field hockey practice that had just been rescheduled. The athletic training student had been drinking since approximately 11 AM with his friends as part of a house party before an afternoon football game. The athletic training student reports to practice out of duty, and the athletic trainer smells alcohol on his breath.

Side 1: Athletic training student is dismissed from the program for showing up to a clinical assignment after drinking.
Side 2: Athletic training student is sent home without any penalty because it was an impromptu, unscheduled practice.

CASE SCENARIO

The supervisor at a clinic recently discovered that an employee leaves 30 minutes early every day to pick up her child at daycare before it closes. A fellow employee agreed to help her out and was treating the remaining patients during that time. No decrease in patient load occurred during this 30-minute period. This employee is a 10-year employee who recently lost her husband in a car accident and is the sole provider for her 20-month-old child.

Side 1: Fire the employee for leaving work early without prior approval.
Side 2: Let her continue to do this as long as the other employee agrees to care for the patients.

CASE SCENARIO

During a lunch break, a fellow employee makes a comment about how "shapely" your legs are in running shorts. You consider this sexual harassment and report the incident to your supervisor.

Side 1: Release the employee for making a suggestive comment because you have a no-tolerance policy on sexual harassment.
Side 2: Do nothing to the employee.

Assessment

A rubric (see Appendix B) designed to evaluate group interaction and participation is most beneficial in this activity. This activity also can be followed up with an individual writing assignment reflecting on the case and the stance taken by the class during the debate and treaty phases.

LEARNING ACTIVITY 9: THINK ABOUT . . .

Objectives

1. To examine personal and professional values from an organizational perspective[2]
2. To clarify the multiple factors that affect an ethical decision
3. To promote critical reflection on perceptions of ethical dilemmas and their resolution

Description

Read the following scenarios (unrelated to athletic training), and respond to them regarding whether you believe the employee acted ethically. Provide a rationale for why you chose the response you did.

Scenario	Ethical or Not?	Rationale
A salesperson accepts a bribe from a customer to reduce the price of a new automobile.		
An employee follows management's directives and fails to inform an auto manufacturer about a faulty component.		
A sales manager authorizes salespeople to give gifts to purchasing agents.		
A worker blames an innocent co-worker for errors.		
A manager authorizes a subordinate to violate a company policy.		
A management decision violates the privacy of subjects during a marketing research project.		
A salesperson gives gifts to customers to increase sales.		
A salesperson asks buyers for information about competitors.		

Next, create scenarios relative to athletic training, and assess whether you believe they are ethical with a given rationale. These situations should be real-life scenarios that you have encountered in clinical experiences. They must somehow affect the organization and profession.

Scenario	Ethical or Not?	Rationale

Next, respond to the following questions:

- Was determining ethical behavior easier in unrelated professions than in athletic training scenarios?
- Did you have difficulty thinking of ethical situations in athletic training? Explain why or why not.
- Does the athletic training profession gain anything from assessing how other professions respond to dilemmas?
- How did these situations link to your professional and personal values identified in previous chapters?

Assessment

The ability to identify ethical or unethical behavior is paramount in this activity. Providing rationales helps clarify the principles, theories, and values that connect to how you consider issues. Group discussion after this activity can be helpful in promoting dialogue about the multiple perceptions of each scenario. A group discussion rubric (see Appendix B) can be used.

LEARNING ACTIVITY I0: RINGS OF UNCERTAINTY

Objectives

1. To reflect on the multiple roles of the athletic trainer in an ethical dilemma.[4]

2. To reflect on the potential interventions in ethical dilemmas.
3. To collaborate to reach a common understanding and resolution.

Description

Figure 18-1 uses concentric rings to represent the varying degrees of uncertainty present in an ethical dilemma. The rings are divided into sectors—communication, resources, ethics, law, and professional competence—to help you sort through the potential options. Use this graphic to process the potential options for resolving an ethical dilemma.

The center ring represents the area of most certainty, and the outermost rings represent areas in which you identify the highest degree of uncertainty relative to the resolution of the dilemma.

As you sort through the dilemma, shade the graphic to reflect the percentage of the issue you believe to be related to the sector (Figure 18-2). (If you believe that resources are the major consideration in resolving this issue, shade approximately 50% of the graph at the resources sector, leaving 50% to divide among the other sectors. The shading of the sectors must equal 100%.)

Place a dot in the concentric rings of each sector to reflect how certain you are that this factor should be considered in the decision-making process.

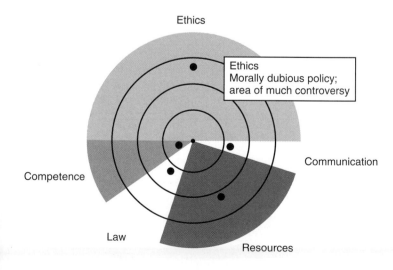

Figure 18-1 ■ Rings of uncertainty. *(Modified from MacClaren P, Seedhouse D: Computer mediated communication with integrated graphical tools used for health care decision making, ASCILITE Conference Proceedings, 2001, p. 111.)*

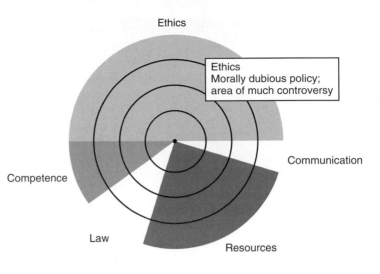

Figure 18-2

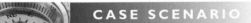

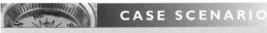

Case 1

A high school athlete sustains a concussion at a practice session. Although he successfully completes a functional return-to-play evaluation with marginally acceptable scores, he reports a continued mild headache. The championship game is tomorrow night, and the coaches push you to return him to play. His parents also are supportive of his return to play.

Case 2

You are an athletic trainer at a clinic and are directed by your employer to administer electrical muscle stimulation to a pregnant woman with back spasms. The patient is a close friend of the owner, who is a physical therapist. You are tentative regarding the modality because you know that pregnancy is a contraindication for electrical stimulation in the lower back or abdominal region. You approach your employer, who says to do it anyway and asks if you are questioning his authority. He tells you to do it or find another place to work.

Assessment

The process of considering options and gaining an appreciation for the fact that many decisions are made with some level of uncertainty is critical. The most effective way to evaluate these concepts is through a journal activity that ties together the activity and the effect on professional decision making. Grading the grid itself is not necessary, although it can be used to spark a group discussion or debate. However, you have the opportunity to reflect on the complexities of decision making from a personal perspective through a journal entry or other individual writing assignment.

LEARNING ACTIVITY 11: ETHICAL GRID

Objectives

1. To promote critical thinking about the multiple layers of any ethical dilemma[4]
2. To encourage reflection on the themes or threads that emerge from completing the grid
3. To develop skills in discerning relevant and irrelevant information in solving ethical dilemmas

Description

Figure 18-3 shows an ethical grid consisting of a set of 20 tiles arranged in four concentric rectangular rings. Each tile declares a statement that is open to interpretation within categories represented by different colors. The outer ring reflects practical considerations, the

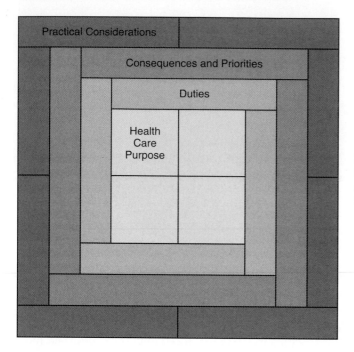

Figure 18-3 ■ Ethical grid. *(Modified from MacClaren P, Seedhouse D: Computer mediated communication with integrated graphical tools used for health care decision making, ASCILITE Conference Proceedings, 2001, p. 110.)*

next ring reflects consequences and priorities, the next ring reflects duties, and the inner ring represents the health care purpose.

Choose one of the following ethical dilemmas, and fill in the grid (Figure 18-4) with the codes in Figure 18-3 to guide your thought processes. Fill the grid as completely as possible while you brainstorm. After you have brainstormed, place an X through any idea that you do not believe is immediately relevant to the resolution of this case. Stop when you believe you have all the relevant information on the grid.

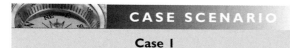

CASE SCENARIO

Case 1

You are working with the women's soccer team and are approached by several members of the team about a player who is binging and purging. You have noticed that the young woman has fluctuated in weight considerably. The girls reporting this incident are contenders for the position that the other player holds, and tension is obvious between the women.

CASE SCENARIO

Case 2

Your employer is involved in research with a nutritional supplement company. This company provides considerable financial perks to the employees in your organization on a regular basis. You are asked to analyze the data for your employer. When you do, you find no significant difference in the subjects who took the supplement from the ones who did not. Your employer asks you to run the data again with different statistical approaches until you find a significant difference.

Assessment

Assessment of this activity should be based on the process of resolution rather than the specific outcome. Consideration of alternative approaches and impact across the multiple constituents in any organization should be reflected in the grid. Feedback in the form of peer evaluation often is insightful, or you may com-

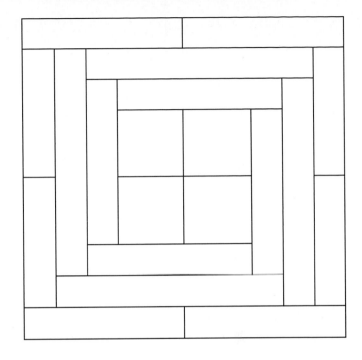

Figure 18-4

plete this activity using a group participation rubric (see Appendix B).

LEARNING ACTIVITY 12: REFLECTION SQUARE

Objectives

1. To describe an initial reaction to a particular case[5]
2. To examine critically the morally salient components of the case
3. To organize your professional position relative to athletic training

Description

Part I: Initial Reflection

After reading the following case, take 5 minutes to record your initial reaction and rationale.

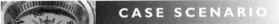

CASE SCENARIO

A collegiate athlete demonstrates a rapid heart rate during practice. He is a first-generation college student who is thought of as a great kid. He is on scholarship and could not afford to attend college otherwise. He intends to become a physician and stays up late to study. He takes an over-the-counter stimulant to stay awake during late study hours. He knows of the risk of a random drug test but is willing to take the chance in the hope he will not be chosen.

Part II: Guided Reflection

After recording your immediate response, begin discussion as a group. Center the discussion on the four dimensions of professionalism as depicted in the reflection square in Figure 18-5.

The instructor or group recorder writes the responses in each of the quadrants as they relate to the

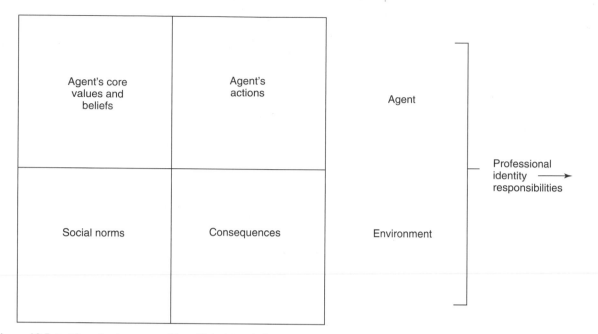

Figure 18-5 ■ The reflection square. *(From Verkerk M, Lindemann H, Maeckelberghe E, et al: An interpersonal exercise in ethics education, Hastings Ctr Rep 36:31-38, 2004.)*

discussion. Discussion should revolve around the four quadrants. If an action is presented and recorded, the next question should be what the consequences or social norms are and what values and beliefs guide that action.

Part III: Mapping Responsibilities

Next, map your responsibilities as a professional in this situation. Depict graphically how your choice is influenced by the organization in which you work. Identification of others' roles in the process may evolve as well, but focus on your role as the health care provider.

After mapping your duties, discuss in a large group the outcomes, issues, and complexities associated with this case, again focusing on the quadrants of the reflection square.

Assessment

This activity is best evaluated from a group participation perspective and/or a personal journal reflection after the large-group activity, with a link in the entry specifically to professional behaviors in a complex organizational setting.

SUMMARY

As you embark on your professional journey, you will see that ethical decision making requires careful consideration of many different factors. These dilemmas demand moral courage and moral character, which require that you understand how to make decisions personally and professionally as well as within an organizational context.

By challenging yourself to think through some of these activities and reflect on the situations you have already seen, you will be better prepared as a professional to address ethical dilemmas. Ethical dilemmas occur more often than you expect. Having the foresight to consider the effect of your decision will help you carefully weigh the alternatives. Each of the dilemmas you face builds your character and shapes you professionally. That is what foundational behaviors for professional practice are all about in athletic training. These behaviors permeate all that professionals do.

REFERENCES

1. Angelo TA, Cross KP: *Classroom assessment techniques: a handbook for college teachers,* San Francisco, 1993, Jossey-Bass.
2. Barnett T, Brown G, Bass K: The ethical judgments of college students regarding business issues, *J Educ Bus* 69:333-338, 1994.
3. Darr K: *Ethics in health services management,* Baltimore, 1997, Health Professions Press.
4. MacClaren P, Seedhouse D: Computer mediated communication with integrated graphical tools used for health care decision making, *ASCILITE Conference Proceedings,* 2001, pp. 109-112.
5. Verkerk M, Lindemann H, Maeckelberghe E, et al: An interpersonal exercise in ethics education, *Hastings Ctr Rep* 36:31-38, 2004.

Level III: Professional Application

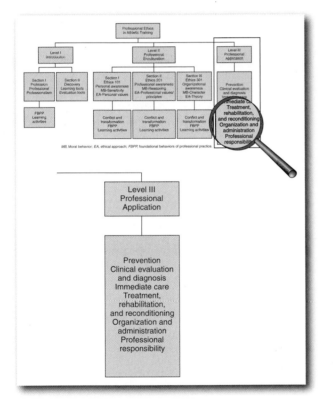

MB, Moral behavior; EA, ethical approach; FBPP, foundational behaviors of professional practice.

Chapter 19: Learning Activities: Linking Content to Practice

This section of the text serves as the culmination of all of the content addressed throughout the text. This chapter is intended to demonstrate that ethical dilemmas permeate all aspects of our profession and can occur in any of the professional domains of practice. Using the *Role Delineation Study* (5th edition) as a template for creating scenarios, you will be challenged by ethical dilemmas from each of the domains.

However, before you get started, we would like to address a few important points. Throughout this text, you have been introduced to the profession of athletic training and what it means to be a professional and reflect professionalism. You have been introduced to the concept of professional enculturation and its role in your personal and professional journey. Additionally, you have been provided a rich background providing the rationale and need for ethical discovery throughout your career. You have read about and participated in activities that encouraged a variety of learning approaches and have challenged yourself as you engaged in activities that emphasized a broad range of ethical decision making models.

As you continued through the text, you learned about professional ethics relative to self awareness, professional awareness, and organizational awareness. You have been entrenched in the theory and application of moral behavior and its impact on moral development. You have been introduced to, and hopefully embrace, the concept of moral character that is sustained by moral courage and integrity. Moral character will be contested throughout your professional life. The greatest learning occurs when you examine and reflect upon all aspects of professional conflict through a variety of ethical approaches (values, principles, and theory) in a genuine attempt to seek the lesson. Allow conflict to transform you.

As you begin this chapter, we challenge you to think critically and reflectively about what you have learned. Take each case scenario seriously, and look at it from multiple ethical approaches. Think about the personal and professional impact of your decisions. Think about who you are personally and professionally and how that may bias your decision. We encourage you to *think*, . . . *think*, . . . *think*. You have a tremendous foundation that will serve as a compass throughout your career. Remember, this is just the beginning . . .

CHAPTER 79

Learning Activities: Linking Content to Practice

Athletic trainers face ethical challenges in multiple contexts throughout their daily work. Although most athletic trainers associate ethical dilemmas with major issues affecting them as a professional, ethical dilemmas are present in all domains of athletic training. In your journey of ethical discovery, you have seen the connection between ethical behavior and foundational behaviors of professional practice.[5] The processes by which you approach, analyze, and resolve ethical situations are rooted in who you are personally and professionally. Although guided by the law, policies, and procedures, values have a tremendous effect on how people act.

Be sure to reflect continually on how you make decisions, a process that will change as you journey through your career. When scrutinizing your professional behaviors, use your conscience as a guide. According to Ray, "A good conscience requires both knowledge of the moral and ethical standards of the profession and awareness of individual circumstances and how they affect your patients" (p. 1).[7] Embrace this challenge on a daily basis. Think about how you perform your job and how that performance may affect others.

The following scenarios were created to help you think about situations that may arise in each of the Board of Certification domains of athletic training.[6] Carefully consider each, and devise your own scenarios; the more practice you have in dealing with these type of issues, the more competent and confident you will become in the ethical decision-making process.

THE BOARD OF CERTIFICATION DOMAINS: APPLYING ETHICAL THEORY TO EVERYDAY DILEMMAS

Prevention

A. Educate the appropriate patients about risks associated with participation and specific activities by using effective communication techniques to minimize the risk of injury or illness.

CASE SCENARIO

As a certified athletic trainer, you are in a position to educate patients about risky behaviors, including substance abuse. You often joke with a student-athlete about suspected use of anabolic steroids, although you are confident that the athlete is not using these substances. Other athletes and athletic training students participate in the joking. Is this ethical?

B. Interpret preparticipation and other relevant screening information in accordance with accepted guidelines to minimize the risk of injury and illness.

CASE SCENARIO

An athlete, who happens to be the only son in the family line, reports to football camp in August. At the preparticipation clearance, the athlete is discovered to have only one testicle; the other was surgically removed in late May. The athlete is adamant about playing and is willing to sign a release to play, understanding the risk associated with the likelihood of a serious injury to the remaining testicle. The parents are adamantly against him playing, fearing for his fertility in the future because it would end the family line if he could not reproduce. As the athletic trainer, you consult the team physician, who must make the decision. What are the legal and ethical issues you must address in this case?

C. Instruct the appropriate patients about standard protective equipment by using effective communication techniques to minimize the risk of injury and illness.

CASE SCENARIO

A football player reports to the office of the athletic trainer and discloses that he has a sexually transmitted disease that is making his protective cup uncomfortable to wear during practice. The athletic trainer verifies he is receiving medical treatment, then advises the athlete to do whatever makes him feel better. The athlete chooses not to wear the protective cup during the practice session and subsequently receives a significant injury to the testicles. Was the athletic trainer practicing ethically?

D. Apply appropriate prophylactic and protective measures by using commercial products or custom-made devices to minimize the risk of injury and illness.

CASE SCENARIO

A high school athlete recently underwent surgery for an injury to the anterior cruciate ligament. He is cleared to return to participation with a custom-fit prophylactic knee brace. The physician directs the athlete to talk to the athletic trainer about which knee brace is best. After consulting the athletic trainer, the athlete is confident that the XYZ brace is the best option, particularly because it is covered by his insurance. The athlete takes his prescription for the brace to a local brace vendor, where the personnel there tell him that brand ABC is similar to the brace recommended by the athletic trainer, but it is flashier and comes in his school colors (whereas the XYZ brace comes only in black). The athlete is excited about the school colors and selects the ABC brand, which costs his parents considerably more as an out-of-pocket expense. After receiving the bill for the brace, the mother of the athlete calls the athletic trainer to discuss how disappointed she was in how he advised the athlete about the brace and discloses that the out-of-pocket expense exceeded several hundred dollars. Did the athletic trainer act ethically?

E. Identify safety hazards associated with activities, activity areas, and equipment by following accepted procedures and guidelines to make appropriate recommendations and minimize the risk of injury and illness.

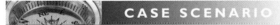

CASE SCENARIO

An athletic trainer works at a clinic that recently underwent a change in ownership. The new owner failed to have the therapeutic modalities inspected at the annual inspection date. Although all the modalities are in working condition, the athletic trainer expressed his concern to the new owner about the inspection dates. The new owner said that at his old clinic, they had their modalities inspected only every other year and they always functioned fine. The owner expresses dissatisfaction with spending that kind of money on an annual basis when all the modalities check out fine each time, yet commits to having the modalities inspected in 6 months. The athletic trainer continues to treat patients with a variety of therapeutic modalities during the 6-month period between this conversation and the modality inspection. Is this ethical?

F. Maintain clinical and treatment areas by complying with safety and sanitation standards to minimize the risk of injury and illness.

CASE SCENARIO

A high school athletic trainer fills the warm and cold whirlpools each morning and allows student-athletes to get in the whirlpools before and after practice without changing the water. Athletes often go in the whirlpools after practice without being prescribed this treatment by the athletic trainer. Many of these athletes are not visually inspected before submerging in the whirlpools. Because the athletic trainer acknowledges the value of hydrotherapy, concern is not great that the athletes often share the tanks. At the end of the day, the athletic trainer appropriately cleans and disinfects the tubs. Is this ethical?

CASE SCENARIO

The head athletic trainer at a local university has a huge dog as a pet. The dog is too big to be bathed at home, so he brings the dog to the athletic training room after hours and gives the dog a bath in the whirlpool tubs. These tubs are sterilized and disinfected each time after use. Is this behavior ethical?

G. Monitor participants and environmental conditions by following accepted guidelines to promote safe participation.

CASE SCENARIO

The assistant athletic trainer assigned to volleyball is responsible for monitoring the weight of each athlete before and after each practice to prevent heat illness. Several athletes are quite conscious of their weight and have been advised by the coach to lose a few pounds despite acceptable weight and body composition measurements recorded during the preparticipation clearance. The athletes are distraught about the coach nagging them to lose weight and ask the athletic trainer to tell the coach that they have lost a few pounds. The athletes have lost a few pounds according to the weigh-ins; however, they also gain them back before the next practice (as recommended during hot weather exercise). The athletic trainer abides by the requests of the athletes and tells the coach that they have lost a few pounds. The coach stops badgering the players at practice, and everyone seems more relaxed. Is this ethical?

H. Facilitate physical conditioning by designing and implementing appropriate programs to minimize the risk of injury and illness.

An athletic trainer for a local college is responsible for the health care of the cross country and track teams. The track coach recently attended a strength and conditioning workshop that emphasized the role of overtraining to facilitate speed. The coach is incorporating overtraining into all aspects of the track program at the school. This track coach comes new to this college with multiple conference and national championships. A sharp increase in injury occurs in the first 2 weeks after the new coach arrived. Many of the injuries are caused by overtraining stresses. After talking with the coach, he states that the athletes need to get used to the process and that he knows how to build champions. Another 2 weeks pass, and even more injuries occur and are of a more serious nature. The athletic trainer expresses concern to the coach once again, who says that he will have her removed from covering this sport if she continues to bother him with her concerns. The athletic trainer then reports her concerns to the athletic director, who advises her to go with the flow. She cannot afford to lose her job. She reports back to practice and never addresses the situation again. Is this ethical?

I. Facilitate healthy lifestyle behaviors by using effective education, communication, and interventions to reduce the risk of injury and illness and promote wellness.

An athletic trainer for a local high school recently read an article that stated ingesting a raw egg with 3 tablespoons of honey before sprinting events increases energy. After trying this concoction several times before her own running, she does see an increase in energy and performance. One afternoon in the athletic training room while the athletic trainer closed down for the day, an athlete sees her ingest this concoction. The athlete inquires about what she is drinking, and the athletic trainer shared what she read and how it affected her performance. Is this ethical?

An athletic trainer at a clinic is evaluating a patient experiencing considerable back pain. The patient is clinically obese, which is addressed during the assessment. During the course of treatment, the athletic trainer and the patient establish a rapport. One morning, the patient brings in her 9-year-old daughter, who is off from school that day. The daughter asks if she can come in to the treatment room with her mother during the initial treatment of heat and electrical stimulation. The athletic trainer allows this. As she checks on the patient, the athletic trainer notices that the child is eating cheese curls and a sugary soft drink for breakfast. By the end of the treatment, the child has consumed 2 sodas and a large bag of snacks. The athletic trainer takes this opportunity to talk to the mother about appropriate nutrition for her child and how obesity runs in families. Was this ethical?

Clinical Evaluation and Diagnosis

A. Obtain a history through observation, interview, and/or review of relevant records to assess current or potential injury, illness, or condition.

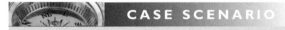

You are taking a history on a patient with upper/mid back spasm and discomfort. In the course of the history portion of your evaluation, the patient discloses that she has had breast implants within the past 5 months. You disclose to her that you have been considering implants as well, and you spend the next 15 minutes discussing the surgery, surgeon, recovery, and cost of this procedure. You thank the patient for the information and return to the evaluation for her condition. Is this ethical?

You are performing a palpation on an athlete who reports to the athletic training room with a suspected groin injury. You are a male athletic trainer assessing a male athlete. You take the athlete into a personal examination area to preserve his privacy and perform your evaluation. During your examination, you follow proper protocol by informing the patient that you will need to palpate the area and ask his permission, which is granted. During the evaluation, the athlete runs out of the examination room, screaming that you were inappropriately touching him and calling you derogatory names. The athletic training room is full of athletes who are receiving prepractice treatments.

B. Inspect the involved area visually to assess the injury, illness, or health-related condition.

D. Perform specific tests in accordance with accepted procedures to assess the injury, illness, or health-related condition.

You are performing an evaluation on a patient who reports to the athletic training room with a stiff neck. During the observation portion of your examination, you notice several suspicious marks around her cervical region that may indicate abuse. You ask the patient about the marks, and she says that she is unsure how she got them and says she was not aware they were there. What do you do?

As an athletic trainer in a clinic, you are performing an evaluation on a patient who reports to the clinic with shoulder instability. You have never felt a true subluxation on a patient. During the special testing portion of the examination, you perform an apprehension test with a little extra vigor (understanding that the patient has no pain with the subluxations) so that you can feel the actual movement out of the socket. Is this ethical?

C. Palpate the involved areas by using standard techniques to assess the injury, illness, or health-related condition.

E. Formulate a clinical impression by interpreting the signs, symptoms, and predisposing factors of the injury, illness, or conditions to determine the appropriate course of action.

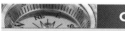

CASE SCENARIO

An athlete reports to the athletic training room immediately before practice when it is packed with athletes. He has a considerable limp and is reporting an inversion ankle sprain incurred during practice. After a brief history, observation, and palpation of the lateral ligaments and a quick anterior drawer test, you indicate that the athlete has a grade 2 ankle sprain. You establish a treatment plan to treat the pain, swelling, and lack of function. Is this ethical practice?

CASE SCENARIO

A patient reports to the clinic for evaluation of her rotator cuff injury. She is referred to you by the orthopedist, who works closely with you on a daily basis. During the history portion of her examination, she discloses to you that she has postpartum depression but she refuses to seek medical attention for fear her husband will think she is not happy about the birth of their baby. She comes to therapy as scheduled but is making slow progress and is quite lethargic during her exercises. She states she is compliant with her home exercises. At the 4-week checkup, the patient demonstrates little progress in her shoulder rehabilitation. The physician asks you why she is not progressing. Do you disclose her postpartum depression as a factor for slow progress?

F. Educate the appropriate patients regarding the assessment by communicating information about the current or potential injury, illness, or health-related condition to encourage compliance with recommended care.

Immediate Care

A. Use life-saving techniques through the use of standard emergency procedures to reduce morbidity and the incidence of mortality.

CASE SCENARIO

After seeing a physician for a sexually transmitted disease, an athlete comes to you to discuss the condition. He asks you what the long-term implications are of this condition. Knowing that the athlete will not curtail his sexual behavior unless the condition is truly serious, you tell him about the documented, yet highly unlikely, serious complications that can arise from this condition. Is this ethical?

CASE SCENARIO

A community member exercising in the university field house has a sudden cardiac arrest while walking one morning. You are in the facility performing your daily exercise. You are called over to help the man. As you arrive, his wife, who was walking with him, states that he has terminal cancer and has a do-not-resuscitate order on file with his physician. What do you do?

G. Share assessment findings with other health care professionals by using effective means of communication to coordinate appropriate care.

B. Prevent exacerbation of non–life-threatening conditions through the use of standard procedures to reduce morbidity.

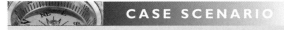

CASE SCENARIO

An athlete reports to the athletic training room with a boil that is not responding to conventional treatment. You once shared with your team physician that when you were a graduate assistant, you saw an athletic trainer use a heated glass bottle placed over the area to extract the core of the boil. It provided immediate relief from the pain and removed the core so that the site could heal. The team physician asks you to try that procedure on this athlete. What do you do?

C. Facilitate the timely transfer of care for conditions beyond the scope of practice of the athletic trainer by implementing appropriate referral strategies to stabilize and/or prevent exacerbation of the conditions.

CASE SCENARIO

An athlete needs a bone scan for a suspected femoral stress fracture. She is unable to return to play until she receives clearance, which will be based on the scan results. You receive the referral from the team physician and have set up an appointment and transportation to the appointment for the athlete. On the morning of the scan, the athlete calls to cancel the appointment 30 minutes before you are to leave to take her there. You reschedule the appointment for the following day; this time the athlete fails to show. When you see her that afternoon, she laughs and said she must have forgotten and asks you to reschedule the appointment. This time when you call to reschedule, you are given an appointment time 1 week away. You typically try to see if the bone scan staff can "squeeze you in sooner," but you do not ask for that favor this time. Is this ethical?

D. Direct the appropriate patients in standard immediate care procedures by using formal and informal methods to facilitate immediate care.

CASE SCENARIO

You are the athletic trainer at a college where emergency medical technicians staff the ambulance at each home football game. You have tried to meet with them to discuss the role of the athletic trainer and how the two groups of professionals can work to best serve the athletes in an emergency situation. The ambulance staff declines any offer to meet and discuss roles. During a game, an athlete dislocates a hip, which requires immediate transportation to the hospital. After approaching the injured athlete, you assume the role of calming the athlete and stabilizing the dislocated limb. Shortly thereafter, the emergency medical technicians arrive and tell you to step back so they can prepare the athlete for transportation. What do you do?

E. Execute the established emergency action plan by using effective communication and administrative practices to facilitate efficient immediate care.

CASE SCENARIO

In the clinic where you are employed as a certified athletic trainer, you are responsible for establishing an emergency action plan and educating the staff regarding proper policy and procedures. Many of the staff are disinterested because they do not suspect life-threatening emergencies will happen in the clinical environment. Many of the staff joke with you about your intensity regarding the plan and attribute it to your previous years as a professional football athletic trainer. Once the plan is established, you hold an in-service to review the policies and procedures to be implemented. Several of the therapists ask the supervisor to be excused from the meeting, stating that you will handle the situation if anything happens. The supervisor excuses them from the meeting. What do you do?

Treatment, Rehabilitation, and Reconditioning

A. Administer therapeutic and conditioning exercises by using standard techniques and procedures to facilitate recovery, function, and performance.

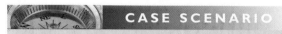

CASE SCENARIO

A junior high school athlete plays elite-level tennis and has been invited to attend a specialized program for the summer. The athlete recently gained approximately 15 pounds as a side effect of puberty but has been able to maintain the level of play necessary to qualify for elite status. Her parents approach you to discuss the training protocol, which would involve strict diet modifications, practice sessions three times per day, and evening weight-lifting programs. This summer program is sponsored by a well-known tennis organization and employs tennis professionals from around the country. The parents ask your opinion on the program. You are concerned about the intensity of the program but do not want to ruin the opportunity for this young athlete by raising concern in her parents as well. What do you do?

B. Administer therapeutic modalities by using standard techniques and procedures to facilitate recovery, function, and performance.

CASE SCENARIO

An athletic training student is assigned to your clinic as part of a clinical assignment. You have worked with this student for the past 3 months and are confident in her abilities. One of the athletic trainers on staff calls in sick at the last minute, and 15 patients are on the schedule for this staff person. You decide to pick up 10 of the patients and allow the student to care for the other five patients, which includes therapeutic modality application and therapeutic rehabilitation processes. Is this ethical?

C. Apply braces, splints, or assistive devices in accordance with appropriate standards and practices to facilitate recovery, function, and performance.

CASE SCENARIO

The volleyball coach approaches you after you have fitted a brace for the starting outside hitter for her patellar tendonitis. The athlete states that the brace helps decrease the pain during practice. The coach explains that you have a key match this weekend and that he would prefer that the athlete not wear the brace because it would highlight the fact that she is not 100%, which may cause the other team to change their game tactics by targeting this "weak link." Without the brace, no one will know that the athlete is in pain. What do you do?

D. Administer treatment for general illness and/or conditions by using standard techniques and procedures to facilitate recovery, function, and performance.

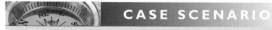

CASE SCENARIO

You are caring for an athlete who has a laceration on his left arm. You are in a hurry and fail to use gloves during the treatment. The athlete reports you the next day to the head athletic trainer and states that you put him at risk by not using gloves during the treatment. Policy and procedures require that you use gloves, but you wanted to respond quickly to control the bleeding and know the athlete well enough to assume he did not present a risk to you. Did you behave ethically? Is the athlete right in complaining?

E. Reassess the status of injuries, illnesses, and/or conditions by using standard techniques and documentation strategies to determine appropriate treatment, rehabilitation, and/or reconditioning and to evaluate readiness to return to a desired level of activity.

CASE SCENARIO

You work for a private physical therapy clinic as an athletic trainer. A worker who was recently injured is nearing time to return to his job. His progress has been fair, but it certainly falls within the marginal range. He has shared with you that during his time off he has been able to help his elderly father care for his mother, who has Alzheimer's disease. He is always on time to the clinic and works hard during his rehabilitation. He states that his father cannot afford to institutionalize his mother and his help creates some relief from the situation. You are writing the report for his follow-up visit for the physician, which will determine whether he returns to work the next week or has his therapy extended another 3 weeks. You know the physician will ask what you think about his readiness to return to work. What do you do?

F. Educate the appropriate patients in the treatment, rehabilitation, and reconditioning of injuries, illnesses, and/or conditions by using applicable methods and materials to facilitate recovery, function, and/or performance.

CASE SCENARIO

A female athlete presents with nonlocalized medial shin pain with an onset of approximately 1 week. The pain is becoming progressively worse. The athlete has doubled her mileage (from 33 to 66 miles per week) in the past few weeks. In addition, she is using heat and aspirin to ease her pain before and after workouts. The coach demands a bone scan; however, the team physician wants to decrease activity and try a more conservative approach before prescribing the test. The athlete is not informed that a potential stress fracture is suspected, but she is informed that a follow-up radiograph will be performed in a week (after reducing activity significantly) and, if needed, a bone scan will be ordered. Did the physician and athletic trainer act ethically?[4]

G. Provide guidance and/or counseling for the appropriate patients in the treatment, rehabilitation, and reconditioning of injuries, illnesses, and/or conditions through communication to facilitate recovery, function, and performance.

CASE SCENARIO

You are working with a high school athlete being treated for a low back condition. She discloses to you that she is seeing a therapist regarding an eating disorder that she has been fighting for the past 3 years. During several of her next treatments, you disclose to her that you, too, had an eating disorder when you were young. You share with her that it never goes away and that you still struggle with it today despite your successful career and family. Is this ethical?

Organization and Administration

A. Establish action plans for response to injury or illness by using available resources to provide the required range of health care services for patients, athletic activities, and events.

CASE SCENARIO

You are a director of a sports medicine clinic that provides services to area high schools. You have 15 high schools that need coverage in the clinic every morning, and you have 10 athletic trainers available for 8 hours per day with any extra time being compensatory. Each school has a full line of athletic teams—boys and girls—and range in distance from 1 mile from the clinic to 25 miles from the clinic.

Your committee needs to decide how everything will be covered, guidelines for compensatory time, and guidelines for coverage at the high school sites to maximize your resources.

B. Establish policies and procedures for the delivery of health care services following accepted guidelines to promote safe participation, timely care, and legal compliance.

A collegiate basketball player has significant pain and weakness with documented degeneration of the spine. The athletic trainer says no participation, but the athletic director, who is also the basketball coach, takes the athlete and an athletic training student over state lines to get cortisone injections so the athlete can play. The athlete does play that evening with release from the out-of-state physician, who is not the team physician. What do you do?

A budget cut has taken place in your department. You have two employees (assistant athletic trainers) who work for you. One assistant has worked for you 1 year longer, has a strong record of performance, and is single. The other athletic trainer also has a strong record of performance and recently found out that her child has cystic fibrosis—a costly, time-intensive medical condition. Who do you terminate and why?

You are the budget committee for a district organization. You have been given the following budget and must determine which projects are to be cut, reduced, or funded based on the following budget information. You must evaluate the budget and cut approximately $10,000 for the next year.

C. Establish policies and procedures for the management of health care facilities and activity areas by referring to accepted guidelines, standards, and regulations to promote safety and legal compliance.

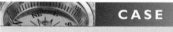

You are serving as the athletic trainer for the women's softball program at a small institution. The weather is becoming increasingly more threatening although there is no lightning. It is raining quite hard, but the coach and umpire declare that if there is no lightning, they are willing to continue to play. You do not want to be wet, so you take the lightning detector and sit in your closed car adjacent to the field. You can still see the field and have the lightning detector with you. Is this ethical?

Line Item	Budgeted Cost
New Projects	
Web consultant	3500.00
Public relations activities	4000.00
Strategic planning meeting	1000.00
Fall meeting	16000.00
Fall meeting executive council travel (10 people) — Only voting members will travel to this meeting — Web, public relations, newsletter not funded	10000.00
Executive council travel to national meeting (14 people) — All members, including nonvoting — Five-night stay	14000.00
Executive council travel to district (14 people) — All members, including nonvoting — Four-night stay	14000.00

D. Manage human and fiscal resources by using appropriate leadership, organization, and management techniques to provide efficient and effective health care services.

Scholarship and endowments	5000.00
Technology replacement	5000.00
Charitable contributions	1000.00
State grants — Money given back to states for projects — 1000 each state	6000.00
Research and education foundation donations	5000.00
Newsletter (three per year, one on Internet) — Paper copies = 8000.00 each — Assembly = 4500.00 — Postage = 3500.00 — Web copy = 1000.00 — Postcard reminder — Minimal mailing	16000.00
Executive council phone (50.00/person × 14)	700.00
Conference call (November) — General meeting — Finance committee	3000.00
District director travel to each state meeting — Six state meetings at 1000.00 each	6000.00
Election costs — Mailing: original and return postage first class	6000.00
Fundraising personnel travel and entertaining — Travel to all meetings: fall, district, national — Entertaining budget = 2500.00 per meeting	10500.00
Income	
Dues	110000.00
Meeting profits	4000.00
Total	114000.00

E. Maintain records by using an appropriate system to document services rendered, provide for continuity of care, facilitate communication, and meet legal standards.

CASE SCENARIO

As the athletic trainer at a large clinic, you see approximately 25 patients per day. You ask the supervisor if you can dictate the records at the end of the day to expedite the recordkeeping process, which will allow you to spend more time with the patients. The physical therapist must sign off on your records and dictation when they come in. Most days, you are able to dictate records at the end of the day; however, sometimes you have 4 days' worth of records piled on your desk to be dictated. Therefore a week or more may pass before the dictation is returned and the physical therapist signs off on the record. Is this ethical?

F. Develop professional relationships with appropriate patients and entities by applying effective communication techniques to enhance the delivery of health care.

CASE SCENARIO

Your employer is conducting a personal relationship outside the office with a colleague of yours. The employer has given significant financial perks to the employee despite her inconsistent performance in the clinic and poor attendance at work. Other employees are coming to you as the unit coordinator to address this situation. You have lost two employees (out of 10) to date, and others are extremely dissatisfied and also are looking for other employment. What do you do? Is this behavior unethical?

CASE SCENARIO

You are responsible for notifying several employees that your employer has reduced its medical coverage from 90% of total cost to 70% of total cost. Several employees have considerable medical expenses because of illness or disease conditions. You decide to send a memo to each person explaining the benefit change without first meeting with the employees to tell them in person. The letters are delayed, and one employee goes to the physician's office, where she is notified of the change by the office personnel. She argues that a mistake must have occurred because she had not been informed by her employer of the change. Is this ethical behavior on your part as supervisor?

Professional Responsibility

A. Demonstrate appropriate professional conduct by complying with applicable standards and maintaining continuing competence to provide quality athletic training services.

CASE SCENARIO

An athletic trainer is registered to attend the National Athletic Trainers' Association Annual Meeting and Symposium in June. The certified athletic trainer has family in the area whom she has not seen for approximately 5 years. The athletic trainer desperately needs the units to complete the continuing education requirements for the reporting period. The athletic trainer picks up her packet and badge on the initial day of registration, then departs for her family's home to spend the next week visiting. She does not attend any sessions at the meeting yet reports the units at the end of the reporting period to maintain her certification. Is this ethical?

B. Adhere to statutory and regulatory provisions and other legal responsibilities relating to the practice of athletic training by maintaining an understanding of these provisions and responsibilities to contribute to the safety and welfare of the public.

CASE SCENARIO

As an athletic trainer for a collegiate athletic department, you identify a student-athlete who is noted to be HIV positive on his participation clearance form. He is cleared to participate in intercollegiate athletics. During a competition, he sustains an open fracture to the lower leg. He is splinted and transported by the emergency medical team on site. You disclose to the emergency medical technicians that he is HIV positive. This comment is overheard by several athletic training students, who were assisting in the immobilization and transport procedure. Is this ethical?

C. Educate appropriate patients and entities about the role and standards of practice of the athletic trainer through informal and formal means to improve the ability of those patients and entities to make informed decisions.

CASE SCENARIO

As the head athletic trainer for a local high school, you are asked to provide a schedule of coverage for the high school events. You recently had a baby and prefer not to work in the evenings. You propose coverage for after-school events, with the exception of football contests, and recommend appropriate policy and procedures for medical issues after work hours. The athletic director asks if this practice is common elsewhere, and you comment that each school has its own policy for coverage. Is this ethical?

CASE SCENARIO

You are working in a collegiate setting where athletic training students are assigned clinical instructors and must work under the direct supervision of a certified athletic trainer. The athletic training education program director has advised that you must be in auditory and visual contact with the students at all times. You are assigned to cover lacrosse and soccer athletes, who practice on fields located approximately 100 yards from each other. You work directly with the students in the athletic training room as they prepare for practice, but on the field you are located on a golf cart approximately half the distance from both fields. The athletic training student is within visual contact and has a walkie talkie to contact you. Is this ethical?

ACTIVITIES FOR APPLICATION: LINKING CONTENT TO PRACTICE

The activities listed below can be used after any of the case analyses performed for the domains to reinforce or support the development of foundational behaviors for professional practice. These activities require you to think reflectively about the case from a different perspective than case resolution, tying the process to professional behavior.

LEARNING ACTIVITY 1: ANNOTATED PORTFOLIO

Objectives

1. To illustrate an understanding of a chosen domain in athletic training[1]
2. To apply the performance domains in athletic training to real-life scenarios
3. To produce a cumulative document reflecting conceptual comprehension

Description

Choosing a central topic from the course (any course related to any of the domains of athletic training),

put together a brief portfolio consisting of two to three artifacts that demonstrate an understanding, comprehension, and/or proficiency in that selected area.

Artifacts may consist of a variety of activities such as audiotaped or videotaped activities, journal entries, research papers, creative projects, presentations, or any other item that reflects your understanding and applications within a given domain.

Assessment

This activity can be presented as an individual project or to the class in a formal presentation. The class presentation is preferred because it allows you to share your ideas and ways of learning that others may not have previously considered. Also, through someone else's artifact, you may learn something new about that topic.

LEARNING ACTIVITY 2: ASSIGNMENT ASSESSMENT

Objectives

1. To promote critical thinking about a specific case[1]
2. To align personal and professional values with a given case scenario
3. To encourage dialogue among peers relative to a given case

Description

After a case review, reflect on index cards the value you placed on the learning activity by using two to three posed questions to elicit responses. These questions can address the methods, outcome, process, or any other factor in the case. The instructor collects these index cards and may use them in class to stimulate further discussion or clarification of the case.

Assessment

Individual responses to case analyses are often personal. This activity allows you to ask questions anonymously regarding any aspect related to the case without fear of peer pressure. If not anonymously submitted, assessment should be based on whether two to three questions were posed and their connection with the case. Another activity using these cards is to create your own scenarios and apply the material in the case to professional development activities and/or behaviors you have experienced.

LEARNING ACTIVITY 3: THE 3-MINUTE PAPER

Objectives

1. To provide an opportunity to address key elements or concerns related to the case[1]
2. To summarize discussion from a case analysis
3. To apply the information from the case to professional behaviors

Description

Answer the following questions in 3 minutes:

- What was the most important point of today's class discussion?
- What important question remains unanswered?
- How can you apply this to your professional development?

Assessment

This activity has no right or wrong answers. Simply reflecting on the case framed in a response to a question helps focus on your personal perception of this discussion. By reflecting on the responses later, you can see how your personal values and professional standards affected your responses. During a case discussion, you may not think about some of these issues or may not feel confident enough to ask these questions. This will help you process concerns.

Tip: Change the questions to the following: What was the most controversial issue related to the case? What was the most convincing argument or counterargument related to the case? What was the most disturbing idea that arose during the case discussion?

LEARNING ACTIVITY 4: MUDDIEST POINT

Objectives

1. To provide an opportunity to address key elements or concerns related to the case[1]
2. To summarize discussion from a case analysis
3. To apply the information from the case to professional behaviors

Description

As with the 3-minute paper, this activity encourages you to think about what is unclear about the case or the discussion. Jot down a response to the following questions: What was the muddiest point about the case? What is unclear? What is troubling? These anonymous cards may be used in the next discussion to provide points of discussion to clarify concerns.

Assessment

Because the cards are anonymous, you can create a database of the questions or most unclear points discussed in class for examination questions or study guides. These also can be collected and used as out-of-class assignments to look again at the troubling areas for discussion or review.

LEARNING ACTIVITY 5: ONE-SENTENCE SUMMARY

Objectives

1. To emphasize the key issue related to a case[1]
2. To foster discernment about discussion points in a case discussion
3. To identify personal interpretations of group discussion aligned with professional behaviors

Description

Write one sentence answering the following question: Professionally, what is the moral to the case?

Assessment

This can be assessed as a journal assignment, or peers can work together to analyze and debate (if appropriate) responses to the question.

LEARNING ACTIVITY 6: WORD JOURNAL

Objectives

1. To facilitate reflection on ethical decisions[1]
2. To summarize content into key terms and issues
3. To provide an avenue to disclose personal perceptions on an activity or reading

Description

Write one word that summarizes the activity or text reading just completed. Provide follow-up elaboration of the reason that you selected that word.

Assessment

Because this activity is highly subjective, assessment should be based on the concept of expression rather than content. Alternative activities that expand this task include identification of one main conflict or theme as the word choice or elaboration to create an abstract from the word journal.

LEARNING ACTIVITY 7: DECISION TREE

Objectives

1. To visualize the processes by which you make decisions[1]
2. To understand the impact of the decisions you make along each path
3. To encourage critical reflection on the reasons that you chose the paths for each decision

Description

Create a decision tree (Figure 19-1) as you progress through a decision-making process. Analyze the case, and create a pathway by which you selected your responses.

Assessment

Consideration of viable alternatives and processing the "payoff" versus the "risk" of each path on the tree is the objective of this activity. Assessing how you complete the chart with consideration of the ability to delve into deeper implications for selected actions is critical. Assigning a point value for the ability to generate viable options with consideration of the cost/benefit ratio is a good approach. Peer evaluation also is helpful because it will help you see what others were thinking and alternatives that you may not have considered.

LEARNING ACTIVITY 8: ETHICAL QUESTIONS

Objectives

1. To encourage critical thinking of the case from a health care perspective[3]
2. To address ethical questions through guided probes
3. To facilitate multiple perspectives on any given case

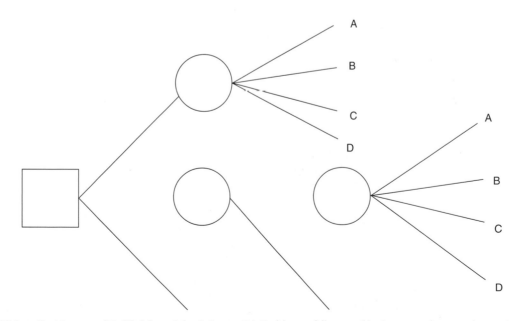

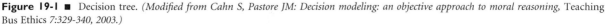

Figure 19-1 ■ Decision tree. *(Modified from Cahn S, Pastore JM: Decision modeling: an objective approach to moral reasoning,* Teaching Bus Ethics *7:329-340, 2003.)*

Description

Provide written responses to the following questions (if appropriate) related to the case activity you just completed.

- What is the right thing to do when you see a health care provider taking a short cut that could potentially harm the patient?
- What do you do when patients are not receiving the care they need or the person administering the care is not properly trained?
- Should you report an action by a co-worker, friend, or colleague that is inappropriate or potentially harmful to a patient?
- What should you do when you believe the physician or a co-worker put you in a position in which you felt uncomfortable professionally?
- What should you do when your co-workers' or patients' lifestyles are not in agreement with your values?
- Do athletic trainers or other health care professionals have the right to know if a patient or athlete is infected with AIDS or another contagious disease?

Assessment

Using these activities as journal reflections encourages personal reflection. The activity should be assessed on the reflection rather than the content. Peer evaluation also can encourage discussion about how to resolve some of these complex issues.

LEARNING ACTIVITY 9: WRITING ABSTRACTS

Objectives

1. To articulate key information about a case concisely
2. To promote scholarly writing skills
3. To acknowledge and recognize personal bias in writing

Description

Write a 150-word abstract on the case just discussed. In this abstract, summarize the case, the issues, and outcomes. Be specific and concise. Direct the issues and outcomes at professional behaviors.

Assessment

An evaluative tool that looks at writing dynamics as well as content is essential. Assessing your ability to extract key information from a case and apply it to the particular summary is the goal of the activity.

LEARNING ACTIVITY 10: THE WHITE PAPER

Objectives

1. To script a proposal relative to a given case or policy
2. To demonstrate professional writing skills
3. To support a position through formal writing

Description

A white paper is a proposal that justifies your position on a specific issue. It is a formally written document that recommends a certain action. The proposal should have the following elements: introduction, proposed action, supporting documentation and rationale, implications of the action or lack of action, and summary. It can range in length from brief (one to two pages) to lengthy (five to six pages). Your instructor will help you select the appropriate length for the assigned case or issue.

Assessment

As with any formal written assignment, writing skills should be included in the evaluation. However, conceptually, identification of the critical elements provides the evaluative structure to this assignment. Peer assessment also is a helpful tool and demonstrates the stances taken by classmates.

LEARNING ACTIVITY 11: DEBATE

Objectives

1. To encourage professional dialogue with supporting facts
2. To address conflicting opinions or positions regarding a case
3. To promote effective verbal and nonverbal communication skills

Description

You and/or a small group of students will be assigned to support and debate a particular stance on a case. You will be given a time frame to debate the issue. Typically, the debate will include opening remarks, two rounds of discussion, then closing remarks from each side.

Assessment

Peer evaluation is extremely helpful with this activity. It should focus on communication, content, and ability to support the case. Self-reflection by a journaling or a written reflective activity can help assess your performance from a strengths and weaknesses perspective.

LEARNING ACTIVITY 12: FLOW CHARTS

Objectives

1. To create a graphic reflecting the process by which decisions are made
2. To analyze the process by which decisions are made
3. To identify any alternative paths for consideration in resolution of the case

Description

Make a flow chart or algorithm of the steps and processes you took to resolve any case. This should reflect the connections among the elements as you progressed through each case.

Assessment

Assessment of flow chart creation should focus on the connections made throughout the process. The content is important, but the consideration of alternative paths and the interconnectedness reflected in the chart are most important. An assessment alternative could include rationalization or explanation (in written form) of the course of action and/or critical analysis of the flow chart if a group performed the activity. Lastly, comparing flow charts among peers and having a reflective activity to critique the other flow charts develop critical thinking skills.

SUMMARY

As you continually grow in the profession of athletic training, you will become increasingly more aware of the complexity of many ethical issues facing you. The activities in this chapter illustrated the depth and breadth of ethical dilemmas facing the profession by immersing you in actual cases related to the specific domains of the profession. Critical analysis of each case is essential to the development of professional behaviors because it addresses the multiple effects any ethical dilemma can pose.

Post-case activities help you prepare for a professional role by encouraging the development of professional skills such as writing and communicating. Although experience with case resolution is important, being able to articulate your position and/or defend your stance becomes more critical as you journey through your professional career. You are encouraged to use these activities frequently throughout your profession as you continue to refine your professional behaviors in the face of the ethical dilemmas you will encounter.

REFERENCES

1. Angelo TA, Cross KP: *Classroom assessment techniques: a handbook for college teachers.* San Francisco, 1993, Jossey-Bass Publishers.
2. Cahn S, Pastore JM: Decision modeling: an objective approach to moral reasoning, *Teaching Bus Ethics* 7:329-340, 2003.
3. Cameron ME, Schaffer M, Park HA: Nursing students' experience of ethical problems and use of ethical decision making models, *Nurs Ethics* 8:432-448, 2001.
4. Colston MA: Informed consent: review and implementation, *Athl Ther Today* 9:29-31, 2004.
5. National Athletic Trainers' Association: *Athletic training educational competencies,* ed 4, Dallas, 2006, National Athletic Trainers' Association.
6. National Athletic Trainers' Association Board of Certification: *Role Delineation Study,* ed 5, Omaha, Neb., 2004, Board of Certification.
7. Ray R: Ethical practice in athletic training: a thing of the past? *Athl Ther Today* 8:1, 2003.

Appendices

A
Athletic Training Compliance and Noncompliance

COMPLIANCE/NONCOMPLIANCE CARDS

This information can be used to create index cards for use with learning activities addressed in Chapter 2, Learning Activity 2.

A head athletic trainer fails to hire an assistant athletic trainer because she uses a wheelchair.

An athletic trainer is not offered a position at a private girls' school because of rumors that she has a lesbian lifestyle.

An African-American student-athlete is not videotaped for practice because he is 5 minutes late for the athletic training room taping hours.

An athletic training student is directed to provide care to an athletic team traveling to an area college.

An athletic trainer provides information regarding an athletes' progress in rehabilitation to a scout for a professional team.

An athletic trainer applies a nontraditional medical ointment to an injured athlete's blister to facilitate healing.

An athletic trainer discloses to the newspaper that an injured athlete is scheduled for surgery.

An athletic trainer refuses to treat a potentially HIV-infected athlete until an HIV test can be performed.

An athletic training student administers ultrasound to an athlete while the athletic trainer is in another room.

An athletic trainer recommends that an athlete seek the services of an acupuncturist for chronic pain.

An athletic trainer who works in a college setting reports suspicion of alcohol abuse by a colleague to the athletic director.

An athletic training student reports to the governing office of NATA that an incident of sexual harassment occurred during a clinical assignment.

An athletic trainer has completed but fails to report continuing education activities during the reporting period.

An athletic training student is dismissed from an academic program after admission into a chemical dependency program.

An athletic trainer dispenses over-the-counter medications from a large, multiunit bottle for an injury condition.

An athletic trainer is on the payroll of a local orthopedic clinic and is compensated for referrals directed from the athletic department.

An athletic trainer attends continuing education activities pertaining to massotherapy.

An administrator encourages an athletic trainer to collaborate with a company that manufactures ankle supports as part of a financial agreement with the athletic department.

An athletic trainer provides laser therapy to an injured athlete.

An athletic director directs a high school athletic trainer to speak directly with college recruits regarding the medical status of each athlete.

An athletic training student works with a faculty member to collect research on student-athlete medical conditions garnered from the medical files.

An athletic training educator expresses dissatisfaction with several required competencies and proficiencies in the curriculum.

An athletic trainer drinks excessively the night before a game but is called at 2 AM to care for an injured athlete who just returned from another contest.

An athletic trainer openly discusses reasons that athletic trainers should not have to be accountable to physical therapists.

An employee at a clinic places the NATA logo on the marketing materials used to promote an upcoming clinic on athletic injuries to the shoulder.

An athletic trainer discloses to a friend that the star basketball player may not be able to play at tomorrow's game for personal reasons.

An athletic training club from a local university uses the NATA logo on the back of a t-shirt that members wear for volunteer events for their organization.

An athletic training student participates in a local pool for the NCAA basketball championships being coordinated with his friends at his residence hall.

APPENDIX B
Assessment Tools

ANALYTIC RUBRICS FOR AN ESSAY RESPONSE OR WRITTEN TASKS

	4	3	2	I	Total
Thesis and organization	Thesis is defensible and clearly stated; appropriate facts and concepts are used in a logical manner to support the argument	Thesis is defensible and clearly stated; appropriate facts and concepts are used in a logical manner to support the argument; although support may be thin or logic is not clear	Thesis is not clearly stated; some attempt at support is made	No thesis or indefensible thesis; support is missing or illogical	
Content/knowledge	All relevant facts and concepts are included and accurate	All or most relevant facts and concepts are included and accurate	Some relevant facts and concepts are included; some inaccuracies	No facts or concepts are included or irrelevant facts and concepts are included	
Writing style and mechanics	Writing is clear and smooth; word choice and style are appropriate for the topic; no errors in grammar or usage	Writing is generally clear; word choice and style are appropriate for topic; there are a few errors in grammar or usage, but they do not interfere with the meaning	Writing is not clear; style is poor; some errors in grammar and usage that interfere with the meaning	Writing is not clear; style is poor; many errors in grammar and usage	
Total					

From Brookhart SM: The art and science of classroom assessment: the missing part of pedagogy, *ASHE-ERIC Higher Education Report,* 27:47, Washington, DC, 1999, The George University Press.

ASSESSING THE INDIVIDUAL

Voice   10 ←→ 1
Clarity of speech   clear _____ vunclear
Intonation   varied _____ monotonous

Nonverbal communication
Gestures   sufficient _____ too many
Eye contact   plenty _____ too
                                              much/little

Name: _____

Group: _____

Voice   5 4 3 2 1
Clarity   good ☐☐☐☐☐ bad
Volume   good ☐☐☐☐☐ bad
Intonation   good ☐☐☐☐☐ bad

Nonverbal communication
Gestures   good ☐☐☐☐☐ bad
Eye contact   good ☐☐☐☐☐ bad

Name: _____

Group: _____

From Brown S, Glasner A, editors: *Assessment matters in higher education: choosing and using diverse approaches*, Philadelphia, 1999, Open University Press, p. 200.

CLASSROOM ASSESSMENT OPTIONS

	Objective Scoring	Subjective Scoring	Most Appropriate Uses	Major Advantages	Potential Pitfalls
Paper-and-pencil tests	Multiple choice, true/false, matching, fill-in-the-blanks	Essays or show-the-work problems judged with rubrics or rating scales	To assess knowledge and thinking over a range of content *or* to assess dispositions and interests (ungraded)	Most reliable way to assess knowledge and thinking in a content area domain; best way to cover a large number of facts and concepts	Require clearly written items that appropriately sample a range of content material; easiest to write recall-level questions
Performance assessments	Judgments of performance on a task by using a checklist	Judgments of performance on a task by using rubrics or rating scales	To assess in-depth thinking in one area or assess skills attained *or* products created	Allow measurement of in-depth thinking, skills, or products not readily assessable by tests	Require clear expectations for tasks and scoring to provide meaningful assessment information
Oral questions	In-class questions with right or wrong answers	Discussions or interviews evaluated with rubrics or rating scales	To assess knowledge and thinking during instruction *or* to assess dispositions and interests (ungraded)	Provide feedback for instruction; identify students' concepts and misconceptions; tap students' interests and opinions	Students may prefer not to speak up or give their honest responses in class
Portfolios	Could use a checklist for portfolio entries but not recommended except for special purposes	Collection of a student's work and reflections over time; entries can be rated separately or as a whole	To document progress or development *or* to showcase complex achievement of a range of skills	Allow assessment of student's development and some ownership and control by student	Require clear purpose, focused construction, and long-term attention to get any more useful information than stand-alone assessments

From Brookhart SM: The art and science of classroom assessment: the missing part of pedagogy, *ASHE-ERIC Higher Education Report*, 27:36, Washington, DC, 1999, The George University Press.

GROUP ACTIVITIES EVALUATION

Assignment: Group Projects in Athletic Training

Group Project: _____   Member being assessed: _____

Instructions

Using the key that follows, circle the number that represents your opinion of the group member's performance of each item.

3 = Outstanding
2 = More than satisfactory
1 = Satisfactory
0 = Less than satisfactory
NA = Inadequate opportunity to observe

Work-Related Performance					
Comprehension: Seemed to understand requirements for assignment	0	1	2	3	NA
Problem identification and solution: Participated in identifying and defining problems and working toward solutions	0	1	2	3	NA
Organization: Approached tasks (such as time management) in systematic manner	0	1	2	3	NA
Acceptance of responsibility: Shared responsibility for tasks to be accomplished	0	1	2	3	NA
Initiative/motivation: Made suggestions, sought feedback, showed interest in group decision making and planning	0	1	2	3	NA
Creativity: Looked at ideas from viewpoints different than usual	0	1	2	3	NA
Task completion: Followed through in completing own contributions to group project	0	1	2	3	NA
Attendance: Attended planning sessions, was prompt, and participated in decision making	0	1	2	3	NA
Work-Related Interactions with Others					
Collaboration: Worked cooperatively with others	0	1	2	3	NA
Participation: Contributed "fair share" to group project given the nature of individual assignment	0	1	2	3	NA
Attitude: Displayed positive approach and made constructive comments in working toward goal	0	1	2	3	NA
Independence: Carried out tasks without overly depending on other group members	0	1	2	3	NA
Communication: Expressed thoughts clearly	0	1	2	3	NA
Responsiveness: Reacted sensitively to verbal and nonverbal cues of other group members	0	1	2	3	NA

Add total score   Total: _____

Divide by number of items scored with number   Average: _____

Comments:

Name of evaluator: _____ Date: _____

From Walvoord BE, Anderson VJ: *Effective grading: a tool for learning and assessment,* San Francisco, 1998, Jossey-Bass Publishers, pp. 202-203.

GROUP ASSESSMENT

Assessing Group: _____

Presenting Information   10 ←→ 1

Variety   sufficient _____ too few

Overhead projector
Clarity   clear _____ unclear
Layout   good _____ bad

Blackboard
Clarity   clear _____ unclear

Handouts
Content   relevant _____ irrelevant
Layout   good _____ bad

Video
Content   relevant _____ irrelevant
Use   sufficient _____ too much

Content of presentation
Content   relevant _____ irrelevant
Clarity   good _____ bad
Pace   well paced _____ poorly paced
Interest value   entertaining _____ dull

Teamwork
Coordination   good _____ bad
Workload   equal _____ unequal

Visual Aids   5 4 3 2 1
Variety   sufficient ☐☐☐☐ too few

Overhead projector transparencies
Clarity   clear ☐☐☐☐☐ unclear
Amount on slide   sufficient ☐☐☐☐ too much

Blackboard
Clarity   clear ☐☐☐☐☐ unclear

Handouts
Clarity   clear ☐☐☐☐☐ unclear
Content   relevant ☐☐☐☐ irrelevant

Content of presentation
Vocabulary   broad ☐☐☐☐ narrow
Interesting   very ☐☐☐☐ dull
Detail   relevant ☐☐☐☐ irrelevant
Topic knowledge   sufficient ☐☐☐☐ insufficient

Teamwork
Workload   equal ☐☐☐☐ unequal
Coordination   good ☐☐☐☐ bad

From Brown S, Glasner A, editors: *Assessment Matters in higher education: choosing and using diverse approaches,* Philadelphia, 1999, Open University Press, p. 199.

GROUP ASSESSMENT SHEET

Directions

After a self-assessment, the group will come together to tally the group scores and agree on individual scores. Record the names of the group members in the grid below with corresponding group agreed-upon scores from the individual self-assessment scores. Each person should not have the exact score because no one does identical work.

   After entering the scores for each individual, tally the group total score by adding all the scores together. Each individual will then be assigned an individual score by using the formula at the bottom of the chart. Each person will receive a group mark and an individual mark based on the group score.

Names of group members				
Categories				
Regular attendance at group meetings				
Contribution of ideas for the task				
Researching, analyzing, and preparing materials for the task				
Contribution to cooperative group process				
Supporting and encouraging group members				
Practical contribution to end product (such as writing, presenting, making materials)				
Total for each student	_____/120	_____/120	_____/120	**Total for the group** = _____/360

Signature of group assessor _____

From Brown S, Glasner A, editors: *Assessment matters in higher education: choosing and using diverse approaches,* Philadelphia, 1999, Open University Press, p. 145.

HOLISTIC RUBRIC FOR ESSAY RESPONSES

Point Value	Explanation
4	Thesis is defensible and explicit; facts and concepts are used in a logical manner to support the argument; all relevant facts and concepts are included and accurate; writing is clear and smooth; grammar is correct
3	Thesis is defensible and explicit; facts and concepts are used in a logical manner to support the argument, although support may be thin in some places or logic is not clear; all or most of the relevant facts and concepts are included and accurate; any inaccuracies are minimal; writing is generally clear and smooth; grammatical errors are few and do not interfere with the meaning
2	Thesis is not clearly stated; some attempt at support is evident; all or most of the relevant facts and concepts are included; inaccuracies are minor; writing is not clear and style is poor; some grammatical errors exist and interfere with the meaning
1	No thesis or indefensible thesis; support is missing or illogical; no facts or concepts are included or irrelevant facts and concepts are used; writing is not clear and style is poor; many errors in grammar and usage

Modified from Brookhart SM: The art and science of classroom assessment: the missing part of pedagogy, *ASHE-ERIC Higher Education Report*, 27:48, Washington, DC, 1999, The George University Press.

JOURNAL AND JOURNAL DISCUSSION RUBRIC

Criteria	LEVEL OF ACHIEVEMENT		
	3 *Sophisticated*	**2** *Competent*	**1** *Not Yet Competent*
Organization	Written work is well organized and easy to understand	The organization is generally good, but some parts seem out of place	Organization is unclear or disorganized to the extent that it prevents understanding of content
Confidentiality	Patient confidentiality is protected throughout journal	Patient confidentiality is generally well protected	Patient confidentiality is rarely or never protected
Content	Journal is clinically relevant	Journal is generally clinically relevant	Journal is not clinically relevant
Grammar and word choice	Sentences are complete and grammatical and flow easily; words are chosen for their precise meaning	For the most part, sentences are complete and grammatical and flow easily; with a few exceptions, words are chosen for their precise meaning	Readers are distracted by some grammatical errors and use of slang; some sentences are halting, incomplete, and vocabulary is somewhat limited or inappropriate
Freedom from bias (e.g., sexism, racism, ageism, etc.)	Both oral language and body language are free from bias	Oral language and body language are free from bias with one or two minor exceptions	Oral language and/or body language includes some identifiable bias
Journal discussion	Student is always engaged and participatory; student is always prepared and enhances the ideas of others	For the most part, student is always engaged and participatory; with a few exceptions, the student is prepared and enhances the ideas of others	Student is distracted and often distracts others; the student is ill prepared to discuss or share issues or potential solutions

Stemmans, Catherine: Unpublished rubric.

ORAL PRESENTATION ASSESSMENT

Dimension	Range	Comments
Content	Knowledge and understanding Applied problem-solving ability Interpersonal competence Personal qualities	
Interaction	Presentation vs. dialogue	
Authenticity	Contextualized vs. decontextualized	
Structure	Closed structure vs. open structure	
Assessors	Self-assessment, peer assessment, authority-based assessment	
Orality	Purely oral vs. orality as secondary	

Modified from Joughin G: Dimensions of oral assessment and student approaches to learning. In Brown S, Glasner A, editors: *Assessment matters in higher education: choosing and using diverse approaches,* Philadelphia, 1999, Open University Press, p. 148.

PARTICIPATION RUBRIC

Student Name		Weeks		Participation % for the Period =	

Date	Topic	Actively Participated, Conceptual Support of Ideas	Actively Participated, Limited Conceptual Support of Ideas	Participated, but Lacked Conceptual Support of Ideas	Did Not Participate
Sum		0	0	0	0
Score		0.0	0.0	0.0	0.0
Key		95%	85%	70%	50%

Total Score: 0.0

Faculty signature _____

From Peer KS: *Participation rubric.* Unpublished course document for Professional Development in Athletic Training, Kent, Ohio, 2003, Kent State University.

PEER EVALUATION FOR COOPERATIVE LEARNING ACTIVITIES

Directions

Record the names of each member of the group, including yourself, in the boxes in the first column. Put a check in each cell in the grid to indicate "fine job, as expected" for each group member for each criteria. For any box in which you have reservations about making a check because a group member did not meet your expectations for a criterion, write a brief comment. For any box in which you would like to comment on truly exceptional performance, please do so. See example below for comments.

Group Members	1 = Worked cooperatively to complete assignments	2 = Attended and participated in scheduled meetings	3 = Supported and respected other members' efforts and opinions	4 = Prepared adequately for sessions	5 = Made substantial contributions to group's understanding; shared ideas, resources, and information

Comments:

Examples:

Group Member Jones: Item 1: Mr. Jones failed to work with the group and always wanted to work independently and do it his way.

Group Member Smith: Item 3: Ms. Smith always told everyone that their ideas would not work. She even made negative comments to several members that I perceived to be derogatory.

From Munson S: *Learning disabilities.* Unpublished syllabus for GSPED 662, Duquesne University, Pittsburgh. In Brookhart SM: The art and science of classroom assessment: the missing part of pedagogy, *ASHE-ERIC Higher Education Report,* 27:54, Washington, DC, 1999, The George University Press.

PORTFOLIO ASSESSMENT CRITERIA

Ability	Description	Excellent (85%)	Very Good (65%)	Good (55%)	Satisfactory (45%)	Unsatisfactory (<40%)
Psychomotor	Can perform complex skills consistently, with confidence and a degree of coordination and fluidity. Able to choose an appropriate response from repertoire of actions and can evaluate own and others' performance.	Always has technical mastery of skills, performing smoothly, precisely, and efficiently. Able to plan strategies and tactics and adapt effectively to unusual and unexpected situations.	Can always perform complex skills consistently, confidently, and with a degree of fluidity. Able to choose from a repertoire of actions. Can evaluate own and others' performance.	Can always perform complex skills consistently, confidently, and with a degree of fluidity. Usually able to choose from a repertoire of actions. Usually able to evaluate own and others' performance.	Usually able to perform complex skills consistently, confidently, and with a degree of fluidity. Limited repertoire of actions to choose from. Usually able to evaluate own and others' performances; sometimes needs assistance evaluating others.	Rarely able to perform complex skills consistently, confidently, and with a degree of fluidity. Very limited repertoire of actions to choose from. Rarely able to evaluate own or others' performances without assistance.
Self-awareness, reflection on practice	Is able to evaluate own strengths and weaknesses, can challenge received opinion, and begins to develop own criteria and judgments.	Always confident in application of own criteria of judgment and in challenge of received opinions in action and can reflect on action.	Always recognizes own strengths and weaknesses against preset criteria. Begins to develop own criteria and judgment and challenge received opinion.	Usually recognizes own strengths and weaknesses against preset criteria. Begins to develop own criteria and judgment and sometimes challenges received opinion.	Usually recognizes own strengths and weaknesses against preset criteria. Begins to develop own criteria and judgment but does not yet challenge received opinion.	Needs assistance to recognize own strengths and weaknesses against preset criteria. Has not begun to develop own criteria and judgment or challenge received opinion.
Problem solving	Can identify key elements of complex problems and choose appropriate methods for the resolution in a considered manner.	Always confident and flexible in identifying and defining complex problems and the application of appropriate knowledge and skills to their solution.	Can always identify key elements of complex problems and choose appropriate methods for the resolution in a considered manner.	Usually identifies key elements of complex problems and chooses appropriate methods for the resolution in a considered manner.	Usually identifies key elements of complex problems. Sometimes needs assistance to choose appropriate methods for the resolution in a considered manner.	Rarely able to identify key elements of complex problems. Always needs assistance to choose appropriate methods for the resolution in a considered manner.

Continued

PORTFOLIO ASSESSMENT CRITERIA—cont'd						
Ability	**Description**	**Excellent (85%)**	**Very Good (65%)**	**Good (55%)**	**Satisfactory (45%)**	**Unsatisfactory (<40%)**
Communication and presentation	Can communicate effectively in a format appropriate to the discipline and report practical procedures in a clear and concise manner with all relevant information in a variety of formats.	Can always debate and produce detailed and coherent project reports on practice issues in a professional manner.	Always communicates effectively in an appropriate format or language in a clear and concise manner. Can use a variety of formats effectively.	Usually communicates effectively in an appropriate format or language in a clear and concise manner. Can use a variety of formats effectively.	Usually communicates effectively in an appropriate format or language in a clear and concise manner. Limited range of formats can be used effectively.	Rarely communicates effectively in an appropriate format or language in a clear and concise manner.
Interactive teamwork skills	Can interact effectively within a professional team. Can recognize or support leadership or be proactive in leadership. Can negotiate in a professional context and manage conflict.	Can work with and within a team toward defined outcomes. Can take roles as recognized leader. Always able to negotiate and handle conflict. Can effectively motivate others.	Always interacts effectively within a professional team. Can recognize and support leadership or be proactive in leadership. Can negotiate in a professional context and manage conflict.	Usually interacts effectively within a professional team. Usually recognizes and supports leadership or is proactive in leadership. Usually able to negotiate in a professional context and manage conflict.	Usually interacts effectively within a professional team. Usually recognizes and supports leadership but is not proactive in leadership. Sometimes needs assistance to negotiate in a professional context and manage conflict.	Rarely interacts effectively within a professional team. Cannot recognize and support leadership. Not able to negotiate in a professional context and manage conflict.

Modified from Brown S, Glasner A, editors: *Assessment matters in higher education: choosing and using diverse approaches,* Philadelphia, 1999, Open University Press, pp. 129-130.

SAMPLE GROUP WORK EVALUATION FORM

1. Overall, how effectively did your group work together on this assignment?

   Poorly   Adequately   Well   Extremely well

   Explain why you selected the response above:

2. Out of the _____ group members, how many actively participated most of the time?

   None   One   Two   Three   Four   Five

   Explain why you selected the response above:

3. Out of the _____ group members, how many were fully prepared for the activity?

   None   One   Two   Three   Four   Five

   Explain why you selected the response above:

4. Give a specific example of something you learned from the group that you probably would not have learned working alone.

5. Give a specific example of something the other group members learned from you that they probably would not have learned otherwise.

6. Suggest one change the group could have made to improve its performance.

Modified from Angelo TA, Cross KP: *Classroom assessment techniques: a handbook for college teachers,* San Francisco, 1993, Jossey-Bass Publishers, p. 350.

SELF-ASSESSMENT

Name: _____ Group: _____

Teamwork $10 \longleftrightarrow 1$
Cooperation with team   good _____ poor

Contribution
Visual aids   a lot _____ nothing
Eye contact   a lot _____ nothing
Presentation   a lot _____ nothing

Name: _____ Group: _____

Teamwork   5 4 3 2 1
Workload   equal ☐☐☐☐☐ unequal

Individual contribution $-2\ -1\ 0\ 1\ 2$
Gathering information   little ☐ ☐ ☐☐☐ a lot
Presentation   little ☐ ☐ ☐☐☐ a lot
Preparation of visual aids   little ☐ ☐ ☐☐☐ a lot
Structuring the talk   little ☐ ☐ ☐☐☐ a lot

From Brown S, Glasner A, editors: *Assessment Matters in higher education: choosing and using diverse approaches,* Philadelphia, 1999, Open University Press, p. 199.

SELF-ASSESSMENT

	Worth 20	Worth 0	Justification for Mark	Mark
Regular attendance at group meetings	Attended all meetings, stayed to agreed end, worked within timescale, active and attentive, prepared to be flexible about meeting times	Missed several or most meetings, always or often late, left early, digressed, giggled, daydreamed, or gossiped most of the time.		
Contribution of ideas for the task	Thought about the topic in advance of the meeting, provided workable ideas taken up by the group, built on others' suggestions, and prepared to test ideas on the group rather than keep quiet	Did not come prepared, did not contribute any ideas, tended to reject others' ideas rather than build on them		
Researching, analyzing, and preparing material for the task	Did what you said you would, brought materials, did an equal share of the research, and helped analyze and evaluate the material	Did no research, did not do what you promised to, did not manage workload, did not get involved with the task, and allowed others to provide all the material		
Contribution to cooperative group process	Left personal differences outside the group, willing to review group progress and tackle conflict in the group, took on different roles as needed, kept group on track, willing and flexible but focused on the task	Did not take initiative, waited to be told what to do, always took the same role (leader, joker, etc.) regardless of circumstances, created conflict, and was not prepared to review group progress		
Supporting and encouraging group members	Keen to listen to others, encouraged participation, enabled a collaborative learning environment, sensitive to issues affecting group members, supported group members with special needs	Sought only to complete the task, spoke over others and ignored their opinions, kept ideas and resources to self, was insensitive to individuals' needs, and did not contribute to the learning process		
Practical contribution to end product	Willing to try new things, did not hog the tasks, made a high level of contribution, took own initiative, was reliable, and produced high-quality work or presentation	Not willing to take on any task, did not take any responsibility, was unreliable so others felt the need to keep checking up, and made a limited, poor-quality contribution		

From Heathfield M: Group-based assessment: an evaluation of the use of assessed tasks as a method of fostering higher quality learning. In Brown S, Glasner A, editors: *assessment matters in higher education: choosing and using diverse approaches,* Philadelphia, 1999, Open University Press, pp. 138-139.

Team Project Evaluation

Assignment: Student teams work with a firm to identify problems and offer recommendations. This evaluation is to be completed by members of the business firms in which student teams work. Students and members of the firm receive this form at the beginning of the project.

TEAM'S CUSTOMER SATISFACTION SKILLS

Punctuality

Some team members missed appointments or did not return phone calls.	All team members arrived on time for appointments and returned all phone calls promptly.	All team members were always early.
0 1 2 3	4 5 6 7	8 9 10

Courtesy

Some team members were not respectful of some firm employees.	All team members were always courteous and respectful of firm employees.	All employees believed that the team members were respectful and courteous and fully elicited their ideas.
0 1 2 3	4 5 6 7	8 9 10

Appearance

Sometimes some team members were inappropriately dressed.	All team members were always appropriately dressed.	All team members adjusted their attire to match the attire used in the firm.
0 1 2 3	4 5 6 7	8 9 10

Enthusiasm

Some team members did not seem interested in the project.	All team members appeared enthusiastic and eager to work on the project.	The enthusiasm of the team members to complete the project was contagious and inspired others at the firm.
0 1 2 3	4 5 6 7	8 9 10

Communication

Some team members did not communicate clearly during meetings or phone calls.	The team members always communicated clearly with employees during meetings and phone calls.	The team members always made an extra effort to make sure they understood us and that we understood them during meetings and phone calls.
0 1 2 3	4 5 6 7	8 9 10

TEAMS PROJECT MANAGEMENT SKILLS

Plan Awareness

No team member ever presented a plan to the firm about how to complete the project.	The team presented a plan, but some team members did not seem to follow it.	All the team members seemed to be aware of the plan and followed it.
0 1 2 3	4 5 6 7	8 9 10

Problem Definition

The team's definition of the problem was absent or vague.	The problem was clearly defined. Data were provided measuring the scope of the problem.	The problem's importance and relation to the firm's goals were clearly stated.
0 1 2 3	4 5 6 7	8 9 10

Plan Feasibility

The plan presented was not feasible.	The plan presented was feasible but needed improvement.	The plan was feasible and was regularly updated as necessary during the project.
0 1 2 3	4 5 6 7	8 9 10

Plan Presentation

A written plan was not presented.	A clear plan with a Gantt flow chart was presented.	The team was able to explain clearly why it collected certain data and did not collect other data.
0 1 2 3	4 5 6 7	8 9 10

TEAM'S DATA ANALYSIS

Data Collection

The team did not use any apparent method to determine which data to gather.	The data were gathered in a systematic manner.	The team was able to explain clearly why it collected certain data and did not collect other data.
0 1 2 3	4 5 6 7	8 9 10

Collection Method

The team's data collection method was haphazard and random.	The team had a clear plan they followed to collect the data.	The data collection methods simplified the data analysis.
0 1 2 3	4 5 6 7	8 9 10

Analysis Tools

The team used no tools to analyze the data, or the tools seemed to be randomly selected.	The team used all the appropriate tools for data analysis.	The team fully explained why it selected certain tools and did not use others for data analysis.
0 1 2 3	4 5 6 7	8 9 10

Results Analysis

The team did no evaluation of the validity of its data analysis results.	The team validated its results by checking with the appropriate staff for their insight.	The team validated its results by conducting a short experiment.
0 1 2 3	4 5 6 7	8 9 10

TEAM'S RECOMMENDATIONS

Clarity

The team had no recommendations, or they were not understandable.	The team's recommendations were reasonable given the problem examined.	The recommendations logically emerged from the problem statement and data analysis.
0 1 2 3	4 5 6 7	8 9 10

Impact

The impact of implementing the recommendation was not examined or was completely wrong.	The recommendations are specific enough to serve as the basis for decisions by management.	The recommendations include an implementation plan that is feasible.
0 1 2 3	4 5 6 7	8 9 10

QUALITIES OF TEAM'S PAPER

Executive Summary

There was no executive summary.	The executive summary was well written and captured key goals, problems, analysis, steps, and recommendations.	The executive summary is as good as those usually presented in our firm.
0 1 2 3	4 5 6 7	8 9 10

Organization

The paper is difficult to follow.	The paper is easy to follow and read.	All relations among ideas are clearly expressed by the sentence structure and word choice.
0 1 2 3	4 5 6 7	8 9 10

Writing Style

The paper is sloppy, has no clear direction, and looks as if it were written by several people.	The format is appropriate with correct spelling, good grammar, good punctuation, and appropriate transition sentences.	The paper is well written and appropriate for presentation in the firm.
0 1 2 3	4 5 6 7	8 9 10

TEAM MEMBERS' PERSONAL SKILLS

Self-Confidence

Some team members' mannerisms made them look as if they were not confident of their abilities.	All the team members always seemed confident.	All team members were confident and would be able to lead in this organization.
0 1 2 3	4 5 6 7	8 9 10

Knowledge

Some team members did not seem to understand what they were doing.	All team members seemed to have adequate knowledge or ability to learn the necessary material.	All team members were proactive; about identifying skills they needed and obtaining them in advance.
0 1 2 3	4 5 6 7	8 9 10

Reliability		
Some team members did not follow through with their commitments.	All team members fulfilled all commitments they made to staff.	The work the team completed more than met expectations.
0 1 2 3	4 5 6 7	8 9 10

SATISFACTION WITH THE PRODUCT

Project Completion		
The team did not do a reasonable amount of work on the project.	The team completed a reasonable amount of work on the project.	The work the team completed more than met expectations.
0 1 2 3	4 5 6 7	8 9 10

Project Recommendations		
The recommendations provide no insight.	The recommendations are useful and will be examined in detail by our firm.	The recommendations will be implemented in full or in part.

Satisfaction		
We are not satisfied.	We are completely satisfied	We are more than satisfied; we are delighted with the team's work.
0 1 2 3	4 5 6 7	8 9 10

Your name: _____

Would you sponsor another team project? _____

What do you recommend that the department do to improve the project?

From Walvoord BE, Anderson VJ: *Effective grading: a tool for learning and assessment,* San Francisco, 1998, Jossey-Bass Publishers, pp. 212-217.

Sample Rubrics for Ethical Decision Making

ETHICAL DECISION-MAKING MODELS

			ETHICAL DECISION-MAKING MODELS: LEVEL I FOCUS ON PERSONAL MORALITY AND VALUES: EVALUATION RUBRIC		
Step	**Concept**	**Evaluative Questions**	**Thoroughly Developed and Conceptually Supported**	**Moderately Developed and Lacks Conceptual Support**	**Unable to Develop and Support Conceptually**
One	Problem perception	Could the student identify the ethical problem? Were the basic values relative to this case identified? Are the values clarified and understood?			
Two	Analyzing, choosing	Are the facts of the case evident?			
Three	Weighing, prizing	Are the facts of the case assessed for truth? Are the facts clarified?			
Four	Justifying	Are the values critical to this case justified?			
Five	Choosing, acting	Is the chosen decision rooted in values?			
Six	Evaluating	Is the value principle in the decision appropriate? Is the values decision tested?			

Modified from Darr K: *Ethics in health services management,* Baltimore, Md., 1997, Health Professions Press.

Step	Concept	Evaluative Questions	Thoroughly Developed and Conceptually Supported	Moderately Developed and Lacks Conceptual Support	Unable to Develop and Support Conceptually
		ETHICAL DECISION-MAKING MODELS: LEVEL II **FOCUS ON THE DECISION-MAKING PROCESS: EVALUATION RUBRIC**			
One	State the moral problem	What is the apparent moral problem? Can it harm others? What are the rights of others?			
Two	Develop alternative answers to the moral dilemma	Are the factual issues resolved? Are personal effects considered? Are the ethical principles of self-interest, personal virtues, religious injunctions, governmental requirements, utilitarian benefits, universal duties, individual rights, economic efficiency, distributive justice, and contributory liberty considered?			
Three	Research moral solutions	Were the benefits (material, financial, and personal) identified? Were the harms (material, financial, and personal) identified? Were the rights (individual and group) identified? Were the wrongs (individual and group) identified? Were the moral problems stated? Were the major alternatives listed? Were the factual issues resolved? Were personal effects acknowledged? Were self-interests acknowledged? Was a moral solution reached? Was the moral solution supported with the first, second, and third most important principles?			

Modified from Hosmer LT: Standard format for the case analysis of moral problems, *Teaching Bus Ethics* 4:169-180, 2000.

ETHICAL DECISION-MAKING MODELS: LEVEL II
FOCUS ON THE DECISION-MAKING PROCESS: CLINICAL DECISION MAKING— EVALUATION RUBRIC

Step	Concept	Evaluative Questions	Thoroughly Developed and Conceptually Supported	Moderately Developed and Lacks Conceptual Support	Unable to Develop and Support Conceptually
One	Collect the clinical data	Are there any alternatives from a medical and health care point of view? What are the constraints independent of medical indications that would affect this case?			
Two	Assessing the responsibilities	What were the specific responsibilities of all involved? Was the patient respected and protected? Were legal and deontological factors considered?			
Three	Identify the ethical problems	Which ethical problems are involved in this case? Are values considered? Are ethical problems ranked according to importance?			
Four	Formulate ethical judgments	Are alternative solutions weighed? Is the values paradigm promoted in the process? Was the decision referenced to the principles of beneficence, autonomy, and justice?			
Five	Elaborating directives for analogous cases	Were values, principles, and virtues addressed? Is it possible to reduce the case to one single ethical issue? Are strategies identified to deal with recurring conflicts? Were the fundamental virtues rooted in the decision?			

Modified from Viafora C: Toward a methodology for the ethical analysis of clinical practice, *Med Health Care Philosophy* 2:283-297, 1999.

ETHICAL DECISION MAKING MODELS: LEVEL III FOCUS ON ETHICAL AND PHILOSOPHICAL THEORY: EVALUATION RUBRIC					
Step	**Concept**	**Evaluative Questions**	**Thoroughly Developed and Conceptually Supported**	**Moderately Developed and Lacks Conceptual Support**	**Unable to Develop and Support Conceptually**
Step One	Problem analysis	Was appropriate information gathered and analyzed? Were problems recognized? Were problems defined?			
Step Two	Establish assumptions	Were personal assumptions established? Were structural assumptions established?			
Step Three	Identify tentative alternative solutions	Were tentative solutions identified? Was additional information collected? Were the tentative solutions accepted? If so, were organizational philosophies considered? If so, were personal ethics addressed? If so, were professional codes addressed?			
Step Four	Decision criteria for evaluating alternative solutions	Will the solution solve the problem? Is the implementation of the solution feasible? Are there other factors to be considered?			
Step Five	Selection of the best alternative solution and implementation	Was an appropriate implementation plan established?			
Step Six	Actual results	Were the results the desired results? If yes, what new problems could result from the solution? If no, were individual and organizational results addressed? If no, were objectives, standards, and expectations understood? If no, were alternative solutions reconsidered and evaluated?			

Modified from Rakich J, Longest B, Darr K: *Managing health services organizations and systems,* Baltimore, Md., 1993, Health Professions Press.

ETHICAL DECISION-MAKING MODELS: LEVEL III FOCUS ON THE DECISION-MAKING PROCESS: EVALUATION RUBRIC					
Stage	Concept	Evaluative Questions	Thoroughly Developed and Conceptually Supported	Moderately Developed and Lacks Conceptual Support	Unable to Develop and Support Conceptually
One	Recognition of the ethical dilemma	Teleological and deontological? Does it involve the ends or consequences? Does it involve the means or duty?			
Two	Generation of alternatives	Teleological and deontological? Do alternatives maximize ends? Do alternatives maximize means?			
Three	Evaluating the alternatives	Teleological and deontological? Does the process determine a comprehensive alternative (good and right)?			
Four	Identifies the ideal alternative to solve the problem	Is the proposed choice the best alternative? Is the synthesis of alternatives to establish the right and good choice evident?			
Five	Act on data gathered independent of free will	Is the best end chosen? Is the best means chosen? Does the choice allow for the most freedom and responsibility?			
Six	Decision to implement or not to implement the ideal decision based on personal intentions	Was the ethical decision comprehensively followed? If not, why?			
Seven	Evaluate the decision from all perspectives	Teleological: was it good? Deontological: was it right? Existential: was it authentic? Was behavior evaluated based on comprehensive ethical behaviors?			

Modified from Rest JR: The major components of morality. In Kurtines W, Gerwitz J, editors: *Morality, moral behavior, and moral development,* New York, 1984, Wiley Press; and Nutt PC: Types of organizational decision making, *Administrative Science Q* 29:414-450, 1984.

Writing about Moral Issues

Writing about moral issues can be complex because it involves expression of ideas that are usually personal and may have created dissonance. It requires careful reflection and thoughtful expression while articulating your main intention in writing. Several suggestions are provided below to help you present your ideas clearly and connect related thoughts as you write responses to moral issues.

1. MAKE YOUR IDEAS CLEAR (CLAR)

The main idea of most papers on ethics is the judgment of morality of the action being considered. Discovery while writing often leads to unclear thoughts and disconnected ideas. Although freewriting or brainstorming is helpful, it should be a preliminary step to the actual formal writing. By thinking through what you want to say before formally writing about an ethical issue, you will be able to specifically articulate your message to the reader. Let someone read your writing before submitting it—if that person can figure out the main idea and/or your position, other readers likely will be able to as well.

2. KEEP SENTENCES AND PARAGRAPHS COHERENT (COH)

Plan before you write and use an outline that organizes your main thought into a connected, logical order. Transition statements are critical because they make the connections and assist in the flow. Use them liberally, and use a variety of transitions to establish relations among your sentences and paragraphs.

An introduction typically is used to identify essential features of the issue and declare your statement of judgment. Introductions should capture the attention of the reader. The body should support and develop your judgment while providing clarification relative to other options you may have considered. Three options will help you organize the body: time order, order of complexity, and order of importance. Lastly, the conclusion should summarize the main idea or judgment and reinforce your position.

3. ACHIEVE EMPHASIS (EMPH)

Achieving emphasis on major ideas is a challenging part of writing. Assign an important idea *more* space and *better* space (statements at the end usually have the greatest impact). Additionally, repeating the statement in a different way (saying the same thing three times but never the same way twice) will emphasize that specific idea.

4. DEVELOP YOUR IDEAS (DEV)

To begin, look at the rough idea sheet you have created and determine which of the ideas listed might create misunderstanding or be disputed by other readers. Then decide which technique of development will clarify the idea. Several strategies exist, such as detailed description, brief or extended illustration, definition, explanation, tracing (presenting a historical perspective), and summarizing. Develop the writing by using the most appropriate strategy listed.

5. WRITING READABLE PROSE (STYLE)

Writing readable prose is based on three common principles: exactness, economy, and liveliness. Exactness is achieved by avoiding empty expressions and using concrete, specific terms to provide clarity. Economy involves word selection that expresses your thoughts, not words that you think will impress the reader. Furthermore, economic writing is brief; the volume of words should be reduced whenever possible without sacrificing the meaning of the writing. Lastly, lively writing involves rhythm and pace. By reading aloud, you can determine if your writing is dull and drags or if it has a rhythm that presents your ideas. Vivid language and varying sentence lengths will contribute to the rhythm and pace of your writing. Be creative.

Modified from Ruggiero VR: *Thinking critically about ethical issues,* Mountain View, Calif., 1997, Mayfield Publishing, pp. 193-200.

APPENDIX **E**

Sample Course Design and Delivery for Teaching Ethics: Multiple-Stage Approach

	Year One	Year Two	Year Three
Activity	Workshops on selected topics or mini-sessions in selected courses	Specific units on ethics integrated into core courses	Reflective essay writing assignments throughout the selected course and/or clinical
Purpose	Students consider what is right and wrong; emphasis on personal discovery	Students consider how they reach decisions and look at their decisions from a professional perspective	Students combine all previous knowledge and apply it to real-life situations as they reflect; focus on the organizational impact, professionalism
Delivery	Multiple modes; see learning activities in each chapter	Multiple modes; see learning activities in each chapter	Multiple modes; see learning activities in each chapter
Examples	Confidentiality, duty, receiving gifts from patients; others from chapters and personal experience	Informed consent, limited resources, truth telling; others from chapters and personal experience	Professional autonomy, disclosure, conflict of interest; others from chapters and personal experience
Feedback	Immediate feedback in multiple forms; see chapters and appendixes for suggestions	Group feedback; continue using multiple forms; see chapters and appendixes for suggestions	More personal, individual feedback needed at this stage; see chapters and appendixes for suggestions

From Agarwal J, Malloy DC: An integrated model of ethical decision making: a proposed pedagogical framework for a marketing ethics curriculum, *Teaching Bus Ethics* 6:245-268, 2002.

APPENDIX F

Summary of Steps or Stages of Practice-Based Ethical Decision-Making Models

Corey, Corey, & Callanan (1998)[1]	Forester-Miller & Davis (1996)[2]	Keith-Spiegel & Koocher (1985)[3]	Rae, Fournier, & Roberts (in press)[4]	Stadier (1986)[5]	Steinman, Richardson, & McEnroe (1998)[6]	Tarvydas (1998)[7]	Tymchuk (1986)[8]	Welfel (1998)[9]
1. Identify the problem	1. Identify the problem	1. Describe the parameters		1. Identify the competing principles	1. Identify the problem	1. Interpret situation	1. Determine stakeholders	1. Develop ethical sensitivity
2. Identify potential issues involved		2. Define the potential issues	1. Gather information	2. Secure additional information		2. Review problem or dilemma		2. Define dilemma and options
3. Review relevant ethical guidelines	2. Apply the ACA Code of Ethics	3. Consult legal and ethical guidelines	2. Consult legal and ethical guidelines	3. Consult colleagues	2. Identify the relevant ethical standard	3. Determine standards that apply to dilemma		3. Refer to professional standards
4. Obtain consultation	3. Determine nature of dilemma	4. Evaluate the rights, responsibilities, and welfare of all		4. Identify hoped-for outcomes	3. Determine possible ethical traps			4. Search out ethics scholarship
5. Consider possible and probable courses of action	4. Generate potential courses of action	5. Generate alternate decisions	3. Generate possible decisions	5. Brainstorm actions to achieve outcomes	4. Frame preliminary response	4. Generate possible and probable courses of action	2. Consider all possible alternatives	5. Apply ethical principles to situation
6. Enumerate consequences of various decisions	5. Consider potential consequences, determine course of action	6. Enumerate consequences of decision	4. Examine possible outcomes	6. Evaluate effects of actions	5. Consider consequence of that response	5. Consider consequences of each course of action	3. Consider consequences for each alternative	

7. Decide on best course of action		6. Evaluate selected course of action	7. Estimate probability for outcomes of each decision	7. Identify competing nonmoral values		6. Consult supervisor or peers	6. Consult supervisor or peers	6. Consult supervisor or peers
8. Make the decision		7. Implement course of action	8. Make the decision	8. Choose a course of action	6. Prepare an ethical resolution	7. Select an action by weighing competing values given context	4. Balance risks and benefits to make the decision	7. Deliberate and decide
				9. Test the course of action	7. Get feedback	8. Plan and execute the selected action	5. Decide on level of review	
	5. Implement best choice and evaluate			10. Identify the steps, take action, evaluate	8. Take action	9. Evaluate course of action	6. Implement the decision	8. Inform supervisor and take action
	6. Modify practices to avoid future problems						7. Monitor the action and outcome	9. Reflect on the experience

ACA, American Counseling Association.

1. Corey G, Corey MS, Callahan P: *Issues and ethics in the helping professions*, ed 5, Pacific Grove, Calif, 1998, Brooks/Cole.
2. Forester-Miller H, Davis T: *A practitioner's guide to ethical decision making* (website): http://www.counseling.org/resources/pracguide.htm. Accessed 1996.
3. Keith-Spiegel P, Koocher GP: *Ethics in psychology*, New York, 1985, Random House.
4. Rae WA, Fornier CJ, Roberts MC: Ethical and legal issues in the assessment of children with special needs. In Simeonsson RJ, Rosenthal S, editors: *Clinical assessment in child and adolescent psychology*, New York, 2001, Guilford Publications.
5. Stadler HA: Making hard choices: Clarifying controversial ethical issues, *Counseling and Human Development* 19:1-10, 1986.
6. Steinman SO, Richardson NF, McEnroe T: *The ethical decision making manual for helping professionals*, Pacific Grove, Calif, 1998, Brooks/Cole.
7. Tarvydas VM: Ethical decision making processes. In Cottone RR, Tarvydas VM, editors: *Ethical and professional issues in counseling*, Upper Saddle River, New Jersey, 1998, Prentice-Hall.
8. Tymchuk, AJ: Guidelines for ethical decision making, *Canadian Psychology* 27:36-43, 1986.
9. Welfel, ER: *Ethics in counseling and psychotherapy: standards, research, and emerging issues*, Pacific Grove, Calif, 1998, Brooks/Cole.
From Cottone RR, Claus RE: Ethical decision-making models: a review of the literature, *J Couns Dev* 78:279, 2000.

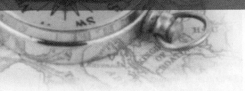

Administrative law. The authority of administrative agencies to regulate practice.

Affective taxonomy. Learning objectives ordered according to the principle of internalization; internalization refers to the process by which a person's affect (emotions) toward an object passes from a general awareness level to a point where the affect is "internalized" and consistently guides or controls the person's behavior.

Arete. Greek word for excellence or virtue.

Aristotle. A fourth-century Greek philosopher whose contribution to philosophy was that the soul was divided into two spheres, a rational sphere (mind) and an irrational sphere; morality emerged as a result of conflict between the rational and irrational spheres.

Athletic trainer. Certified athletic trainers are health care professionals who specialize in preventing, recognizing, managing, and rehabilitating injuries that result from physical activity. As part of a complete health care team, the certified athletic trainer works under the direction of a licensed physician and in cooperation with other health care professionals, athletics administrators, coaches, and parents.

Autonomy. The principle that respects the individual's rights to self-determination and self-governance.

Beneficence. The principle that refers directly to the covenant that all health care providers are obligated to use their skills in the best interests of the patient.

Bentham, Jeremy. A nineteenth-century philosopher who advanced the theory of utilitarianism, along with John Stuart Mill, and argued that the right act or policy was that which would cause "the greatest happiness of the greatest number."

Board of Certification. The governing body that certifies athletic trainers and identifies the quality of health care professionals through a system of certification, adjudication, standards of practice, and continuing competency programs.

Boundaries. The limits of fiduciary and therapeutic relationships.

Case analysis. The use of real or simulated events to facilitate the application of theory in the learning process.

Character. One of the attributes or features that compose and distinguish an individual.

Clinical ethics. Ethics rooted in the actual practice of health care professionals.

Clinical model. A decision-making model that emphasizes the resolution of ethical dilemmas by using case studies that move from specific details to generalizations.

Clinical pragmatism. A prospective decision-making model that focuses on collaboration and consensus when addressing moral conflicts.

Code of ethics. Guidelines of a professional body that convey a moral tenor; designed to govern the conduct of members when acting alone, interacting with one another, and caring for the people they serve in the professional role.

Collaborative model. An ethical decision-making process based on the values of working together through cooperation and inclusion that emphasizes sequential steps to resolving dilemmas.

Commitment model. A system that reflects deep-seated, shared values, attitudes, and beliefs that sustains itself with little surveillance.

Compliant model. A system that uses policies, procedures, rules, and regulations to guide behavior that requires surveillance.

Consensus model. An ethical decision-making process that highlights the critical role of considering the personal and professional in consultation with all members of the health care team in deciding on the desired action and striving toward and/or reaching agreement on the outcome.

Constitutional law. The essential principles of a nation or society.

Cultural competence. The state of being conscious, sensitive, and attentive to a group's distinctive qualities; for example, values, beliefs, attitudes, and behaviors.

Cultural responsiveness. The application of cultural competence to practice; being aware of, and capable of functioning in, the context of cultural difference.

Culture. The shared values, beliefs, traditions, customs, and practices of a particular group of people.

Decision modeling. Creating an objective flow of alternatives while approaching moral reasoning.

Deontology. The Greek word for duty; an action-based moral theory that considers that the means justify the end.

Descriptive ethics. A branch of ethics that does not advocate a particular moral outlook (as prescriptive, normative ethics does) and does not seek to determine the rightness or wrongness of moral actions but simply describes what people actually do and how people think or have thought about morality.

Ethical discovery. The process of uncovering a person's values and principles that guide ethical practice.

Ethical engagement. The different applications of ethics in teaching and learning that immerse the student in active discovery through didactic and clinical activities that translate into practice.

Ethical standards. Professional values that guide, and interpersonal skills that convey, appropriate professional conduct.

Ethics. A systematic inquiry and judgment about the moral dimensions of human conduct or morality.

Ethics education. The part of an athletic training education program that integrates the development of ethical behaviors in students throughout the curriculum.

Ethics of care. A model that emphasizes the human notion of the developing moral agent as well as a balance between the prevalent existing theories of actions and consequences; also known as *humanism.*

Ethics of justice. A model that focuses on fairness; equality; rational decision making based on rules and principles; and autonomous, impartial decision making.

Ethics training. Formalized training programs designed to facilitate ethical discovery.

Existentialism. A philosophy that asks "Who am I?" and is concerned with the examination of the "authentic" and "inauthentic" self in human life.

Experiential learning. Learning rooted in engagement in field experiences similar to the experiences characteristic of the profession.

Fiduciary relationships. The trusting relationships that health care providers establish with patients.

Foundational behaviors of professional practice. Basic behaviors, identified in the fourth edition of the *NATA Athletic Training Educational Competencies,* that are incorporated into instruction in every aspect of the educational program.

Four principles model. A decision-making model that contextualizes ethical dilemmas in health care by using the four principles of beneficence, nonmaleficence, justice, and autonomy.

Gaming approach. An approach to learning in which a person is actively engaged in a process that involves some type of reward—not only for the person's own case deliberation but also in assessing the merit of other case presentations. The process of ethical discovery in a "play-based" environment.

Hermeneutic method. A method rooted in the philosophy that anything (e.g., a written document, a morally relevant situation or action) can be best understood when placed in a larger context.

Humanism. A philosophical theory that affirms the dignity of all people and emphasizes the compassion in developing the moral agent.

Identity trust. Trust that emerges from being a member of a profession in which a patient-athlete expects a certain level of care through predictable and acceptable foundational behaviors of professional practice.

Integrity. The conviction to hold on to truth and honesty and readiness to carry out duty simply because it is the right thing to do.

Interpersonal skills. The verbal and nonverbal behaviors involved in the relationship between the certified athletic trainer and the patient-athlete and other colleagues.

Judicial law. Law that is decisional in nature and has courts (trial, appellate, supreme) that interpret and wrangle over legal issues.

Justice. The principle that cultivates the fairness and equity in the treatment of the individual or group.

Kant, Immanuel. A Western philosopher who advanced the theory of deontology by suggesting that reason is the highest principle that ultimately concludes in goodwill.

Kohlberg's theory. A theory that outlined six stages within three different levels; extends Piaget's theory, proposing that moral development is a continual process that occurs throughout the lifespan.

Learning activities. A series of tasks designed to facilitate personal and professional discovery.

Linked learning activities. Learning activities designed to bridge across groups to increase interaction and dialogue to develop citizenship and social skills.

Management model. An ethical decision-making process similar to business models that is comprehensive in addressing the clinical and administrative dimensions of each situation.

Metaethics. The branch of ethics that seeks to understand the meaning of moral language.

Mill, John Stuart. A nineteenth-century philosopher who advanced the theory of utilitarianism, along with Jeremy Bentham, and advocated that the right act or policy was that which would cause "the greatest happiness of the greatest number."

Moral behavior. Behavior composed of moral sensitivity (which incorporates moral motivation), moral reasoning, and moral character.

Moral character. The last step in the development of moral behavior yielding strength to persevere against adversity while attending to moral duties.

Moral courage. Courage reflective of the willingness to risk disgrace, as well as social ridicule and disapproval, for attending to moral duties.

Morality. The values, principles, and judgments applied to guide right or wrong conduct and based on cultural, religious, and philosophical concepts.

Moral motivation. The process of prioritizing moral action (behavior) when confronted with conflicting values; incorporated into moral sensitivity in the development of moral behavior.

Moral reasoning. The second step in the development of moral behavior; the ability to distinguish right from wrong and to interpret, judge, and make a decision.

Moral sensitivity. The first step in the development of moral behavior; the ability to recognize and identify ethical issues.

Moral values. Values that focus on human rights, integrity, and welfare; how others ought to be treated.

Narrative ethics. Emphasizes the role of communication in the analysis of ethical dilemmas.

NATA Code of Ethics. The athletic training profession's guide to rules of right conduct; developed, monitored, and enforced by the National Athletic Trainers' Association.

NATA Strategic Plan. The National Athletic Trainers' Association plan that identifies its mission and short- and long-term goals.

Nijmegen model. A prospective decision-making model that focuses on prospective ethical case deliberation in clinical practice and aims for a justified decision.

Nonmaleficence. The principle that requires the health care provider to do no harm.

Nonnormative ethics. A branch of ethics consisting of descriptive ethics and metaethics.

Norm. Principle of right action that serves to guide members of a group.

Trust. To have faith in the honesty, integrity, and competence of another.

Utilitarianism. A doctrine that states doing the greatest good for the greatest number is the most useful.

Value analysis. A systemic way to evaluate a values conflict.

Value conflicts. Competing values that struggle for primary consideration.

Value tension. A no-win situation in which none of the options that will resolve the particular dilemma is satisfying because some dissonance in the values emerges throughout the process.

Values. Ideals that may have a moral disposition or simply depict relative worth, utility, and importance; when learned and developed by repeated experiences, they are the source of consistent patterns of behavior.

Values clarification. A process of identifying and prioritizing moral values.

Values-driven model. A model that focuses on incorporating the person into the decision-making process by considering the value system and/or preferences of the individual decision maker.

Values education. The process of helping students see how people differ and what they share to become more sensitive to others while promoting understanding; recognition of implications of individual differences is key to the process.

Virtue. Moral disposition; cardinal virtues of courage, prudence, temperance, and justice; spiritual virtues are faith, hope, and charity.

Virtue ethics model. An ethical decision-making process that emphasizes the importance of self-responsibility in making ethical judgments and focuses on the person making the decision rather than the decision itself.

Workplace bully. A member of the workforce who targets another.

Workplace politics. A complex organizational culture described as power or influence that is illegitimate, informal, and dysfunctional.

Page numbers followed by *f* indicate figures; *t,* tables; *b,* boxes.